# Studies in
# Health Technology and Informatics

*Editors*
Jens Pihlkjær Christensen, CEC DG XIII/C-AIM, Brussels
Tim De Dombal, University of Leeds
Jaap Noothoven van Goor, EFMI WG III, Brussels
Antonio Pedotti, Politecnico di Milano
Viviane Thévenin, CEC DG XII/F BIOMED-I, Brussels
Christoph Zywietz, Medizinische Hochschule Hannover

## Volume 9

ISSN: 0926-9630

# Rehabilitation Technology

## Strategies for the European Union

Proceedings of the 1st TIDE Congress,
6 – 7 April 1993, Brussels

Edited by

E. Ballabio, I. Placencia-Porrero and
R. Puig de la Bellacasa
(DGXIII, CEC, Brussels)

*IOS Press*
*1993*
Amsterdam • Oxford • Washington • Tokyo

ISBN 90 5199 131 2
ISSN 0926-9630

*Publisher:*

IOS Press
Van Diemenstraat 94
1013 CN Amsterdam
Netherlands


*Sole distributor in the UK and Ireland:*

IOS Press/Lavis Marketing
73 Lime Walk
Headington
Oxford OX3 7AD
England


*Distributor in the USA and Canada:*

IOS Press, Inc.
P.O. Box 10558
Burke, VA 22009-0558
USA


*Distributor in Japan:*

Kaigai Publications, Ltd.
21 Kanda Tsukasa-Cho 2-Chome
Chiyoda-Ku
Tokyo 101
Japan

LEGAL NOTICE
The publisher is not responsible for the use which might be made of the following information.


PRINTED IN THE NETHERLANDS

# FOREWORD

Welcome to the 1st TIDE Congress on Rehabilitation Technology Strategies for European Union. The Congress is being held in Brussels on 6 & 7 April 1993. It offers a unique opportunity to gather people from inside and outside Europe to share the results of the projects and discuss critical issues and possibilities for the future of Rehabilitation Technology in Europe, a future with an enormous market of between 60 and 80 million people concerned.

The Congress will last two days and consists of 3 parallel streams of sessions as well as an exhibition running in parallel. The subjects addressed are :

*The Results from R&D Programmes.*

Under these topics contributions were selected to cover the benefits for Rehabilitation Technology coming from basic and applied industrial research carried on in Community or national R&D programmes. Also considered was the impact on RT of the results of Information Technology R&D projects in areas like Microelectronics, Communications, Bioengineering, Computer Hard- and Software and suggestions for targets and development profile in RT to be explored by TIDE.

*The Methodology of R&D Programmes.*

Within this topic, contributions have been selected to approach the analysis of the aspects that influence the orientation of R&D and to identify specific requirements arising from the interaction between elderly or disabled persons and the various scenarios of life. Challenging areas were also considered from the point of view of their technical complexity or the innovations in general technical production processes as well as the implication of the involvement of multidisciplinary fields, human factor techniques, or complex evaluation and verification methodologies in the RT.

*Market and Service Delivery.*

For this topic contributions have been selected on subjects dealing with market issues such as technology transfer, information dissemination, legislation, consumer involvement, if possible based on empirical data, cases or field studies.

In the exhibition, the 20 TIDE Pilot Action projects will demonstrate their results and achievements, displaying the prototypes developed during the projects lifetime. The exhibition, which is open to the general public, also shows innovative contributions from other companies and organizations active in the RT field.

The exhibition offers an excellent opportunity to acquire comprehensive knowledge about the results obtained in all areas of the TIDE Initiative programme and it shows the contribution it makes to the economic and social life of disabled and elderly people in the Community.

I would like to thank everyone who has contributed to the Congress: the Programme Committee in charge of selecting papers; the authors and reviewers of the papers themselves; the chairmen, speakers, the project teams which set up the Exhibition demonstrations, the TIDE Office team and the TIDE Secretariat MC-Consultancy.

E. Ballabio
TIDE OFFICE

## ORGANIZATION

TIDE Office
CEC DG XIII C.3
Rue de la Loi 200
BU-29 3/10
B-1049 Brussels
Tel. +32.2.29.90.244
Fax +32.2.29.90.248

MC Consultancy
Stationsstraat 38
NL - 3511 EG Utrecht
Tel. +31.30.31.10.38
Fax +31.30.32.19.67

### Steering Committee

R. Puig de la Bellacasa
I. Placencia Porrero
L. Bos

TIDE Office
TIDE Office
MC Consultancy

### Programme Committee

Dr. P. Cornes — Disability Management Research Group (UK)
Prof. K. Fellbaum — Technical University Berlin (D)
Prof. H. Funakubo — Medical Precision Engineering Institute (Japan)
Mr. R. Foulds — Univ. of Delaware (USA)
Mr. J.L. Lindström — Swedish Telecom/infologics (S)
Mr. O. Lorentzen — Sentralinstitutt for Industriell Forskning (N)
Mrs. M. Lundman — Handikappinstitutet (S)
Mr. M. Martin — Royal National Institute for the Deaf (UK)
Prof. A. Newell — Dundee Univ. (UK)
Prof. A. Pedotti — Fondazione pro Juventute "Don Gnocchi" (I)
Prof. P. Rabishong — INSERM Un. 103 (F)
Prof. A. Spaepen — Katholieke Universiteit Leuven (B)
Mr. E. Winterberg — Datch (DK)
Dr. W. Zagler — Arbeitsgemeinschaft für Rehab. Technik (A)

**Photographs** of the cover by Nestor Peixoto - Noya

# Contents

# Invited Speeches

Session 1:  Results from R&D Programmes

M. Millner:
(Director Ontario Rehabilitation Technology
Consortium, past President of RESNA)
Rehabilitation Technology: Exploitation of
R&D and Current Technologies.

Session 2:  Market and Service Delivery

R. Worsley
(Director of Community Affairs, British
Telecom):
The Provision of Services for Disabled and
Elderly Customers

# Rehabilitation Technology: Exploitation of R & D and Current Technologies

Morris (Mickey) Milner

*The Hugh MacMillan Rehabilitation Centre and University of Toronto*
*350, Rumsey Road, Toronto, Ontario, M4G 1R8, Canada*

**Abstract.** This paper summarizes the contributions made by all of the authors in Session (1) of the 1st TIDE Congress and highlights the potentialities for exploitation of research and developments in areas of technology relevant to aspects of interfaces relating to visual perception, facilitation of human communication, prosthetics and orthotics, robotics and signal processing. Means by which promising technological developments can be expedited for more widespread availability are discussed together with aspects of consumer involvement and teamwork through consortia of relevant expertise.

## 1. Introduction

The author considers it a distinct honour to make one of the opening presentations for this 1st TIDE congress, for it provides a special opportunity to gain wider perspectives of developments in rehabilitation technology internationally, while affording opportunities for the sharing of relevant experiences. The programme pertinent to this section is extremely exciting as gauged through a review of the submitted abstracts in order to facilitate the relevance of this presentation. It is divided into six sections as follows:

1. Interfaces to compensate for visual perception.
2. Enabling communication.
3. Daily support.
4. Motor enhancements.
5. Robotics.
6. Signal processing.

The various contributions address a wide variety of human impairments and related disabilities, including those affecting people who are blind and partially sighted, people with speech impairments, people with locomotor and mobility problems, those requiring artificial upper extremities and those who might benefit from robotic applications, and finally, the profoundly deaf. Aspects concerning elderly persons and those with multiple impairments are included.

Striking observations relating to the contributions are:
- The many papers with multiple authors.
- The involvement of consortia of researchers and developers with common interests.

- Considerable advantages arise from the availability of tools to conduct the R & D efforts, particularly computers.
- A call for standardization in certain areas such as testing protocols and computerized information.
- The importance of user testing, and the appropriate involvement of consumers.
- The need for defined quality of life measures.
- Thrusts relating to modularization.

In the material to follow, highlights of the problems and potentialities of the technologies presented in the various areas alluded to above are discussed along with some examples of recent Canadian activity.

## 2. Interfaces to compensate for visual perception

The developments in computer interfaces such as the mouse and graphical user interfaces, which provide enormous speed advantages and simplifications of considerable benefit to able-bodied people to facilitate their access to, and operation of, computers, regretfully, have negative effects on the accessibility for persons with physical disabilities, and those who are blind and partially sighted. Several papers emphasize related issues. A contribution relating to fast optical icon and character recognition [1] addresses issues of significant concern to blind and partially sighted people. Pertinent developments and a thrust towards the provision of a universal aid have considerable promise for the exploitation of the technology involved. A paper relating to standardisation efforts [2] emphasises the need for a computer independent, standardised system for text formatting to ensure accessibility by a large group of reading impaired people. The print disabled group includes people who are blind, visually impaired, deaf-blind, dyslexic or with physical impairments in regard to paper handling or computer access. Relevant reference materials and findings are to be presented.

A most intriguing paper on multimedia interfaces for blind computer users [3] describes methods and specialised hardware developed to transform visual information into acoustic information along with tactile output if required. An application is described in which a user controls, interactively, the translation to a verbal description of a photorealistic computer graphic. The potential of this development is considerable and immediate questions that spring to mind relate to usability issues from the user's perspective, especially in regard to cognitive loading.

A contribution on project IRIS - an infrared orientation and information system which transmits coded information to persons equipped with an appropriate receiver - is described [4]. Received information is converted to synthetic speech in the user's language. Using a pair of photodetectors provides stereophonic signals which guide the user towards the transmitter. The system has applicability to those with visual and physical mobility impairments. Some perspectives on the possibilities of using digitally stored maps and methods of optical 3D scene analysis are to be presented. This product has potential for a substantial international market.

SYMBOL [5] is an interactive C-D based multicode, multilingual language training system designed for all people who have language communication difficulties. A prototype has been produced by a European consortium involving consumers, scientists, sign language experts and university faculty with expertise in auditory deficits and computer science. Each C-D is to embrace symbols relating to a specific theme. The first prototype contains more than four hundred of the most frequently used symbols connected to the theme of the house. Each concept is accessible in seven languages written or spoken in an international phonetic language. They are also translated simultaneously into specific languages for the deaf, currently including two French types. The user can choose several modes for navigating the program: spatial; attributive; functional; and, generic. The technology exploits a commonly used audiovisual medium and incorporates an interactive element which has considerable potential economic value for the home C-D market.

## 3. Enabling communication

A fascinating approach for the teaching of lipreading to persons who are hearing-impaired [6] proposes to use computer animated pictures of an abstracted speaker's face. Research work to provide data for German speakers shows promise for the potential of this approach. Digital signal processing capabilities have aided this project significantly.

Multi-Talk II, a memory-resident IBM compatible program connected to an Infovox speech synthesizer has been evaluated in five subjects [7]. Data for these evaluations will be provided.

The COMSPEC project [8], initiated in 1989, links ten institutions in the five Nordic countries, the UK and the USA, with a view to developing common architecture, relevant software modules and configuration tools of considerable flexibility for widespread use in the development of alternative and augmentative communication devices. The rationale for the project and examples of the developments indicated above will be presented.

## 4. Daily support

This segment of the Congress programme emphasizes technologies in the home and the workplace while stressing certain needs for the elderly.

A consortium embracing researchers, consumers and manufacturers relating to the AUDETEL (AUdio DEscription of TELevision) Project [9] is working towards the development of technology needed to provide an additional speech service for existing television transmissions to provide a narrated description of their important visual elements appropriately interspersed with the existing speech information. Progress to-date and relevant technological and commercial considerations are to be presented. This is an area with significant commercialization potential if the technology can be fully developed.

The TECAD (TEaching the Elderly CAD) Project [10] is developing a system of computer assisted learning for elderly workers to enable them to keep pace with new technologies being introduced to the workplace. The focus is on exploring the cognitive gaps of the selected population having little or no computer experience so as to bridge those gaps using on-line accessible teachware modules. A tutorial concept to provide for the organizational framework of the specific enterprises involved is to be realized. This is an interesting aspect of adult education.

A study on the utilization of videotelephony, in the homes of elderly persons, and incorporating the perspectives of users and their caregivers [11], suggests that the implementation of a videotelephony-based social support service has potential to impact positively on both the quality of life and service support of these people. With the growing elderly population technological support with dignity can make enormous societal contributions.

## 5. Motor enhancements

The use of hybrid functional electrical stimulation and orthotic systems for the restoration of gait in persons with paraplegia is under investigation [12] with a focus on automatic control methods, the minimization of fatigue and utilization of biomechanical modelling studies for optimizing systems for individuals on the basis of acquired gait data. An overview of this work is to be provided and its most innovative aspects appear to be in respect of the hybrid system. This is a challenging area of work and, in general, developments have been painstaking. Of major concern are issues associated with system complexity and hence reliability and wide user acceptance.

The paper on the TIDE MECCS (Modular Environmental Control and Communication System) project [13] reflects the efforts of a consortium of three groups who have developed a prototype system embracing a wheelchair mounted laptop PC, a digital radio link and a home environmental control system. From the wheelchair via keyboard, mouse or custom switches, control can be exercised over the environment system, telephone access and monitoring of the front door. A modular approach has been used. Extensive user testing and design iterations of the interface were undertaken. The provision of flexibility in the choice of components by the user and concomitant minimization of costs are important attributes in getting this technology to users.

A project on an information prosthetic for severely physically handicapped children conducted by a multidisciplinary team [14] has attended to the development of relevant computer applications including hardware and software while ensuring computer accessibility. Explorations are to be conducted on the children's development with respect to independent activity, initiative, concentration, attention span and colour and pattern recognition. Some work in these areas is to be reported. In particular, concentration is enhanced by computer use as compared to pencil and paper exercises. Work in the Microcomputer Applications Programme at The Hugh MacMillan Rehabilitation Centre (HMRC) has been along somewhat similar lines, and exciting innovations have emerged which can have great benefit for the special populations involved [15].

A project entitled "One Switch Control M3S" [16] aims to specify and develop a new flexible and open interface method for systems to be used by disabled and elderly people to control their mobility and their environments. It is intended to ensure that different types of input devices can interface to different types of end-effectors to achieve economies in purchasing different systems which, with current technologies are ordinarily incompatible. Two demonstrations are planned to reflect the efforts of a team of thirteen participating organizations involving a wheelchair, a manipulator and a variety of interface controls. Some early work on mobility for pre-school children with physical disabilities, conducted at HMRC reflected the value of this approach in regard to providing systems that were user-friendly for therapists and others who do not need to acquire detailed knowledge of the technical systems involved.

## 6. Robotics

The first of the papers in this area relates to an open control architecture for an intelligent omnidirectional wheelchair [17] to afford individual adaptation to meet the needs of people with a wide range of disabilities. Essentially, the system of concern is modular, with each unit being provided with local intelligence so as to be highly independent of other modules. Among the advantages of this control concept are: robustness because of the decentralized intelligence, and the ability to act on different levels of abstraction while supporting the user with several operational modes not only for control of the wheelchair, but for other devices including robotic arms and special user interfaces.

The MARCUS hand [18] is being developed by a consortium of four partners in the UK and two in Italy. It possesses two degrees of freedom - finger flexion and thumb flexion. The differential flexion of the fingers and thumb yields fast prehension and a powerful grip. The hand geometry is considered to be more anthropomorphic than conventional prostheses. Since the thumb partly adducts as it flexes and the fingers curl progressively with flexion the hand is able to open more widely than other prostheses and with the added ability to pick up larger objects and those with irregular shapes more securely. The control method employed requires simple user commands to open, close, hold, squeeze or release objects. The detailed task of hand shape or grip tension is devolved to a computer system such that on touching an object, the hand automatically adopts one of a set of generic shapes which is adjusted to maximize the contact area between the hand and the object while minimizing the grip force. If the object slips, this is detected and the force increased until sliding ceases, all without the user's intervention. User commands can take on many forms so long as they can be translated to analogue voltage changes. Thus, myoelectric or switch control systems and the variants on these systems can be deployed. Users appear to have found the hand easy to use and trials are designed to compare the control system with conventional schemes to assess ease of operation and to gauge the hand's functional capabilities. A major challenge with systems of this sort relates to reliability.

A soft assistant robotic arm for safe use by people with tetraplegia [19] is constructed of six foam rubber segments each of which can bend at 30-degree angles in two orthogonal directions. Two independent movements are provided at each junction and the independent control of each segment enables the arm's hand to reach about the individual's environment. Control is achievable through voice recognition or joystick. Refinements to the control method to assure smoother movements are being pursued. The idea of flexibility for safety is notable and has considerable promise for the enhancement of this technology.

A consortium involving eight partners is working on the RAID (Robot for Assisting the Integration of the Disabled) project [20]. Problems and findings relating to the acquisition of user requirements are of concern. The target application is CAD-based work. The methodology involves: selection of an appropriate reference group; group and individual discussions to identify specific needs; presentation of possible solutions through visual aids; investigator experience; and, hands-on exercises when possible on prototypes and other devices. Other factors of concern relate to environmental factors including the availability of support from other system users. Of importance here is the very direct involvement with a group reflective of the ultimate users of the system.

A second paper from the RAID project is concerned with the development of functionally flexible end-effectors for the RAID workstation [21]. User requirements are regarded as paramount and issues relating to robot tasks, layout and execution lead to a technical solution based on two end-effectors - book gripper and page turner. Tests with prototypes have been done and will be presented. Considerations relating to the integration of sensors for enhanced control reliability and speed will be discussed. It is interesting to note the parallel in thinking here with the MARCUS hand project.

## 7. Signal processing

This contribution from project STRIDE [22] is to provide results of speech identification scores, comparing modified speech with optimally amplified speech, when stimuli were presented auditorially, or, as a supplement to lipreading, in persons with profound deafness. After analysis of several speech pattern elements, they were manipulated digitally, then recoded as acoustic signals and matched to individual characteristics. Elements included were voice pitch/fundamental frequency, loudness/intensity, frication/aperiodicity, and vowel formants. Results will also be provided on the relationship of psycho-acoustic properties of profoundly impaired hearing to speech perception. The power and effective use of computer systems is again apparent in this work.

The paper on multi-modality aids for people with impaired communication [23], summarizes a research proposal to the CEC with the primary aim of investigating the feasibility of a prototype modular communication aid based upon a portable computer which can address the main methods of communication, i.e. oral, auditory, visual and tactile. The proposed impaired-speech research is to build on state-of-the-art tools for multilingual normal speech recognition. Emphasis will be placed on techniques which are not language specific. Post-doctoral researchers will benefit from training and education to be made available by the interdisciplinary team of researchers and educators drawn from five countries.

The paper on the brain-computer interface [24] reflects results using electroencephalographic signals, passed through an analogue-digital converter to a personal computer, which is programmed to extract and classify features of the signal, using an artificial neural network. Initial experiments, with electrodes over the left and right sensorimotor cortex, reflect an ability to move a cursor to the left or right on a monitor screen with 80% accuracy after three days of training. The system has potential for switch control for people who are unable to communicate by any other means.

In the STRIDE project on speech analytic hearing aids for profoundly deaf people [25], a specially designed wearable signal processing aid has been developed and made in first prototype quantities for all the patients in the present four country (England, France, Netherlands and Sweden) trials. The essence of these devices is to use pattern recognition algorithms to extract information about particularly important speech components from the speech signal even in normal conditions of noise and reverberation, and matching each aid to the user.. Carefully designed, common standard fitting, training and evaluation procedures are in use in each of the four language environments. This project serves to emphasize the importance of a concerted international approach to common problems and the value of standardization at an appropriate phase of enquiry and technological development.

## 8. Conclusion

Areas of commonality and of importance amongst the many papers as well as for future pursuits are discussed in what follows.

### 8.1 Multiple authors

The many papers with multiple authors is reflective of the teamwork approach and the diversity of disciplinary skills required for an effective address to the problems of concern. This will, in the author's view, be an ingredient of growing importance in realizing the benefits of current and future technological innovation and therefore the effective exploitation of technology.

*8.2 Consortia*

Many of the projects presented involve consortia of committed individuals and organizations. This is a factor of considerable importance, especially when one realizes the limitations of resources available for the work that is needed, together with the requirement to eliminate unnecessary duplication of effort. It is suggested that utilization of research results may be accelerated by the interactions promoted by appropriately structured consortia. It may be of some interest to describe briefly the Ontario-based Rehabilitation Technology Research and Development Consortium with which the author is connected:

The Ontario Ministry of Health supports the provision of assistive devices by providing 75% of the cost of a wide range of devices and currently expends about $100-million per year in the province whose population is about nine million. The Ministry has funded a Rehabilitation Technology Research and Development Consortium from the beginning of 1992, with a ten year commitment at the level of $1.5-million per year (which the Consortium must augment by $750,000 per year). The Consortium is designed to link universities, clinics, consumers, manufacturers and marketers across the province to address the rehabilitation technology needs of consumers, while building a stronger research base to effectively transfer relevant technology to the industrial sector. The Consortium is addressing problems relating to seating, mobility, prosthetics, orthotics, hearing, communication, vision and respiration through teams in each of these areas. It includes also a Psychosocial Evaluation Team (to facilitate meaningful ways of consumer participation and measures of issues such as quality of life) and a Technology Transfer Unit. The creation of the consortium is an innovative step in addressing the needs of persons with disabilities and offers a sincere effort to work in partnership with them, clinicians and industry.

*8.3 Tools including computers*

Considerable advantages arise from the availability of tools to conduct the R & D efforts, particularly computers - mainly microcomputers - which provide the benefits of growing power and speed concomitant with valuable and flexible software developments. Many authors have exploited microprocessors for achieving adaptive control.

*8.4 Standardization*

An emphasis for standardization emerges on a number of fronts. Appropriate standardization of protocols for usability studies and related experimentation, and formats of data could facilitate and accelerate some areas of project work, thus realizing an earlier exploitation of developed and developing technological innovations. It should be appreciated that for areas of activity in the formative phases, early standardization could have a detrimental effect.

*8.5 Usability testing*

The science of usability testing will require more attention in the future to aid in ensuring the effectiveness of technologies developed for specific groups of users, while ensuring appropriate involvement in a partnership vein.

*8.6 Quality of Life*

Quality of life is referred to in many of the papers and it appears that some formalization or standardization of definitions and measures is indicated. This is an issue which the present author considers can best be developed in close and early collaboration with potential users of devices and systems. Several contributors have stressed the value of interaction and definition of needs in collaboration with users. Unfortunately, with few exceptions, little information is provided in regard to the numbers of people involved and the nature of the collaboration.

*8.7 Modularization*

In several areas modularization is stressed. This should be recognized as an important economic element of considerable benefit to persons with disabilities. At The Hugh MacMillan Rehabilitation Centre this has been emphasized and practised to good effect in the areas of postural support and seating, and powered upper extremity prosthetics where it is of special importance to keep costs as low as possible for technology for growing children.

*8.8 Training*

Many of the technologies developed will require users to be trained appropriately for their fullest exploitation.

*8.9 Final words*

The very significant and sincere efforts of all of the contributors reflect superb levels of achievement which point to effective exploitation of the results of research and development with current and developing technologies. The sharing of these efforts should add greatly to the success of the 1st TIDE Congress.

**References**

[ 1] R.J. Whitrow and N. Sherkat, Fast Icon and Character Recognition for Providing Universal Access to WIMP Environment for the Blind and Partially Sighted.
[ 2] J.J. Engelen and B Bauwens, Large Scale Text Distribution Services for the Print Disabled: The Harmonisation and Standardisation Efforts of the TIDE-CAPS Consortium.
[ 3] K. Fellbaum, K. Crispien, M. Krause, T. Strothotte, M. Kurze and J. Emhardt, Multimedia-Interfaces for Blind Computer Users.
[ 4] W.L. Zagler, P. Mayer, F.P.Seiler and N. Winkler, Technical Possibilities for the Improvement of Orientation and Mobility for Disabled Persons.
[ 5] SYMBOL - Systeme d'apprentissage lexical multicode et multilingue sur environnement CDI.
[ 6] H-H. Bothe and F. Rieger, Developing a Computer Animation Program for Teaching Lipreading.
[ 7] P. Raghavendra and E. Rosengren, Effectiveness of MultiTalk II as a Voice Output Communication Aid.
[ 8] M. Lundalv and D. Svanaes, Comspec - Towards a Modular Software Architecture and Protocol for AAC Devices.
[ 9] Helping Visually Impaired People to Gain More from Television - The AUDETEL Project.
[10] M. Collet, Innovative Concept for Teaching Elderly CAD - The TECAD Project.

[11] T. Erkert and S. Robinson, Videotelephony: Support for Elderly People.

[12] P.H. Veltink, H.J. Hermens, B.F.J.M. Koopman, H.M. Franken G. Baardman, J.A. van Alste, G. Zilvold, H.J. Groetenboer, and H.B.K. Boom, Restoration of Gait in Paraplegics by Functional Electrical Stimulation and Orthoses (Hybrid Systems).

[13] B. Redmond, Mobile Communications and Environment Control for Wheelchair Users.

[14] R. Voort, E. Hoenkamp, W. Hulstijn and J. de Moor, The Information Prosthetic for Severely Physically Handicapped Children.

[15] Annual Reports, Rehabilitation Engineering Department, The Hugh MacMillan Rehabilitation Centre, 1987-1991

[16] J.A. van Woerden et al, One Switch Control M3S.

[17] H. Hoyer and R. Hoelper, Open Control Architecture for an Intelligent Omni-Directional Wheelchair.

[18] P. Kyberd, R. Tregidgo, O. Holland, P. Bagwell, P. Chappell, S. Marchese, M. Bergamasco, R. Sachetti and H. Schmidl, The MARCUS Intelligent Hand Prosthesis.

[19] A. Casals, R. Villa and D. Casals, A Soft Assistant Arm for Tetraplegics.

[20] G. Bolmsjo and L. Holmberg, RAID User Requirements and Test Results.

[21] G. Bolmsjo and H. Eftring, RAID Robotic End Effector Developments.

[22] A. Bosman and G.F. Smoorenburg, Speech Processing for the Profoundly Deaf.

[23] P.A. Cudd, M.S. Hawley, P. Dalsgaard, L. Azevedo, S. Aguilera and B. Granstrom, Multi-modality Aids for People with Impaired Communication (MAPIC).

[24] G. Pfurtscheller, J. Kalcher and D. Flotzinger, A New Communication Device for Handicapped Persons: The Brain-Computer Interface.

[25] STRIDE, Speech Analytic Hearing Aids for the Profoundly Deaf.

# Morris (Mickey) Milner Ph.D. P.Eng. C.C.E.

Morris (Mickey) Milner was born and educated in Johannesburg, South Africa. He received the B.Sc.(Eng) and Ph.D. degrees, respectively in 1957 and 1968, in the Department of Electrical Engineering, University of the Witwatersrand. His Ph.D. thesis was entitled "Models of nerve excitation and propagation with special reference to multifibre peripheral nerve." From 1958 through 1968 he served on the faculty in that department and moved through the ranks of Junior Lecturer through to Senior Lecturer. Dr. Milner has held academic and research appointments in Cape Town, South Africa, Canada, and the USA. As a visiting professor or lecturer he has visited many institutions in Canada, the USA, and Australia. He has made numerous presentations in many countries including China, Hong Kong, Japan, Estonia, Finland, Russia, Sweden and the UK.

He is Vice-President, Research and Development, The Hugh MacMillan Rehabilitation Centre, Toronto, Ontario, Canada, where he has responsibilities as Director, Rehabilitation Engineering and Research Departments. This includes responsibility for the overall direction of Variety Ability Systems Inc., a non-profit manufacturing facility in Toronto. Since 1991 Dr. Milner has been Director, Ontario-based Rehabilitation Technology Research and Development Consortium which links rehabilitation facilities, academic centres, consumers, and manufacturers. He is a member of the International Centre for the Advancement of Community Based Rehabilitation, headquartered at Queen's University, Kingston, Ontario.

He has academic appointments as Professor at the University of Toronto (U of T), Queen's University, Kingston and the University of Western Ontario. His appointments at U of T include the Departments of Mechanical Engineering, Rehabilitation Medicine, and Surgery, the Institute of Biomedical Engineering and the Institute of Medical Science.

Dr. Milner is associated with the following professional organizations:

> **Registered Professional Engineer**, Association of Professional Engineers, Ontario.
> **Fellow**, Institution of Electrical Engineers (London).
> **Senior Member**, Institute of Electrical and Electronics Engineers Inc.
> **Member**, Canadian Medical and Biological Engineering Society.
> **Member**, Biological Engineering Society (United Kingdom).
> **Active Member**, American Congress of Rehabilitation Medicine.
> **Member**, International Society for Electromyography and Kinesiology.
> **Member**, Association for the Advancement of Medical Instrumentation.
> **Fellow**, Rehabilitation Engineering Society of North America.
> **Member**, Canadian Standards Association.
> **Certified Clinical Engineer** by the Certification Commission.
> **Fellow**, American Academy of Cerebral Palsy and Developmental Medicine.

Dr. Milner has served on numerous committees relating to rehabilitation and rehabilitation technology, locally, nationally and internationally. Many relate to funding of grant applications and policy relating to rehabilitation technology and assistive devices. He served as President of RESNA (1982-1983) and was Chairman of the International Commission on Technical Aids of Rehabilitation International (1984-1988). He has been the recipient of a number of awards which recognize his contributions to his field of endeavour.

# "THE PROVISION OF SERVICES FOR DISABLED AND ELDERLY CUSTOMERS"

RICHARD WORSLEY
Director Community Affairs, BT
BT Centre, 81 Newgate Street, London EC1A 7AJ, England

This paper offers an introduction to the session of the Congress concerned
with "Market and Service Delivery". It does so by reference to the experiences
of the author's company, BT, of providing products and services to disabled
and elderly people in the UK.

## 1. Introduction

I am delighted and honoured to have been asked to be the opening speaker in this session of
your congress. I have been asked to speak about the provision of services for disabled and
elderly customers. I do so from the perspective of my company's involvement in this type
of work over the last decade and I will seek through my talk to bring to your attention the
main lessons we have learned during that time in a way which I hope will be helpful to
others. I make no pretence that we have got all the answers but, with a great deal of help
from many quarters, we have developed a service in which we take some pride.

My own role is to direct and be responsible for BT's activities in the community -
that is to say making sure that we fulfil our company's commitment in its mission statement
"to play a fitting part in the community in which we conduct our business". That involves
us in addressing a wide variety of issues, including economic regeneration, education, the
environment, people in need, support for the arts and, of most relevance today, people with
disabilities. As part of our work under that last mentioned heading we have since 1984 run
a programme called Action for Disabled Customers, to which I shall return as the main
subject of my talk. However let me say at this stage that I am quite frequently asked why
that service is placed, in organisational terms, alongside our charitable and community
activities. The reason for this is that we seek to address the needs of people with
disabilities in two distinct ways - first as a distinct and identifiable section of our market
which we need to serve with particular consciousness of the special requirements which
disability can bring about. Secondly we seek to address issues of disability in the
community at large, often working with voluntary organisations and charities. We see the
two types of work as entirely complementary - not least because we are frequently working
with the same organisations in both contexts. I am aware that there is a school of thought
which suggests that disabled people should be provided with the services they need as of
right and not as a voluntary or charitable gesture. The view we take is that those needs are
best addressed in both ways - indeed the reality is surely that people with disabilities would

be very much worse off in lots of ways if they were not supported on a large scale by voluntary and charitable organisations.

I should add that my company is slightly atypical in that, although we are a public limited company, we have reached that status from a history of once being part of government and then a nationalised industry. The terms under which we were privatised in the early 80s included the establishment of a licence which imposes restrictions and obligations upon us. Some of those relate to disability but I would just like to emphasise that what I am about to describe goes very substantially beyond our licence obligations.

## 2. The "Action for Disabled Customers" Programme

The essence of our work for disabled customers is based on the premise that we should do all that we reasonably can to make sure that the products and services we provide take into account the needs of disabled people. How do we set about ensuring that objective is fulfilled? I will describe the organisational aspects first and the illustrate our work with a number of examples.

One of the operational units which reports to me is the Action for Disabled Customers unit (ADC). This is a small team of 6 full-time people employed in the company's headquarters to manage the work which I will be describing. They in turn work with 11 locally based ADC liaison managers whose task it is to provide at local level the special expertise which this subject calls for and to help make sure that it is built in to our ordinary operational activity. What we seek to achieve is to make sure that all our employees who deal with customers, whether it is in sales or billing or installation, do have a basic knowledge of the special ways in which we serve disabled customers. The specialist staff are available to back-up that broad knowledge with individual and expert help where it is needed.

One of my tasks is to act as the chairman of a directing committee which oversees this work. It is an unusual body in that it comprises not only people from within all the relevant parts of BT, including research and product development people, but also five representatives from outside the company who bring special knowledge of disability and help to keep us on our toes. These are dedicated people whose contribution is enormously beneficial to us and I cannot underestimate it.

## 3. Examples

Let me next illustrate some of the things that we are doing by examples. Certainly the largest scale operation we have entered into has been the establishment of what is now known at Typetalk. This is the relay service for deaf and speech impaired people which we fund and which is run by the Royal National Institute for Deaf People which is the major organisation of its type in the UK. We have worked with the RNID over many years to bring up the standard and scale of this service from a very limited operation in their London headquarters to what it is now. The service, as many of you will know, provides a means for deaf and speech impaired people to use the telephone through text access to a central exchange, talking through operators completing the other side of the conversation on their behalf and responding to the deaf person in text. The service, which is based at Speke near Liverpool, now operates seven days a week 24 hours a day and has been recognised as a major step forward in serving the needs of deaf people in the UK. It is the result of a partnership between the private and voluntary sectors which has worked particularly well.

This is a service which we have been very happy to undertake on a voluntary basis and we have funded virtually the whole of its operating costs over its first three years of operation - some £4m. We are now embarking on the second four year period at the end of which we envisage that there will be some 20,000 customers registered with Typetalk compared with today's 5000.

Last year, our regulator, the Director General of Telecommunications, decided, in our view unnecessarily, to make the provision of this service an obligation under our licence. No doubt this gave him satisfaction at the time and perhaps reassured the public but there has never been any question about our withdrawal from this service.

The service is backed-up by the Text Users Rebate Scheme which recognises that it takes a deaf person maybe five or six times as long to have a conversation using a text telephone than an ordinary conversation. TURS addresses this by providing for a rebate of 60% of the call charges for the customers concerned up to a maximum of £160 per year. Behind that provision is a principle which is very important to us - namely doing whatever we can to put our disabled customers on an equal footing with other customers. For the same reason calls through Typetalk are charged to the customer on exactly the same basis as if it was an ordinary call between two points, with no extra charge simply because the call is in fact relayed through the exchange at Liverpool.

Our work with blind people includes some simple but very important developments. For example we have completed arrangements for our bills to be available in braille and large print for blind customers and there are now some 4000 customers who have applied for this service. At an even more basic level, we have arranged for all our phonecards to have a little notch on one side so that a blind customer can make sure that it is inserted correctly.

## 4. Product Development

An important aspect of our work is product development. I have available a budget for special funding of development work at our research laboratories on products and services for disabled people. This means that we are able to keep disability issues at the forefront of technological development. Using this budget for example, we have been able to develop and bring to the market last year a brand new range of two telephone instruments, known as Converse, which have been developed with disability in mind - for example they provide inductive coupling for hearing aid users, in coming and outgoing speech amplification, full loudspeaking and additional earpiece and headset capability. Similarly we are working on a development of the videophone which will be specially geared to providing a telephone facility for deaf people using sign language. We are particularly pleased when, as with Converse, we are able to get included in the design of a product features which will benefit disabled people but will also be attractive to a much wider market. There are now around 80,000 Converse telephones in use after only 10 months of availability.

Another product which is playing a very useful role is Claudius. This is a device which enables speech impaired people to converse either face to face or by telephone using pre-recorded messages simply by pressing buttons on the instrument. We are now drawing to the end of testing a second model of this device which has proved particularly useful to speech therapists and their patients.

## 5. Conclusion

Let me sum up and conclude with some themes which I believe are particularly important.

The first of these I have already touched on - the way in which service to disabled customers can sit in a very complementary way alongside voluntary support for disability issues in the community generally. That is why, for example, we have been very pleased to provide extensive support and sponsorship for a very wide range of community activities aimed specifically at helping disabled people and including employment and training initiatives.

Secondly I cannot overstate the importance of partnership in the service of disabled people. Although many aspects of our life as a company are concerned with competition, this is an area where it is much more important for us to collaborate with others, to learn from each other and to bring together the different sorts of expertise that we each possess. We also do this on an international scale through the mechanism of COST 219, an advisory committee which, as many of you know, is concerned with European co-operation in the field of scientific and technical research on behalf of disabled people.

Equally important is the need to listen. We have learned over the years that, whether as providers or researchers, there are so many aspects of disability which it is hard for us to imagine. That is why we spend a lot of time listening to voluntary organisations representing different aspects of disability, and to disabled people themselves. Quite a sizeable proportion of my budget is spent on market research for products and services.

Next I would mention the task of providing information. Disabled people are not the easiest of audiences to address, not least because their circumstances are so diverse, so that no single means of informing them is satisfactory on its own. We produce a guide - known as the Blue Guide - which is revised annually and describes all the products and services which are available to disabled people in the UK, with information on how they can be obtained. We then go to considerable lengths to distribute and advertise the existence of the guide which is also available in braille and on audio tape, as well as holding exhibitions, conferences, briefing our own employees in the way I have described and making sure that other information providers know what we have available.

Let me conclude by saying that the results from this type of work do not come overnight. It needs committed attention on a long term basis, working out what the requirements are for the sort of organisation which you are. In the world of communications, issues of disability are clearly of the greatest importance and I am very pleased and proud to have had the necessary backing and support from my own company at the most senior level to make sure that these issues are never neglected.

# Session 1:

## Results from R&D Programmes

# Fast Icon and Character Recognition for Universal Access to WIMP Interfaces for the Blind and Partially Sighted

S Harness, K Pugh, N Sherkat, R Whitrow
*The Nottingham Trent University, Burton Street, U.K - Nottingham NG1 4BU*
*e-mail rjw@uk.ac.trent.doc*

**Abstract** As the usage of WIMP interfaces increases, the accessibility of software to the blind and partially sighted diminishes. Research and development is underway (TIDE project VISA*) to provide universal access to these interfaces. Systems are monitored in real-time and icon and character recognition interpret the output into suitable audio or braille form. This paper describes Fast Optical Icon and Character Recognition. The fundamental requirements are analyzed. The way in which environmental and contextual information such as layout and "surrounding history" can be used to achieve the required accuracy and speed of recognition is reported.

## 1. Introduction

For most users WIMP (Windows Icons Menus and Pointers) systems are more convenient than conventional text based ones. (Fig. 1) For the blind and partially sighted they present a barrier. To use a WIMP system the user must be able to manipulate windows, icons, menus and control buttons in order to invoke applications. Once invoked the user must be able to interact with the application's local environment.

Special hardware enables blind users to interact with existing text based systems. Screen contents are examined by direct access to the ASCII values which make up the screen memory map. Interaction is possible using speech synthesis, auditory signals and touch.

*This project is funded by the European Tide Initiative, Project no. 135

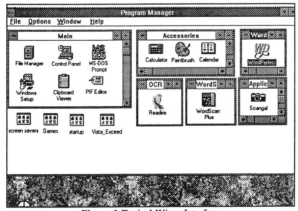

**Figure 1** Typical Wimp Interface

With a WIMP based system the screen image is graphically stored as a bitmap. In order to provide useful information about the screen it is necessary to locate and identify the objects and text contained in this bitmap.

## 2. The Universal Approach

### 2.1. The Aim

There are two main ways in which the problem of screen analysis can be tackled. The simple solution is to internally access the target WIMP interface. The drawback is the need for a dedicated solution for every system. More acceptable is a universal solution to interface to **any** WIMP based system.

### 2.2. The System Concept

A general overview of the proposed system is given ( Fig. 2)

The *application Computer* will be the user's system running the GUI[1] software.
The screen image data will be passed, in Tiff file format[1], to the *Icon Recognition/OCR* software, running on a second system.
The *Current Screen Model* (CSM) will track the latest screen analysis.
The *GUI database* contains all the GUI object information required.
The *User Interface module* generates tones/speech to inform the blind user of the screen contents. It also generates the appropriate mouse and keyboard inputs.

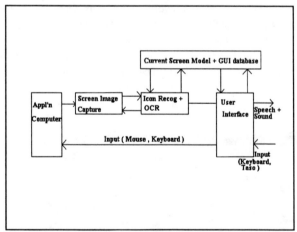

**Figure 2** Overall System Concept

---

[1]GUI - Graphical User Interface

## 3. The Need for Speed

### 3.1. The Aim

Such a system is on-line and interactive. Analysis is performed unobtrusively in real time with processing times of typically 3 seconds considered as satisfactory.

### 3.2. Icon Identification

Object finding software scans the screen image for WIMP objects and text. Edge following routines locate the position and size of visible windows. The window title and controls are identified quickly because their positions relative to the window frame do not change. Window objects are scanned for and classified according to size, shape, colour and location. Encoding routines[2] identify icons by comparison with a database of known icons.

Since many icons have the same or similar shape, the method employed utilises all the data within an icon. For each row of icon pixels a count of all non background-colour pixels is made. This is repeated for each column. The icon_row_counts and icon_column_counts are stored in the icon database.

To uniquely identify an icon, the above encoding is applied to screen icons and compared with the database until a match within an acceptable tolerance is found. Identification is confirmed by character recognition of the icon text and reference to the GUI database. (section 4.1.)

The encoding/identification method appears simplistic. In practice however, it proves extremely effective, resulting in 100% identification of icons

### 3.3. Curtailed Analysis

There is no need to analyze the complete screen every time as the recognition module will be informed about the parts of the screen image that have changed. The revised areas will be concentrated on by the recognition routines. The change may be minor, for example text entered by the user may have appeared. On the other hand, the change may be quite substantial, a window opening for example. Maintaining a current screen model cuts down the amount of processing required. (Section 4.2.)

## 4. Surrounding History

The GUI database and Current Screen Model[3] provide a way of tracking and anticipating the users route through the system.

### 4.1. GUI Database

For each GUI object in the database a list of attributes will apply:

*Visual attributes* relate to the object's appearance on the screen.

Location:       An object cannot exist without having a location on the screen.
Size:           For some objects the size is fixed, other objects are resizeable.
Graphics:       This attribute indicates which objects contain graphical symbols.
Orientation:    "Scroll bar" objects can have a vertical or horizontal orientation.
Default:        Object's value. e.g value indicated by "dials".

*Manipulation attributes* describe the way in which an object can be manipulated; For example Selecting, Activating, Dragging, and Editing.

*Referential attributes* link an object to its child-objects. For example, a dialogue box object will have links to its component buttons, dials, menus, etc.

The database anticipates the screen changes prompted by user actions. Selection of an 'open-file' option triggers the appearance of a dialogue box. All the recognition software has to do is to locate the frame of the dialogue box. The screen location of objects within it can then be calculated using positional information in the database. The box remains until the user 'clicks' the mouse pointer on one or more of the 'buttons' within.

### 4.2. Current Screen Model

When a new window is opened, it will appear as the top screen object. Some of the objects that were previously on the screen 'disappear' underneath the new window; some become partially hidden; the rest are unaffected. Only the window that has just appeared is analyzed. This saves on analysis time as the user goes 'deeper' into the system.
The Current Screen Model (CSM) keeps track of the screen contents in terms of layers. The active window is located in the top layer, the desktop in the bottom. All other inactive windows are located between the top and bottom layer (Fig. 3). Screen analysis on return to inactive layers is now unecessary.

### 5. Icon Recognition

### 5.1. Maintaining the Database

It is possible for the user to move screen objects. He may wish to rearrange the order that the icons appear in a group window. In this case, the information in the database regarding the positions of the Icons will be incorrect. The recognition software provides the ideal way to realise that the database is no longer up to date. The new icon locations can be reported to the database,which can then be altered accordingly.
The window size and location information is also subject to alteration by the user. Again the Icon Recognition software can keep the database informed.

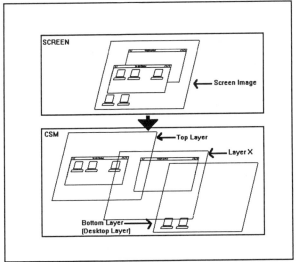

**Figure 3**   Screen to Current Screen Model Conversion

## 5.2. *Speeding up the OCR*

As a rule, a limited number of fonts is used whenever text is generated. Building a history of these fonts allows a more optimal classification of characters during recognition in that the OCR routines initially search a limited and prioritised set of fonts. This naturally reduces execution times, especially within text processing applications.

## 6. Discussion

The problem of location and classification of objects has been largely solved. The routines have been written with execution time in mind. The Current Screen Model and GUI database go a long way to ensuring that only as much processing as is absolutely necessary is performed. Work in progress is now bringing all of the functions together into an integrated system.

**References**

[1] TIFF, A Tag Based File Format to Promote the Interchange of Digital Image Data, Issue 5.0, Aldus/Microsoft Technical Memorandum, August 1988.
[2] K. Pugh, S.J. Harness, N. Sherkat, R.J. Whitrow
Icon Recognition for Providing Access to WIMP Interfaces for the Blind and Partially Sighted. Proceedings of the First Workshop on Iconic Communication, University of Brighton, December 1992.
[3] L.H.D Poll, R.P.Waterman ,Object Library Software Engineering documents, Institute for Perception Research, P.O. Box 513, 5600 MB Eindhoven.

# Large Scale Text Distribution Services for the Print Disabled: The Harmonisation and Standardisation Efforts of the TIDE-CAPS Consortium

Jan J. ENGELEN, Bart BAUWENS

*Kath. Univ. Leuven-CAPS, Kard. Mercierlaan 94, B-3001 Leuven*

**Abstract** The CAPS consortium starts from the idea that the access to the information society by a significant group of handicapped and elderly persons, who have difficulty in accessing the printed word and/or electronic information (reading impaired persons) should be guaranteed as much as possible.

Within TIDE's CAPS project a system independent, ISO-standardised document architecture (the European Interchange Format based on SGML) has been developed to increase text accessibility for a large group of reading impaired persons.

In this paper details will be given on all CAPS results and they will be treated within the context of other related initiatives (ICADD, Electronic libraries).

## 1. Who is active in this field?

The CAPS consortium is working together with many related groups. Here is a brief overview of the most important ones:

### 1.1 The "International Committee for Accessible Document Design (ICADD)".

The main purpose of this group, who originated at the first "World Congress on Technology for the Disabled" (Washington, Dec. 1991) is the definition of a universal text format for the large amounts of textual information that will be available soon.

Some of the technical ideas which have lead to the formation of this Committee, are strongly influenced by the ideas which are developing within the European TIDE-CAPS project.

The USA's impulse was given by the urgent need of harmonisation in this field, particularly as a consequence of the regulating issues in the Americans with Disabilities Act .

Meanwhile three other ICADD meetings took place. During these meetings a workplan for future actions has been set up. We quote from this document [1]:

*The purpose of the International Committee for Accessible Document Design is to develop and encourage the document transformations that print disabled persons are working toward. We do not intend to define standards. Rather, we intend to enable the current standards systems to meet the needs of print disabled persons. Additionally, we intend to clarify what is needed by the print disabled reader.*

Three CAPS participants are member of ICADD. The list of key people involved in this committee's board is quite impressive [2]. The CAPS consortium currently tries to organise a long term co-operation with ICADD, but the necessary financial support is still under discussion.

## 1.2   Digital Newspapers for the visually impaired.

Since 1985 several groups in different countries have set up special services to provide reading impaired persons with the text of daily newspapers. The CAPS project members recently produced a report on these services [3]. It is the first scientific report —and up till now the only one— that is exclusively dealing with the subject of Electronic Newspapers' State of the Art. It gives an overview of the following systems, often described by their developers:

(a)   The Belgian system, report by Jeroen Baldewijns from **Infovisie** and Henryk Rubinstein from **Textalk**

(b)   The situation in the Commonwealth of Independent States (CIS)

(c)   The Finnish system, report by Juha Sylberg from the **Finnish Federation of the Blind** and Henryk Rubinstein from **Textalk**

(d)   The French system, report by Jean-Paul Anton from the **Université Paul Sabatier**

(e)   The ETaB system in Germany, the report was written by Uli Strempel from the **Stiftung Blindenanstalt.**

(f)   The Hong Kong system, information collected by Jeroen Baldewijns from **Infovisie**

(g)   The Dutch system, based on a note by **H. Michels** and reported by Jeroen Baldewijns from **Infovisie** and Henryk Rubinstein from **Textalk**

(h)   The Russian and ex-USSR systems

(i)   The Swedish system, report by Henryk Rubinstein from **Textalk**

(j)   The British system, report by Keith Gladstone, P.Ainley and Richard Orme from **RNIB**

(k)   The American system, report by Keith Gladstone from **RNIB**

(l)   The Canadian system, report provided by Keith Gladstone from **RNIB**

Several elements for a critical analysis and evaluation of existing systems can be found in this work (see also [4]) but many realisations still lack sufficient user evaluation.

## 1.3   Other groups

Several groups, mainly USA based, are setting up large text databases that will be available through electronic mail [5], on CD-ROM or on diskette.

Following is a brief and far from exhaustive list of the most interesting ones. Some archives are accessible by FTP, the electronic mail File Transfer Protocol that can be used on many nodes of the Internet email network.

| name | address | type |
|------|---------|------|
| Project Gutenberg | quake.think.com (ftp) | ASCII |
| EASI archive | easi@educom.edu | ASCII |
| Handicap archives | handicap.shel.isc-br.com (ftp) | ASCII |
| Etext archive | mrcnext.cso.uiuc.edu (ftp) | ASCII |
| Text Encoding Initiative | tei@oxford.ac.uk | SGML |
| SBA (Frankfurt) | CD-ROM | proprietary |
| Macintosh archives | sumex-aim.stanford.edu (ftp) | Hypercard |

## *1.4 The CAPS consortium*

In the **CAPS consortium** following groups are co-operating:
The Royal National Institute for the Blind (London), The University of Bradford, Infologics (Swedish Telecom), the Swedish Handicap Institute, Sensotec (Brugge) and the Katholieke Universiteit Leuven as co-ordinator.
In the first phase of the project (up to March 31, 1993) three more partners (Stiftung Blindenanstalt Frankfurt, Université Paul Sabatier-Toulouse and Elan Informatique-Ramonville-Ste-Agne) were involved together with 6 subcontractors (AGATE [F], FIDEV[F], INFOVISIE[B], STR[S], TEXTALK[S], VUBIG[B]).
Details on CAPS are grouped in the next chapter.

## 2. The objectives and results of the CAPS work

### *2.1 CAPS objectives*

The *primary rehabilitation problem* with which CAPS is concerned is that the amount of written information easily available to the print disabled is extremely small compared to that which the non disabled population takes for granted. Easy access to this information is essential if disabled and elderly people are to play a full, active, useful and satisfying part in society.
The *primary technological problems* to be solved are how to automate the production of information available in accessible forms for the print disabled and by linking it to the normal commercial processes, significantly increase its availability.
CAPS does not pretend that it can completely solve both the rehabilitation and technological problems. However, CAPS is making major contributions towards solving these problems.

### *2.2 CAPS results*

The main objectives reached in the CAPS Pilot Phase (TP 136, ending on March 31, 1993) are:
* the definition and implementation of the European Interchange Format (EIF) using the ISO Standard Generalized Markup Language (SGML). This will enable the European exchange of electronic newspapers for the print disabled as the format is in the public domain [6].

- the description of the necessary legal context and recommendations for full access to documents for people with special needs, with particular emphasis on electronic information.
- the development of better human computer interfaces for the print disabled. By the use of a special I/O card a combined use of specialised input/output devices can be achieved. In addition, multilingual speech synthesis boards with a harmonised command language have been developed.

The main objectives for the CAPS Extension (TP 218, started on April 1,1993) are :

- to develop a Pilot System that will test the concepts of an Information Access Model for the print disabled. This Model is technologically based on the use of *standardised structured electronic documents*. It is designed so that it can link directly into the normal commercial information provision and thus provide a significant improvement in information access.
- to develop the mechanisms by which the print disabled can have access to documents encoded in (or easily convertible to) SGML. Such documents could include for example newspapers, books, magazines and information databases such as catalogues.
- to develop a Telephone Access System, which will enable the print disabled to access information using the most universally available and simplest high technology device— the telephone hand set.
- to lay the foundations for further improvements in access provision by continuing the investigations of the ISO document architectures, such as SGML, its related standards and ODA (Open Document Architecture) together with technology transfer to Small and Medium-size Enterprises.

## 2.3 CAPS "deliverables"

### 2.3.1 Overview of existing projects for digital document distribution.

The CAPS project members produced two reports on current digital data distribution services. In the first one, all systems have been described, in the second their technicalities (media, transmission standards) have been catalogued and discussed.

A report on the social and legal aspects of large scale text distribution services has been produced by the French group AGATE, in a subcontract with the CAPS consortium.

### 2.3.2 Structured text encoding: the European Interchange Format

In order to have a system capable of browsing efficiently through electronic documents, all texts should have built in a system of encodings to specify the logical structure of the document. After preliminary studies of the Standard Generalized Markup Language (SGML) and another encoding scheme, the Open Document Architecture (ODA), the CAPS consortium has produced the European Interchange Format for digital newspapers as a publicly declared Document Type Definition (DTD) conforming to SGML.

*2.3.3   Prototype reading workstation*

The CAPS consortium did not only study document architectures. A prototype reading machine (accessible by blind, low vision, dyslexic and severely motor impaired persons) and capable of reading digital newspapers in the EIF format has been produced and will be demonstrated during this Tide Congress. Conversion software from other national standards into the EIF will also be shown.

*2.3.4   State of the Art Reports*

Following extensive studies and several discussions at major conferences [7], the CAPS consortium produced the *SGML State of the Art Report* . The use of ODA in a similar context is reported in the *ODA State of the Art Report*.
Finally, a *Future Strategy Report* on the use of these document architectures (for the extension phase as well as on a much longer time scale) has been developed.

## 3.   Conclusions

We hope it will be clear that the availability of large quantities of texts for the reading impaired requires a careful determination of formatting issues if these texts are to be made accessible for this group.

It appeared from our study work that logical formatting, using ISO standards (SGML and ODA) is the only viable way in the long run.

As a first step an SGML DTD, adapted to specific problems of the reading impaired, has been developed and technically tested within the CAPS project.

A fully elaborated evaluation of the workstation, the software and methods for transferring text from newspaper publishers into our system has been undertaken.

We think that the actual implementation of the ISO standards should be promoted by all persons concerned by the problems of the reading impaired, especially by those who are running services for text distribution.

We will be glad to have your comments on these ideas and we welcome input from any group or individual who wishes to contribute to this important matter of harmonisation and standardisation.

# References

[1]  An updated electronic version is available from the authors (email: engelen@cc1.kuleuven.ac.be or ask for a diskette version)

[2]  George Kerscher (Recording for the Blind), Tom Wesley (University of Bradford), Uli Strempel (Stiftung Blindenanstalt, Frankfurt); Mike Paciello (Digital Equipment), David Holladay (Raised Dot Computing), Joseph Sullivan (Duxbury Systems Inc.), Jolie Mason (Paramax Division of Unisys), Greg Vanderheiden (Trace Center), Yuri Rubinski (SoftQuad), Maureen Eddins (American Printing House for the Blind), Larry Skutchan (American Printing House for the Blind)

[3]  Contact the authors or other CAPS partners if you are interested.

[4]  J.J. Engelen and J. Baldewijns: *"Digital information distribution for the reading impaired: from daily newspapers to whole libraries"*, Schriftenreihe der Oesterreichische Computer Gesellschaft, Band 48, pp. 155-162 (Vienna, 7-9 July 1992)

[5]  The use of electronic mail by the handicapped community is increasing rapidly. An overview article with descriptions of practical situations has been published:
J.J. Engelen: *"Electronic Mail as a Telematic tool for Disabled People"*, in **Issues in Telecommunication and Disability**, pp. 271-277, ed. by Stephen von Tetzchner, Office for Official Publications of the European Communities for COST219, ISBN 92-826-3128-1 (Luxembourg 1991), (also available electronically).

[6]  This means that copying and using this DTD is encouraged. Details can be obtained from the authors.

[7]  More information can be found in:
* Jan Engelen, *"Information Dissemination on Technology for the Visually Handicapped in Europe"*, **Proceedings of the World Congress on Technology**, Volume III, pp.588-597, 1991, Washington.
* Jan Engelen and Tom Wesley, *"SGML: A Major Opportunity for Access to Information.* **Proceedings of Technology and Persons with Disabilities Conference**, California State University, Northridge, March 18-21, 1992, Los Angeles.
* Tom Wesley and Nick Ayres, "Open *Document Architecture - An opportunity for Information Access for the Print Disabled"*, **Proceedings of the Third International Conference on Computers for Handicapped Persons**, Vienna, July 8-10, 1992.
* Daniel Cotto, Guy Perennou and Nadine Vigouroux, *"Consultation de documents électroniques pour des personnes handicapées de la vue"*, presented at "Interface des mondes réels et virtuels", Montpellier, March 23-27, 1992.

# Multimedia-Interfaces
# for Blind Computer Users

Thomas Strothotte, Martin Kurze

*Free University of Berlin,*
*Department of Computer Science,*
*Takustr. 9, D-1000 Berlin 33*

Klaus Fellbaum, Manfred Krause, Kai Crispien

*Technical University of Berlin*
*Inst. of Telecommunications and*
*Inst. of Communication Sciences,*
*Einsteinufer 25, D-1000 Berlin 10*

**Abstract:** This paper deals with selected aspects of blind peoples' access to graphical user interfaces of modern computers which are addressed by the GUIB Project. A new device for two-dimensional sound output to enable users to locate the position of a screen object acoustically is described. In a prototypical application, blind people are given access to a class of computer-generated graphics using the new device in an interactive process of exploration.

## 1. Introduction

Over the past decade, blind persons have been able to enter numerous new jobs and careers through the prevalence of computers in offices and educational settings. The work of blind users with computers has been based on methods and output devices which convey the information displayed to the blind user. So-called screen readers output the contents of a text-based computer screen on tactile (Braille) displays or via speech synthesis devices.

Together with the up-and-coming graphical user interfaces like MS-Windows, the situation has changed dramatically. Because conventional screen readers depend on a text-based representation of information which is provided by text-based applications, they are not capable of presenting the contents of a bit-mapped graphical screen to a blind person (see Fig. 1).

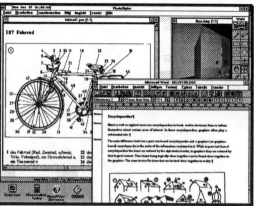

Fig. 1    A typical screen of a graphical user interface (GUI)

To re-enable blind persons to work together with sighted colleagues in one working environment, new devices and methods had to be developed. The problem is being addressed by the GUIB-Project (Textual and Graphical User Interfaces for Blind People), a TIDE Pilot Action.

While our partners are concentrating on the extraction of relevant information out of the data flow within GUIs, the restructuring and treating of the contained text-information as well as the presentation of this information to the blind person via a new device (the *GUIDE*-display), we are looking deeper into two fields of problems that are touched in this context (see also [1]):

- Since the screen is a two-dimensional output device and regular sound-representation (monophonic or stereophonic) offers only poor spatial capabilities, an acoustic technique had to be developed to present the 2D-positional information of objects displayed on screen. This was solved by designing and constructing a 2D-*SoundScreen*; a solution involving a headphone is currently under investigation.

- A graphical user interface not only displays interaction objects like windows, icons, menus and pointing cursors, but increasingly often also contains graphics. Several classes of graphics can be distinguished, of which one - the photo realistic images - can be presented to the blind person using a new tool, the *Image Description Machine (IDM)* which optionally uses the SoundScreen.

Both of these new developments are presented in this paper. They form the basic components for multimedia dialogue systems for blind users.

## 2. Two Dimensional Acoustical Representation of Screen Contents

We now turn to describing general ideas and developments for transforming visual information applied to graphics-based computer user interfaces (GUI's) into acoustic information, leading to an *auditory interface* for blind people.

The screen is transformed into a two-dimensional *acoustic area*, the contents of the screen (windows, icons, buttons, menus, text, and the mouse cursor) is represented by tones, complex sounds and speech (see also [2]). These *acoustic screen elements* are assigned to a two-dimensional spatial acoustic area according to their screen position. A blind person thus can acoustically detect where screen elements are located [3]. Changes in position (e.g. by the mouse cursor) are marked as sounds which are made to move across the acoustic area. If the mouse-cursor is crossing a screen element, a specific acoustic signal is audible. A mouse-click can either be used to specify the screen element using speech output (after the user presses the right mouse button) or to activate the information (usually with the left mouse button). Distance information - represented by artificial reverberated sounds - can be used to specify inactivated screen elements (e.g. overlapped windows).

Digital storage of sound allows a widely flexible access to all parts of acoustical information in high playback quality, without any remarkable delay even by harddisk-, or optical disk (CD-ROM) storage, using direct-memory-access (see also [5]).

The technical solution of the acoustical representation of spatial sounds can be realised by two general techniques, namely by multichannel loudspeaker arrays or headphones. For the *loudspeaker-based approach* we designed a five channel loudspeaker array system, named *Sound-Screen* system (see Fig. 2). Placed in front of the system user, directional acoustic cues are produced by setting the intensity of the single loudspeakers using a digital controlled amplifier matrix (DCA). The fixed control voltages are stored in a memory and can easily be computed in real-time .

The intensity settings of the loudspeaker-channels are based on algorithms derived from the *intensity-stereophony* technique, which precisely describes intensity-depending positioning of sound sources in the *horizontal* plane. In addition, the *vertical* plane was integrated in these algorithm to develop a two dimensional representation of an acoustic area. This technique is currently being evaluated in listening tests carried out at the Royal National Institute for the Blind in London and at the Technical University of Berlin.

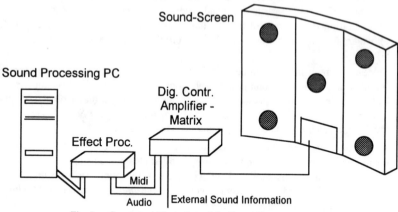

Fig. 2      Conceptual illustration of the *Sound-Screen* system

For the *headphone-based approach* we are experimenting with two different technical solutions: One headphone-based solution is the simulation of a three-dimensional *binaural* - sound field by processing direction-depending filter coefficients according to the human outer ear response functions. If these coefficients are convoluted with the signal function a certain directional cue is percepted by the listener. For the movement of sound sources, the processing has to be carried out in real-time, which requires a very high computational load.

The second headphone-based solution is based on the mechanical positioning and electrical equalisation of the transducers within the headphone shell. Every single transducer on each side of the headphone is assigned to represent a general direction which is needed for producing  a two dimensional acoustical area (left/right, below, above). A certain directional cue can be produced by setting the intensity of the single transducers. This can also be carried out by using a digitally controlled amplifier matrix (DCA), as described for the Sound-Screen system.

The current status of this work is that a demonstrator of the Sound-Screen is working while the headphone-solutions are under development. We shall now tun to a new kind of dialogue system which makes use of the Sound Screen.

## 3. Conveying Graphics to Blind Users

To give blind users a multimedia-tool for the exploration of graphics, a prototypical dialogue system has been developed which provides blind users access to selected photo realistic images. We called this system an *Image Description Machine* (IDM).

With this IDM, the blind user interacts with the computer using the new device developed in GUIB (GUIDE). Furthermore, the user is able to obtain 2D sound output using a first prototype of the SoundScreen. Using these interaction methods, a blind user is able to explore graphics showing scenes with real objects which a sighted user can see on screen.

The dialogue system consists of four logical components (see Fig. 3):

- A scene description is usually the starting point for the production of computer graphics (for more details see [6]).
- The scene description is processed by a separate program, the *Hyper-Renderer*[5], which was adapted to the applications at hand. The result of this processing is an image description, which is stored in a file, the image description file (IDF).
- The IDM uses this file to describe the image to the blind user. This description is an interactive process and requires the GUIDE-device and uses the Sound-Screen.
- The keyboard is used for user input to determine the area of the blind user's interest; 2D-tactile output gives additional feedback about the area of description being described.

Originally, the *Hyper-Renderer* was developed by Jürgen Emhardt to receive a regular text-based scene description as used by the PIXAR *RenderMan* [7]. The output is graphics which is presented using a conventional renderer. In addition, the Hyper-Renderer provides information about the graphics displayed. Using the program's application program interface (API), a special application was developed to write the information obtained thus to another text-file which forms the input for the IDM.

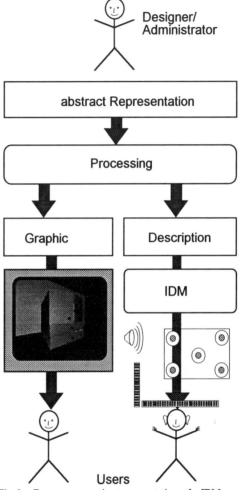

Fig. 3    From representation to presentation - the IDM

Within the GUIB-project, the IDM and its interfaces to the other above mentioned components are being developed. At this time, a first prototype has been implemented in C++. The IDM runs under Windows and uses the advanced interaction functionalities provided by this environment.

Using the image description file, the IDM describes the image to the user. The user can listen to the description spoken by the Sound Screen and get information at various levels of granularity. The position of the part of the graphics being described is displayed using the horizontal and vertical arrays of Braille modules. The user can move the area of the image being observed (the "viewport") using the arrow-keys of a standard keyboard.

To make the appearance more friendly (mainly for the sighted user) and for debugging purposes, the IDM displays the graphics while it is describing it. The "current viewport" is displayed and the (sighted) user can watch it moving over the screen as he (or the blind person) explores its contents (see Fig. 4). All commands are available from menus as well as via key-

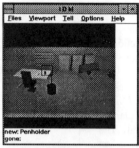

Fig. 4    Screen-Dump from the Image Description Machine (IDM)

strokes. Thus one can choose between these two methods of interaction. The blind user will need the software developed in other parts of GUIB to use the menus, although he can still perform all operations using the keyboard.

## 4. Conclusions

The work described in this paper demonstrates that our new approach has the capability to enhance blind users' interaction with modern graphical user interfaces and applications. Obtaining speech output from the IDM which can be localised in 2D has a very positive effect on the user's subjective interpretation of the scene being explored. Our first experiments indicate that this is superior to conventional speech output.

Our initial results show that it is worthwhile to carry out more work in terms of training and evaluation to enhance the usability of both the IDM and the SoundScreen. This may be done by intensifying the work on the headphone-solution which will enhance the commercial viability. In addition, more investigation in nonspeech-audio will be carried out to enhance the 2D-Sound-output and the scenes being described by the IDM.

## 5. Acknowledgements

We would like to thank Andreas Korthe and Tobias Behrendt for implementing the software driving the SoundScreen. Peter Binner implemented the IDM. Daniel Faensen adapted the interface for the Hyper-Renderer, and Andreas Raab's hints concerning MS-Windows-programming helped a lot. Finally, we wish to thank all our partners in the GUIB-consortium whose invaluable suggestions and comments helped to make our part of the project a success.

**References**

[1] Fellbaum, Klaus ; Crispien, Kai ;. Krause ; Strothotte, Thomas ; Kurze, Martin ; Emhardt, Jürgen : **Tactile and acoustic computer output for blind users** (in German). 7th Workshop on Medical Technology, September 17-18, 1992, Berlin.
[2] Gaver, W. W. : **The Sonic Finder: An Interface that Uses Auditory Icons** . Human Computer Interaction, Vol. 4, 1989, pp 67-94.
[3] Blauert, J. : **Räumliches Hören** . S. Hirzel Verlag, Stuttgart 1974.
[4] Wenzel, E. M. ; Wightman, F. L., Forster S. H. : **Real Time Synthesis of Complex Acoustic Environments** . Customer Information by Crystal River Eng. Inc., 1990.
[5] Emhardt, Jürgen ; Strothotte, Thomas : **Hyper-Rendering** . Proc. Computer Graphics '92, Vancouver, Canada, May 13-15, 1992, pp. 37-43.
[6] Foley, James D. ; van Dam, Andries ; Feiner, Steven K. ; Hughes, John F. . **Computer Graphics - Principles and Practice** . (2nd ed.) Reading, Massachusetts, Addison-Wesley 1990.
[7] Upstill, Steve . **The RenderMan Companion** . Reading, Massachusetts, Addison-Wesley 1990.

# Technical Possibilities for the Improvement of Orientation and Mobility for Disabled Persons

W.L. Zagler, P. Mayer
*'fortec'- Rehabilitation Engineering Group*
*Institute for Electronics, University of Technology Vienna*
*Gusshausstrasse 27/359/1B, A-1040 Vienna, Austria*

**Abstract.** Blind or visually impaired persons as well as persons suffering from severe motoric impairments face various problems when it comes to independent travelling. This paper will shortly review the state-of-the-art technical solutions and show what future improvements could be achieved by using up-to-date technology like GPS (Global Positioning System), optical 3D scene analysis or digitally stored maps. The paper is also a call for European R&D cooperation to make these new technologies available to disabled users as soon as possible.

## 1. Introduction

Different groups of disabled persons face various difficulties when it comes to the necessity of independent and unaccompanied travelling in either familiar or unfamiliar environments. Blind and visually impaired persons do not have direct access to all the commonly used visual landmarks and cues that their sighted peers use (very often unconsciously) to identify their position, to find the correct directions and to avoid collisions with obstacles.

Severely motorically impaired persons using an electric wheelchair or a scooter have access to all the visual orientation information but might encounter problems in converting their navigational decisions effectively and in good time into appropriate steering commands for the vehicle used. This is especially true if the motoric impairment is affecting the upper limbs also and the usual joystick controls have to be replaced by alternative input methods like head-pointers, suck-puff switches, eye-movement sensors or even by speech recognition devices.

The two above mentioned groups of handicapped persons can profit a great deal from electronic navigation aids to improve their independence, flexibility and safety.

## 2. State of the Art

The general navigational task to move from point A to point B can be divided into five distinct jobs by which answers to the following questions have to be found:

o Where am I? What is my present position?
o In which direction do I have to walk or drive to approach location B?
o Are there any obstacles in the path which could cause collision or other dangerous situations?
o If there are obstacles in the direct path, how can they be avoided?
o If the obstacles cannot be avoided are there alternative routes to reach position B?

State of the art devices for blind and visually impaired travellers can commonly only give answers to single questions from the above catalogue.

## 2.1 Obstacle Detection

The most simple and yet unmatched obstacle detector for blind and visually impaired persons is the white cane. Correctly used, this purely mechanical device is able to provide a multitude of travel information which, if the user is familiar with his/her surroundings, in most cases will suffice for safe walking. But, as a matter of fact, the cane will only provide information from an area near the floor. Therefore, protruding obstacles which start higher than say 0,5 m from the floor represent a high risk for the chest and head.

For this reason various ultrasonic and optical collision warning devices have been developed, which can be worn on the chest, attached to the cane, integrated into glasses or hand-held, and issue a signal if any object is detected in front of the user [1]. Obviously devices of this kind will deliver little or no information about the type of the obstacle and where to find a clear path. Directionality is often reduced to walking from one detected obstacle to another [2].

## 2.2 Position Determination

The only available positioning system which does not require any modifications to the environment is the satellite-based GPS (Global Positioning System) which is - at least in non-urban areas - capable of displaying longitude and latitude with an accuracy of 25 meters. Unless this system is combined with some kind of prestored map to interpret the practical meaning of the coordinate and unless the accuracy is not increased by some fine tuning or metering relative to some calibration marks, the practical use for blind and visually impaired pedestrians is rather small [3].

Less sophisticated systems are harder to install as they require the installation of receivers or transmitters at all locations at which a position should be reported to the user [4]. The most simple solution is the mounting of some kind of acoustical beacon, e.g. for the location of a crossing or a specific entrance. There are also methods to switch on these sound sources, which can also issue spoken messages, only if they are triggered by a credit card sized transmitter worn by the blind or visually impaired pedestrian [5].

Over the last few years several attempts have been made to use infrared transmitters to announce the whereabouts to a receiver carried by the blind or visually impaired pedestrian.

I.R.I.S. the Infrared Information and Orientation System developed at our laboratory uses transmitters which broadcast coded infrared information [6]. Using predefined codes for different pieces of information instead of prerecorded speech messages makes I.R.I.S. language independent as these codes are turned into speech by a synthesizer implemented in the receiver. Therefore, the language of the message is determined by the language the receiver is set to. In order to transmit proper names which should not be translated language invariant phoneme-coding is used [7].

Identification bits embedded in the coded signal indicate the class of information a specific message belongs to, (e.g. information about the name of the street or crossing, status of a traffic light or information about public transport). A selector switch at the receiver makes it possible for the user to mask out all information he or she presently is not interested in. By listening to the transmitted information and by comparing this information with the mental map of the street-environment or building the blind user will know his or her position.

### 2.3 Direction Finding

The most popular method - and in many cases the only one possible - to find a direction is the comparison of the path with the orientation of the earth's magnetic field. Using some kind of tactile or audible compass a blind or visually impaired person can get his/her bearings [8].

All the acoustically operating beacons mentioned in 2.2 not only serve as indicators for marking a specific position, but by using the fact that human hearing is a directional sense also communicate information about directions. Thus, acoustical signals (e.g. mounted on traffic lights) help the blind or visually impaired pedestrian to cross the road and arrive at the opposite curb at the desired location.

This directional-hearing capability is also used by the I.R.I.S. system even though nothing can be acoustically heard at all without the receiver device. The prototype I.R.I.S receivers have been equipped with two infrared sensors mounted on a frame of glasses frame. As the optical axes of the two receivers subtend an angle, a synthetic stereophonic effect can be achieved. The wearer of these glasses has the impression that the infrared transmitter is "sounding" from a certain direction and is able to walk toward the target as if approaching a real sound source.

In addition to this, I.R.I.S. supports direction finding by providing verbal descriptions of how to approach possible targets relative to the present position of the transmitter he or she is listening to.

### 3. Future Aspects in Orientation and Navigation

The discussion of the state of the art shows that there are different approaches to solve single orientation and navigation problems. With these methods plus further technical refinement combined with improved user interfaces could, in the near future, result in universal orientation and mobility devices from which not only blind and visually impaired users but also motorically disabled persons could benefit.

As satellite navigation systems like GPS are too coarse and electronic sound and infrared transmitters cannot be installed everywhere it will be necessary to work out a system which is able to exploit the existing optical cues of the environment.

### 3.1 Blindness, Visual Impairment and Navigation

First approaches to use visual information provided by a television or CCD camera tried to map the visual information to the skin by using an array of vibro-tactile stimulators. Even the reduction of the complexity of the image by means of image preprocessing did not lead to the desired results as the spatial resolution of the skin is not sufficient for this task and there is no way to represent any range information. The only way out of the dilemma seems to be to replace the use of vibro-tactile images by more meaningful descriptions and interpretations of the environment obtained by computer-vision procedures [2],[9].

### 3.2 Motoric Impairments and Mobility

Many a person using a powered wheelchair encounter problems in steering by conventional methods. The use of headpointers, suck-puff-switches or speech input can be very tedious or risky if it takes the user too much time to give the appropriate commands [10],[11].

A future intelligent wheelchair could use a similar computer-vision system as proposed for the navigation device for the blind. If this computer-vision system is combined with a prestored map of the user's environment, a simple destination command could be sufficient to make the wheelchair move to the desired place.

If the wheelchair is steered by the user in a direct way, however, a built in computer-vision system could act as collision-detector, recognize hazardous situations and in this case overrule the user's commands to bring the wheelchair to a safe standstill.

### 4. Areas for Cooperation in R&D

The method of directly stimulating the skin with vibro-tactile images placed all the load of picture interpretation on the user. The computer system only had the task of reducing the image resolution and to perform some image preprocessing tasks.

The experiments with computer-vision try to use the computer system for image understanding and interpretation. To the user, only easy to understand descriptions of the scene should be conveyed.

Neither method brought a breakthrough as either the computer or the human being had been overloaded with the image understanding task. The ideal situation would be to find a compromise between these two extreme approaches and to find a way to effectivly share the entire process of image perception, preprocessing and understanding between computer and user without overloading either party.

For this reason our group has recently started a study to find out if there are chances for this third approach [12]. By using LDC-screen-eyeglasses (as used in Virtual Reality experiments) which will present preprocessed (e.g. filtered, feature extracted) images of the environment or a simulated scene, we want to study the behaviour of sighted and visually impaired persons.

The project goal is to find out which principles sighted and visually impaired persons use to extract orientation relevant information from their environment. By a step by step reduction of the complexity of the displayed images it will be studied how sighted and visually impaired persons (with and without orientation and mobility training) can cope with the reduced visual information. Thus we intend to assess which optical cues are relevant and necessary for human orientation.

This being a very complex interdisciplinary task, experts from at least the following fields are needed: Human perception and cognition, artificial organs, implants, neurology, physiology, computer vision, low vision and orientation & mobility.

We feel that making progress in computer assisted navigation and orientation device is a challenge for international cooperation.


## 5. Conclusion

In 1950 P.A. Zahl had already put forth the challenge: "A civilization with such skills should be able to develop guidance aids for the blind more knowing then the cane, more dependable than the dog" [13],[14]. Despite forty more years of development, science and technology has not yet met this challenge in a satisfactory way.

This paper does not claim to offer a concise discussion of the topic nor offer any ultimate solution for the problem. Its main intent is to point out the similar demands of blind and motorically impaired persons when it comes to orientation and mobility, to create awareness for the need of further investigation and to stimulate the European rehabilitation engineering community to undergo this task more ambitiously

## References

[1] A.G. Dodds, The Sonic Pathfinder - An Objective Evaluation. In: International Journal of Rehabilitation Research, Vol. 6, No. 3, pp. 350-351, Heidelberg, 1983
[2] M. Adjouadi, A Man-Machine Vision Interface for Sensing the Environment. In: Journal of Rehabilitation Research and Development, Vol. 29, No. 2, 1992

[3] D.A. Brusnighan, M.G. Strauss, J.M. Floyd, B.C. Wheeler, Orientation Aid Implementing the Global Positioning System. Bioengineering, Proc. of the Northeast Conference, IEEE, Piscataway, 1989

[4] L.A. Brabyn, J.A. Brabyn, An Evaluation of "Talking Signs" for the Blind. In: Human Factors, Vol. 25, No. 1, pp. 49-53, 1983

[5] R.G. Main, A Data Base and Sensing Device for Use by the Blind in Providing Location Information. Report issued by the California State University, Chico, 1989

[6] P. Mayer, M. Busboom, W.L. Zagler, I.R.I.S. - An Infrared Orientation System for the Visually Impaired. In: Precision Machinery, Vol. 3, pp. 93-97, 1991

[7] P. Mayer, M. Busboom, A. Flamm, W.L. Zagler, I.R.I.S. - A Multilingual Orientation and Information System for the Visually Impaired. In: W.L. Zagler (Ed.), Computers and Handicapped Persons, Proceedings of the third international conference, Oldenbourg, Vienna, 1992

[8] R. Priemer, J. Trimble, A Portable Navigational Aid for Blind Persons. In: Rehabilitation R&D Progress Reports, Vol. 25, No. 1, pp. 393-394, Veterans Administration, Baltimore, 1987

[9] M.F. Deering, Real Time Natural Scene Analysis for a Blind Prosthesis. Mountain View, Fairchild Corporation, Technical Report No. 622, 1982

[10] M.A. Regalbuto, J.B. Cheatham, T.A. Krouskop, A Model-Based Graphics Interface for Controlling a Semi-Autonomous Mobile Robot. In: Proceedings of the 11th Annual International Conference of IEEE Engineering in Medicine & Biology Society, 1989

[11] T. Komeda, The Development of a Mobile Robot with Visual Sensor Designed to Aid the Daily Life of the Bedridden. In: Precision Machinery, Vol. 3, pp 17-50, 1990

[12] F.S. Seiler, P. Mayer, W.L. Zagler, 'VISION' - Untersuchungen zur Substitution des Sehsinns für Blinde (Investigations in Vision Substitution for the Blind). Proposal for a basic research project on human vision an orientation, Federal Ministry for Science and Research, Vienna, 1992

[13] P.A. Zahl, ed., Blindness: Modern Approaches to the Unseen Environment. Princeton University Press, 1950

[14] J.S. Hauger, The Creation and Innovation of Electronic Travel Aids and Reading Machines. In: Technology and Disability, Vol. 1, No. 1, pp. 69-86, 1991

[15] W.F.E. Preiser, C. Kemper, Tactile/Electronic Orientation Devices for the Visually Handicapped - A Selected Bibliography. Vance Bibliographies, Monticello, 1983

# SYMBOL

## Multilingual and multicode lexical learning system on CD-I environment

*Georges RENSONNET*
*Association Nationale des Parents d'Enfants Déficients Auditifs*
*10 quai de la Charente, 75019 Paris, France*

The project SYMBOL has been developed within the framework of the European Community program in support of technological initiatives for handicapped and elderly persons. It is positioned at the intersection of two areas : development of new technologies and application of pedagogic innovations for the purposes of rehabilitation.

## 1. Concept

SYMBOL involves the creation of a lexical learning system for all target groups experiencing communication distress due to an inability to link the signified (images ...) to their signifiers (words expressed or written in spoken or sign language). The two primary groups concerned are thus aphasics and the deaf. Although these persons control language with difficulty, they nonetheless possess a non-verbal representation of objects and actions which condition their world and their lives. By extension, the project will hold interest for all individuals learning a language, including young children, the illiterate, and people learning a foreign language.

With the interactive procedure incorporating the signified (pictures of objects) and the signifier (words, gestures, pictograms), users are able to acquire new vocabulary or to extend their existing lexical base within a user-friendly database.

## 2. Prototype

The prototype consists of a CD-I disk including an image bank of still pictures involving the home environment : "The Home". The user is able to access these images either through the path set by the system, or through itineraries which he or she can choose individually. For each object or action selected, which remains visually displayed in a window on the screen, the user finds a spoken and written representation, in a choice of 7 European languages : the pronunciation in audio, the common spelling, and the phonetic transcription (International Phonetic Alphabet). The complementary database offers other signifier choices. For the time being, these are limited to their equivalents in French Sign Language (FSL) and the visual form of French words in Cued Speech (CS).

The technological innovation resides essentially in the creation of a universal system of navigation in a CD-I program to establish the base for a true "author system" through a network of European co-producers. A CD-I configuration has been chosen over a PC (DV-I) environment in order to open access to the widest public possible.

The psycho-pedagogical innovation lies primarily in the possibility of triple access to this "pictionary" : by logical choice, by cumulating or eliminating attributes, and by visual selection. For the user, this means new independence and freedom to create his own itineraries, thus further enriching the contents. Although research in vocal synthesis is very active, the development of non-verbal languages has so far been confined to the production of specific local and partial language dictionaries, which are available in printed form or, at best, on computer.

For the first prototype, an interactive compact disk for the learning of the signified (images ...) and their signifiers encountered in the microworld Home has now been designed and produced. It was developed in the following main stages :
. creation of modes of access to the signified contained in the "pictionary", built up from pictures of objects and actions organized in a tree structure;
. creation of the preliminary VO prototype from a model;
. in-situ validation leading to the final prototype V1.

## 3. Extention

The project has now reached a new stage :
. extension of the product to include an applications generator enriched by the user.

This extension of the product is aimed at the creation of a lexical generator of CD-I applications allowing users, via their institutions, to co-produce learning environments. The project will supply a learning kit including an applications **executor**, the "Home" environment CD-I, and an accompanying guide for the use and the creation of applications.

The CD-I author system will be composed of the standardized generator BALBOA, of an editor, and of a "learner mode" executor designed to pilot the future re-inscribable CD-I. The user-producer network will make it possible to pool and thus optimize experience and knowledge through a proximity tutoring device.

The extension will involve the following main steps, in consecutive order :
- creation of a linguistic, graphic and technical architecture, and an arborescent navigation path that can be modulated to all microworlds of real objects;
- technical development of the CD-I author system;
- pressing of a final version of the "Home" universe created on the first prototype;
- writing of the User's Guide;
- development of the Teaching Kit to be distributed throughout the user-producer network;
- longitudinal evaluation of the "socialization" of the CD-I "The Home".
The industrialization of the product will benefit, on the one hand, from the marketing policy planned for the CD-I by Philips and Sony, and on the other hand, from the contacts that will be established with specific target groups in international networks to demonstrate the educational value of the system. The constitution of a "user network" for production and distribution will ensure an attractive market.

This lexical learning system offers two key advantages. For one, it takes into account specific particularities (individuals experiencing communication difficulties) while operating with a general public technology (CD-I environment). Secondly, it permits an enrichment of the contents by the users, who thus mutualize their knowledge and optimize their experience through auto-production.

## 4. Consortium

The consortium is composed of an organisation of parents of deaf children developing and providing educational support for children, industrialists specialised in CD-I production, and research institutions with a strong background in linguistics and system development :

- Computer Science Corporation (CSC Brussels/Belgium) - in charge of technical development, together with Philips;

- Centre d'Etudes Pluridisciplinaires en Langue des Signes (CEPLUS Liège/Belgium) -
structuring of data from a linguistic viewpoint;
- Facultés Universitaires Notre-Dame de la Paix (FUNDP Namus/Belgium) - study
covering the pedagogic aspects of the products, the exploitation of tracks and the
evaluation of the learning system;
- Système Expert Communication et Intelligence Artificielle (SECIA Paris/France, sub-
contracted by ANPEDA) - production of the media base (graphic chart, image base);
- Association Nationale des Parents d'Enfants Déficients Auditifs (ANPEDA
Paris/France) - project leader in charge of coordination, management, and development
of a marketing plan.

The product will be validated through the following user institutions :

L'Institut Royal pour Handicapés de l'Ouïe et de la Vue (IRHOV Liège/Belgium)
Die Gehörlosen Schule (Bremen/Germany)
L'Association Régionale pour l'Intégration des Enfants Déficients Auditifs (ARIEDA
Montpellier/France)
L'Ecole J. Anspach (aphasic children) (Brussels/Belgium)
Le Centre de Fraiture (aphasic adults) (Belgium)

The educational program will be assessed by the Institut National de l'Audiovisuel (INA
Paris/France)

However, an effective strategy of marketing and distribution must also be applied, to
ensure that the product may fully meet the aims for its intended use.
It will thus certainly contribute to the creation of a single market in rehabilitation
technology in Europe, which constitutes the final objective of the TIDE program.

# The Development of a Computer Animation Program for the Teaching of Lipreading

Hans-Heinrich Bothe, Gerhart Lindner and Frauke Rieger
*Technical University of Berlin, Einsteinufer 17, D-1000 Berlin 10 (W)*

**Abstract.** In March 1991 a new interdisciplinary research project was launched at the Technical University of Berlin (TUB). The aim is to design a computer animation program showing realistic movements of an abstracted speaker's face. For this purpose, video tapes with prototypic speakers have been recorded and analyzed. The investigations lead to the fundamental correlation between phonetic sequences of given German text and corresponding visual movements of the articulation organs. The animation program is designed to be a training aid for lipreading for hearing-impaired people and is based on an open vocabulary. First performance evaluations at a hard-of-hearing school show that after a short-term crash-course the recognition of long single words increased by approx. 15% for a natural speaker. Involved in this project are the Departments of Electronics and Linguistics of the TUB as well as the Department of Special Education (in the field of Rehabilitation) of the Humboldt-University, Berlin. The project is based on various preliminary studies of the participating departments.

## 1   Articulation and Coarticulation

Articulation movements are intended to produce acoustical speech signals in order to establish verbal communication. With respect to achieving efficient interpersonal communication, our society is very much dependent on this kind of human interaction. People with a decreasing sense of hearing, or respectively complete deafness, increasingly lose the ability to communicate through language.

Those concerned have a good chance to compensate for their hearing loss by reading and interpreting the articulation movements together with the distorted sound signal. It is a basic ability of the human brain to allow a combined perception of this kind; the use of which is also important to people with a normal sense of hearing who have to differentiate between sounds in a noisy environment. Whereas, for instance, the acoustical signal gives little help to distinguish between /m/ and /n/, the difference is clearly legible from the speaker's lips.

The ability of the hearing-impaired to garner spoken information from the visual signals alone is dependent chiefly on the lip and jaw movements. Both elements must be separated for the computer simulation, wherein lies the difficulty because the active and passive lip movements are interconnected and interdependent.

The control mechanism relating to the lip movements and by which every phone is produced, is not sufficient to produce sound phone by phone, but rather only in the course of a fully overlapping phonal coarticulation. From the experimental work of Menzerath, together with de Lacerda [1] it is known that the movements of the speech organs are structurally interrelated within the spoken context. And the speech organs needed for the formation of upcoming phones, even though currently not engaged, take up position relatively early to their actual use.

With respect to the general articulation process speech gives rise to different results; only the acoustic and visual ones effective over distance due to the limited capacity for movement of the vocal organs. The smallest meaningful speaker-independent units derived from the acoustic signal are the phonemes. The smallest units of the visual articulatory movements being the visemes.

Owens and Blazek [2] give a good overview of the examination and determination of the consonantal visemes in English, while Alich's dissertation [3] can be viewed as a work of key research concerning the German language.

## 2    Animation on the Basis of Key Pictures

Naturally one wishes to develop an all-encompassing articulations model for the German language, thereby integrating the possible individual expressions of coarticulation. A realistic appraisal of the research effort leads to a necessary limitation due to the high number of influencing factors (e.g. speech-specific facial physiognomy, dialect, speed of delivery, sentence and word stress). On the one hand the word material on which the movement analysis is based had to be fixed so that the phonetic sequences, which exist in German, are sufficiently represented. On the other hand, the investigation was limited to the articulatory movements of two speakers with fairly standard German pronunciation.

For the following analysis the speech and movement data were stored on videotape. To facilitate the extraction of characteristic visual features in the face of the speaker from the video-frames in an automatic, i.e. non interactive, process, several points on the chin, nose and forehead, as well as the contours of the lips, were marked with a contrasting color. From this, according to figure 1, are derived the six indicators;

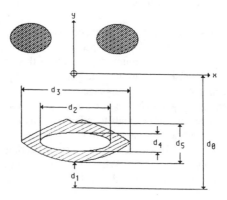

**Fig. 1.** Feature extraction from the speaker's face in single video-frames.

Distance from Chin to Nose $d_0$ and Distance Chin to Lower Lip $d_1$, Width of Inner and Outer Lips $d_2$ and $d_3$, as well as Height of Inner and Outer Lips $d_4$ and $d_5$.

According to a phone-oriented classification, clusters were indicated and representative pictures marked. To reduce the number of these key pictures, the corresponding feature sets were themselves re-clustered to provide definitive representatives. This reduction of information limits the number of key pictures to a quantity which makes the synthesis possible on a small computer (PC).

The test material consists of 470 frequently-used, short-syllable, single words and corresponds mainly to the word material described by Alich [3]. The phonetic transcription was adapted to the actual pronunciation.

As hardware an analysis-synthesis system (see figure 2) developed by the Institute for Electronics of the Technical University of Berlin and described by Bothe [4] was available. The analysis system is based on an IBM compatible PC with integrated expansion cards and makes possible the extraction of the key pictures from the videorecordings. The phonal characteristic pictures were marked with the help of both the acoustic and visual material. To define the optical characteristics within the video frames the user can set points or contours either interactively with a mouse or with the help of an automatic contrast-search program.

The information serves as original material for computer-animation on a synthesis machine. There is an entry version of an existing commercial home computer (Atari ST), which converts any given text in phonematic transcription into a cartoon of a moving face on the screen. The lips, the lower incisors, and the tongue are seen to move. Key pictures corresponding to the text input are chosen for the film; seven interim frames are calculated with the help of an interpolation algorithm.

Two different selection processes were implemented. With a 1:1 depiction every phone was integrated with a set key picture, requiring a corresponding classification during the analysis. To counteract a monotonal movement the frame rate of the single pictures can be fixed for each phone. With this method, however, the already mentioned error arises if single phones appear several times in different contexts.

The second speech model implemented, when selecting the key picture, takes into account the preceding neighboring phone. And in the case of the first vowel of a diphthong it also takes into account the second vowel.

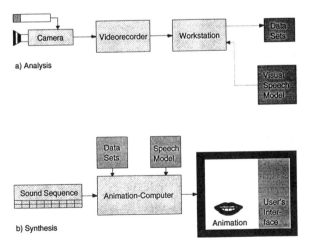

**Fig. 2.** Block-diagram of the analysis-synthesis system.

The phonetic text to be depicted is divided into overlapping diphones whereby the choice of the second phone depends on the first. Of course, in the accompanying video analysis the classification of the features and formation of representative pictures has to be undertaken correspondingly. On the basis of Alich's 1961 viseme model the phones are combined into 14 groups corresponding to Table 1.

| Consonantal group of sounds | | Vowel group of sounds | |
|---|---|---|---|
| $C_1$ | /p, b, m/ | $V_1$ | /a, a:/ |
| $C_2$ | /f, v/ | $V_2$ | /ɛ, e:/ |
| $C_3$ | /s, z/ | $V_3$ | / i, i:, e, e:/ |
| $C_4$ | /t, d, n/ | $V_4$ | /o, o:, ø, ø:, |
| $C_5$ | /l, r/ | | u, u:, y, y:/ |
| $C_6$ | /k, g, x, ŋ, ʀ/ | $V_5$ | /ɔ, œ/ |
| $C_7$ | /ç, j/ | $V_6$ | /ə/ |
| $C_8$ | /ʃ, ʒ/ | | |

**Table 1.** Eight groups of consonants $C_1$-$C_8$ and six groups of vowels $V_1$-$V_6$ for the classification and depiction of key pictures.

There are 14×14=196 possible clusters, so a combining of the representative pictures is necessary, especially with the use of cheap home computers. The set of representatives implemented in the diphone model consists of 38 single pictures. The use of the diphone model offers the possibility to calculate the average phonal time distance between the two marked single-phone points of the diphone, and thereby imitate the movement approximately in real time. Greater accuracy is achieved by calculation of the relative single-picture stand-times on the screen, which result from the distribution of the corresponding distances between the key indicators on the single pictures.

This method, too, gives rise to errors in the depiction in cases of fully overlapping phonal coarticulation. An improvement over the 1:1 selection method is, however, clearly visible, resulting from considerably less dispersion in the corresponding characteristic-clusters, and which has been confirmed by use of the syntheses computer at the School for the Hearing-Impaired in Gotha/Germany (also see [5]).

The screen display of the current syntheses is depicted in figure 3. In the memory at present is a still picture of a face. The range of movement results from a sequential fade-in of visual elements. The lips are moveable, as is the position of the tongue and the lower incisors, as well as the nostrils and eyebrows. The speed of depiction can be set in several steps from slow motion to time lapse. The phone sequences to be practised are entered by keyboard or mouse and can be combined according to content to form corresponding lessons. The sequence to be depicted from the contents of the chosen lesson can also be selected with the help of a random sequence generator. This method offers the student the advantage of learning actively and not to get used to the contents sequentially. Depending on the level of difficulty, the indicator of success is given either by a simple display of the textual solution, or the entry of a proposed solution by a change in the mimic expression on the speaker's face.

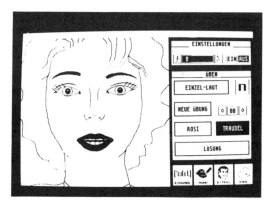

**Fig. 3.** Screen-display of the current synthesis.

## 3 Research Program

With the realization of the diphone-synthesis-system the foundation is laid for the use of a computer as an educational tool. Further development and improvement of this version will be achieved in the context of the research project by taking much greater account of coarticulation phenomena. Therefore the syllable, as the smallest articulatory unit, should form the basis of further research and synthesis. It seems plausible that coarticulation effects within this unit are stronger than outside the unit. In as much as there is influence from preceding or following syllables, they will above all concern the beginning or end border of a syllable.

Since for the listing of data, which means the analysis of visible speech movements, only a small selection of syllables that exist in German can be examined, for the time being a hybrid model is the goal. This means that analysed speech syllables or parts of speech are integrated into the existing diphone model. The comprehensive examination of the optical expression and the changes in the parameters of articulation, depending as well on the stress as on the phonal or syllable environment, are essential for embedding the known parts of the spoken syllables, by interpolation, in the key picture environment. For this reason, with the aid of a similarity-analysis, we can try to isolate core areas of the same syllables in different contextual sounds, in which the development of the movement of the syllables does not change at all or changes very little. Whereas at the beginning and end border of the syllable concerned the influence of the neighboring sounds might, circumstances permitting, be stronger. Also for syllable groups that differ only slightly in the sequence of phones, and thereby in the sequence of visemes, a comparable pattern of movement could be applicable and so a simplification in the frame of the synthesis will be possible.

**References**

[1]   P. Menzerath and A. de Lacerda: Koartikulation, Steuerung und Lautabgrenzung. Berlin 1933.
[2]   E. Owens, E. and B. Blazek: Visemes observed by hearing-impaired and normal-hearing adult viewers. Journal of Speech and Hearing Research (1985) 28, 381-393.
[3]   G. Alich: Zur Erkennbarkeit von Sprachgestalten beim Ablesen vom Munde (doctoral thesis). Bonn 1961.
[4]   H.-H. Bothe: Lippenlesen lernen mit dem Computer. InfoTech 2 (1991), 49-52.
[5]   H.-H. Bothe, G. Lindner and F. Rieger: Forschungsschritte zu einem computergestützten Absehtraining. Sprache-Stimme-Gehör 16 (1992), 139-144.

# Effectiveness of Multi-Talk II as a Voice Output Communication Aid

Parimala RAGHAVENDRA and Elisabet ROSENGREN
*Department of Speech Communication and Music Acoustics*
*KTH, Box 70014, S-100 44 Stockholm, Sweden*

**Abstract.** Multi-Talk II, a voice output communication aid (VOCA) is currently being evaluated by five adults who are physically disabled and users of augmentative and alternative communication (AAC) systems. This paper presents findings from three subjects and describes their communicative interactions with their regular communication system and Multi-Talk II. For one subject, communication rate increased with Multi-Talk II but there were more communication breakdowns, whereas for the other two subjects rate of communication increased with Multi-Talk II and there were no breakdowns.

## 1. Introduction

Multi-Talk was the first portable, multi-lingual voice output communication aid (VOCA) to be developed in Sweden [1]. Long term follow-up investigations of use of Multi-Talk resulted in the development of Multi-Talk II [2]. Multi-Talk II, an updated version of Multi-Talk consists of a communication program that can be installed on any IBM or IBM-compatible computer and an Infovox speech synthesiser. Currently, the program is available in Swedish, English, German and French, and the Infovox synthesiser is available in 10 languages.

Multi-Talk II contains the features of the first Multi-Talk such as text-to-speech, access to pre-programmed expressions with single keystrokes, and a user's lexicon. There are two ways to store and retrieve messages; one is the "quick store", wherein messages that are commonly used are stored under each key and only one keystroke is needed to retrieve a message. The second store is called the "sentence store" where messages can be stored under combinations of two letters or numbers or a letter and number. In addition, the memory demands on the user are reduced as the codes and the messages stored under each code can be easily displayed on the screen. Another advantage is the flexibility of using a personal computer for communication as the user can interrupt any running program to switch into the communication mode of Multi-Talk II.

The importance of evaluation of the effectiveness of devices or programs cannot be stressed enough. The literature in the AAC field has innumerable technical descriptions of augmentative devices, some research on users' satisfaction with devices [3] and consumer-based criteria for the evaluation of assistive devices [4]. However, there is limited research in the area of long-term, functional evaluations with multiple users that would provide us with information on the effectiveness of the device, suggestions for future design, and factors that would help in selecting suitable devices so that a device prescribed would not be abandoned.

## 2. Objective

The aim of the project is to evaluate the effectiveness of Multi-Talk II as a VOCA using single-subject ABAB design, and supplementing it with social validation measures. The evaluation is being conducted with five adults who are physically disabled, have near normal linguistic and adequate literacy abilities and are currently using letter/word boards, Blissymbols, dysarthric speech, Polycom or Canon Communicator for communication. This paper will present the communicative interaction behaviours of three subjects SA, PT and CR with their regular communication system and with Multi-Talk II.

## 3. Method

### 3.1. Subjects

Subject SA is a 28 year old female with cerebral palsy who uses an electric wheelchair for mobility. She is severely dysarthric and uses speech, vocalisations, gestures, and letter/word board for communication. She points to letters or words using her left thumb tucked inside her palm and has been using the communication board for the last 10 years. She has completed high-school education and has basic training in the use of computers. She is currently working at an army museum making an inventory of museum pieces on a computer with other employees who are also disabled. She lives by herself with round the clock assistance.

Subject PT is a 25 year old male with cerebral palsy and he uses an electric wheelchair for mobility. He has no speech and uses vocalisations, eye pointing, facial expressions, and a Polycom (an electronic communication device) for communication, and a Canon communicator outside his residence. He types his messages using a head pointer attached to an ice hockey helmet, and has fairly good spelling skills. He has completed equivalent to a high school education at a special school and has some work experience in computer data entry. He has been without a job for few years now. He lives on his own, but shares a recreational area with other residents who are also disabled.

Subject CR is a 38 year old female with quadriplegia resulting from cerebral haemorrhage 5 years ago. She refuses to use an electric wheelchair and wants to be pushed around in a manual wheelchair. She is anarthric and uses vocalisations, her own signs for "yes" and "no," and a Polycom for communication. She types with her right index finger and has excellent spelling and writing skills. She studied to be an architect and worked as a journalist before her illness. She lives by herself with round the clock assistance. CR has not accepted her disability completely, and had refused to use a VOCA before this investigation.

### 3.2. Procedure

The objective and the procedure of the study was explained to all the subjects and they consented to participate. The subjects were asked to select a normal speaker with whom they felt comfortable interacting to be their familiar partner (FP). Subject SA and PT chose their personal assistants and CR chose her occupational therapist. The subjects and their FPs were videotaped, first having a general conversation and later with subjects describing a pre-read news item 1 to their FPs. The subjects used their communication system described above to communicate. The FPs did not know the content of news item 1. The communicative behaviours measured from these tasks was taken as the baseline measure (A) of the subjects' communication.

Following this, the subjects were trained on the Multi-Talk II by their speech pathologists for several sessions, each session lasting for about an hour. Earlier, the speech pathologist had been trained on Multi-Talk II by the investigators. The speech pathologist followed a training program developed by the investigators. The program introduced the different features of Multi-Talk II, and provided immediate opportunities for the subjects to use each feature in a communicative context. As part of the training, scripts were used to role-play contexts such as going shopping, and calling for a taxi on the telephone using Multi-Talk II. The subjects had access to Multi-Talk II only during the training sessions.

At the end of the training period, the subjects were videotaped with the same FPs describing news item 2 with Multi-Talk II (B, first treatment) and news item 3 with their regular communication systems (A, second baseline). Currently, the subjects have the Multi-Talk II with them and they are being encouraged to use it in various contexts. They use the Multi-Talk II installed either on a Texas Instruments TravelMate 2000 or a Sharp PC-6240 286 laptop computer connected to an Infovox miniVoxbox synthesiser which is mounted on the back of the laptop screen. SA, PT and CR will be videotaped after 3 months with the same FP, narrating another news item (B, second treatment). At that point, the subjects, their FPs and their speech pathologist will complete a questionnaire providing feedback and comments on the effectiveness of Multi-Talk II as a VOCA.

## 4. Analysis

Five minutes of the videotaped interactions between the subjects and their FPs were transcribed in detail for the above contexts. The interactions were transcribed by adapting the notation system developed by Bailey and Shane [5] and also by developing new notations for the current project. The following measures were calculated:

Communication rate in words: As a measure of efficiency; total number of words in a message divided by a sum of time taken to access a board or a device plus time taken for the message to be transmitted.

Communication breakdowns: As a measure of effectiveness; number of breakdowns divided by total number of opportunities provided where a breakdown could have occurred multiplied by 100.

Amount of participation: Number of words spoken by the familiar partner and number of words spoken, pointed to on the letter/word board or typed by the subjects. These were converted to percentages.

## 5. Results and Discussion

Figure 1 shows the baseline communication rate when describing news item 1, and during conversation for the three subjects with their regular communication system. It also shows the communication rate with Multi-Talk II describing news item 2 . For all three subjects, the rate was higher with Multi-Talk II than with their regular communication system. CR showed the biggest increase from 4.8 to 18.8 words/minute, followed by SA who showed an increase from 12.4 to 18.8 and PT whose rate increased from 6.6 to 11.3 words/minute. CR used the sentence store to narrate her news item and retrieved sentences easily, but made a monologue presentation of the story. PT also used the sentence store, but he also typed some appropriate comments and questions and the communication interaction was more natural. SA's rate during conversation was 29.3 words/minute, the highest as she spoke mostly and used her letter/word board only few times. However, when describing news item 1, she chose to point to words or spell words resulting in a slower rate of communication. For all three, their rate was higher during conversation than when presenting new information with their regular system. This could have been due to the familiarity of topics and vocabulary used during conversation.

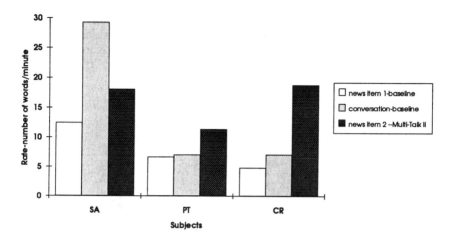

Figure 1. Communication Rate for Current Communication Systems and Multi-Talk II

At baseline, only SA had 10% breakdowns in conversation and none during description of news item 1. This could be because she used speech for conversation, and her FP found it difficult to understand her occasionally. When SA used her board, there were just occasional errors by her FP in identifying a letter or a word due to pointing, or predicting a wrong word. These were corrected with feedback from SA or self corrected by FP and the conversation flow was maintained. PT and CR used Polycom to type their new and old information and their partners also only had occasional letter or word identification errors.

With Multi-Talk II, the communication breakdowns increased to 38% when describing news item 2 for SA. This could be because her FP was hearing the synthetic speech for the first time and had some difficulty in understanding it. SA's FP laughed as soon as she heard the first sentence. The first 3 sentences had to be repeated several times, and finally the FP changed modes and looked at the screen to understand the message. Since SA had not used Multi-Talk II extensively, she could not use the strategies that she had learned to repair breakdowns. Interestingly, PT and CR's partners did not have any problems in following the synthetic speech. One reason could be that the subjects worked with their speech pathologists in improving the pronunciations of certain words by using the user's lexicon and also the way PT and CR presented the new information.

Figure 2 shows the amount of participation by subjects and their FPs during baseline description of news item 1 and during description of news item 2 with Multi-Talk II. The amount of participation during baseline showed that the SA contributed 37% during description of the news item 1 and 23% during conversation. SA was more in control during news description as she knew the information. With Multi-Talk II, SA spoke 27% and FP talked continuously while AB was retrieving messages which was a slow process for SA due to difficulties in accessing the keys. PT's amount of participation in terms of number of words spoken was similar during the baseline and when using the Multi-Talk II (33% and 35%). His FP was patient and waited till he completed his messages and never held on to her turn for too long. CR's FP dominated the interaction during the baseline interrupting CR constantly and contributing 87% to the conversation. However, there was a dramatic change when CR used Multi-Talk II to describe news item 2. Her FP was distracted by how CR used the device and contributed only 39%. The second baseline measures are currently being analysed .

PT mentioned after the videotaping that he really enjoyed using Multi-Talk II and it was easier for him to describe new information with Multi-Talk II. PT's partner also commented that it seemed natural with voice output and everyone could hear PT without peering over his shoulders. CR's familiar partner was impressed with the way CR could retrieve complete sentences with few keystrokes. CR has not rejected the device and is willing to try the VOCA outside the therapy situation.

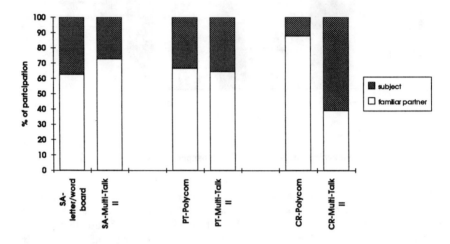

Figure 2. Amount of participation by the subjects and their familiar partners during news item narration at baseline and with Multi-Talk II

## 6. Summary

Initial findings show that the subjects communication rate increased with Multi-Talk II and they seem to participate more with Multi-Talk II. Currently the subjects are using Multi-Talk II outside the clinic situations. Long term use of the device in a variety of situations would provide us with clearer picture of the effectiveness of Multi-Talk II as a VOCA.

## 7. Acknowledgement

This project has been supported by the Swedish National Board for Industrial and Technical Development (NUTEK).

References

[1] Fonema AB (1986): Multi-Talk. Färgargårdstorget 24, S-116 43, Stockholm, Sweden.
[2] K. Galyas and E. Rosengren, Experiences with Multi-Talk in Sweden since 1987, *Proceedings of the European Conference on the Advancement of Rehabilitation Technology* (1990) pp. P.11. Maastricht, The Netherlands.
[3] A.F. Jinks, Consumer satisfaction with AAC devices, *ASHA*, (1992, October) 130.
[4] A.I. Batavia and G.S. Hammer, Towars the development of consumer-based criteria for the evaluation of assistive devices, *Journal of Rehabilitation Research and Development*, 27 (1990) 425-436
[5] Bailey, P. & Shane, H. (1983). Interactional strategies used by subject and adult communicators. In A.Kratt, (Ed.), (1985), *Communication interaction between aided and natural speakers- An IPCAS report* (pp.295-297). Toronto: Canadian Rehabilitation Council for the disabled.

# Comspec - Towards a Modular Software Architecture and Protocol for AAC Devices

Mats Lundälv, DART - Bräcke Östergård, Sweden
Dag Svanæs, University of Trondheim, Norway

**Abstract.** This paper presents research on the development of a software architecture for users with special needs. One of the aims is to gain experience with modular and versatile communication aids and access systems. A software architecture has been specified that incorporates some of the requirements of technical aids for disabled users. To be able to evaluate its feasibility empirically, an interactive design tool based on this architecture has been developed. It includes an Interface Builder, a Configuration Editor and a Vocabulary Editor. Existing software is integrated by way of a communication protocol that implements an abstract application. Trained therapists have already used the tool successfully to construct new applications from existing software components.

## 1. Introduction

The COMSPEC project was started in January 1989 based on a growing consciousness of the increasing difficulties in Alternative and Augmentative Communication (AAC) system development. We had by then gathered some experience in both the development and practical use of these systems. We saw clearly the rapidly growing complexity in AAC systems due to the increasing demand for more flexible and adaptive systems. We started to appreciate the huge efforts needed to maintain and further develop systems, and to transport them from old hardware platforms to new ones, or from one language and cultural environment to another. We saw similar systems being developed repeatedly from scratch, sometimes with some new valuable features added, but at the same time missing out some equally important old ones. We saw an increasing number of development projects not progressing from idea to product due to insufficient resources in terms of money or competence nor finding a broad enough market to support maintenance and further development of the product. At the same time we were aware of the great opportunities offered by the rapidly developing hardware and software platforms.

## 2. The COMSPEC Phases

The project aims to evolve a design in which the next generation of communication aids can be built from software modules which fit into a common architecture. The long term objective of the project is to produce: (1) A well-defined protocol and a set of programming tools to enable software developers to use existing modules and to create new ones. (2) A library of software modules to be made available to developers. (3) A user-friendly design tool for non-technical designers such as teachers and therapists, enabling them to build or adapt communication aids for individual users. The editor will be icon-based using metaphors and structures that are comprehensible and easily accessible to the non-technical designer.

## 2.1 Phase 1

Phase 1 of the project was funded by the Nordic Council for Handicap Issues (NNH) and ran from 1989 to 1990. During this phase, a questionnaire was produced to gather views on the functional design of a modular communication aid. It was distributed to individuals and institutions in the UK and the Nordic countries. The thirty replies were analysed, summarised and disseminated. Subsequently, working group members met to formulate the rationale for the design, and to produce a preliminary architecture and an initial set of protocols. The group met representatives from projects working along similar lines at the Hugh MacMillan Centre in Toronto and at the AI DuPont Institute in Delaware. Our conclusions have been influenced by their work, and we consequently aim to continue discussions and share ideas with these groups.

## 2.2 Phase 2

Phase 2 of the project ran from 1991 to 1993 and was funded by the Nordic Development Centre for Rehabilitation Engineering (NUH) and the Swedish Handicap Institute. Among the goals fulfilled in this phase were: (1) The design and implementation of a prototype COMSPEC system in Smalltalk/V on the Macintosh computer. It includes an Interface Builder, a Configuration Editor and a Vocabulary Editor. This prototype has been put in the public domain and made available for interested third parties and research centres. Details can be found in [5]. (2) The integration of existing and new systems through the COMSPEC inter-application protocol. We have so far been experimenting with the CALL Centre Smart Wheelchair, HyperCard and the popular drawing tool KidPix. Details can be found in [2].

## 2.3 Phase 3

We are currently seeking funding for a third phase of the project. The overall aim of this phase is to further develop the COMSPEC prototype and transfer it into a close-to-product form. A detailed evaluation by a wide range of technical and non-technical users will be performed, in readiness for the final production phase.

## 2.4 Phase 4

We see phase 4 as the implementation phase for the complete COMSPEC system. In the final system, new COMSPEC components will be distributed as DLL/XCMD files that will automatically be integrated into the software environment. This feature makes it possible for third party developers to extend the available set of COMSPEC components without having to alter the COMSPEC software environment.

## 3. Related Work

The COMSPEC project was inspired by work at the Hugh MacMillan Medical Centre in Toronto [4]. The aim of their project was to come up with guidelines for developers of alternate access systems. They structured their guidelines around an architectural model of alternate access systems based on a data flow model. This framework consisted of 12 interconnected components in a fixed structure. A prototype was implemented for demonstration purposes, but to our knowledge the full architectural model has never been applied directly to any large-scale project. It has, on the other hand, worked very well as an abstract model of current systems and has thus helped increase the general awareness and understanding of this class of problems.

HyperCard and its clones and spin-offs have made it possible for non-programmers to create and modify their work environment to an extent that was not imaginable only a decade ago. We have been much inspired by these systems and by its ancestor SMALLTALK-80. The separation we make in our architecture between Control, Presentation and Linguistic Content has borrowed much from the MVC-paradigm of SMALLTALK-80 [1].

## 4. The COMSPEC Architecture

We judged the Hugh MacMillan architecture to be too limited for the following reasons: Its fixed structure does not allow for multiple input and output channels. New modules cannot be easily integrated into the structure. Due to its static nature it does not allow for novel combinations of the modules. The data flow model makes it hard to implement semantic feedback. The symbol set and language skills of the end user are not made explicit.

The need for encapsulation and object specialisation (inheritance) in their architecture makes it natural to try an object-oriented solution. Unfortunately, object-orientation alone does not solve the problem. As Wegner points out in [6]: "..concerns of classification are complementary (orthogonal) to those of communication...". A software architecture must always be worked out in detail.

In the current COMSPEC architecture a running application consists of three parts: a configuration of functional components, screen layouts, and a language module. The latter is capable of storing a model of the user's vocabulary and linguistic skills. Our architecture is similar to the one proposed by the Hugh MacMillan group in that a running system is a configuration of interconnected functional components, but it is more open in the sense that we allow for the components to be interconnected more freely. Each component has one or more connection points that may be "wired" to one or more connection points in other components according to certain rules. We currently distinguish between connections of two kinds: unidirectional signal connections and bi-directional navigation connections. Connection points are either output points or input points of either signals or navigation. Connections can only be made from output points to input points. Signals allow for many-to-many connections, while navigation connections only allow for one-to-many. The structure of an application cannot be changed at runtime. The communication between the components is asynchronous and the execution is event-driven. Activities are either triggered by external events or by internal clock events.

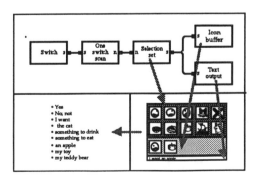

Figure 1. Application = Configuration + Layout + Language.

Figure 1 shows the three parts of a running COMSPEC application. The configuration has the visual appearance of a hi-fi system. We use this metaphor in the current version of the Configuration Editor in the design tool. Each box corresponds to a module in the resulting application and the wires reflect their interconnections. S-sockets are used for signals and N-sockets are used for navigation. The flow of information goes from left to right (i.e. output points are on the right side of the boxes and input points are on the left side).

The screen layouts define the size and position of a set of graphic objects. Some of these objects are referred to by the functional components of the configuration (e.g. text-editor components refer to text-area objects).

All components in a configuration automatically have access to a language module that contains the vocabulary of the end user with the available representations of the language items (symbols/words/phrases). This module can also incorporate syntactic and semantic rules. The language module is not a functional component as such. It resides at a level below an actual configuration and provides its components with the necessary lexical, syntactic, and semantic information.

*4.1. Signals*

Signal connections are unidirectional and allow for the transmission of event objects (signals). If a connection is branched to more than one receiving component, copies are automatically made of the signal objects. Signals are produced by hardware devices, internal clocks, and external sources (e.g. other applications or systems). Signals can be filtered, transformed and translated by appropriate COMSPEC components. This low-level control of the input devices is important for most communication aids and alternate access systems.

*4.2. Navigation*

Olsen [3] has argued that browsing activities take up a considerable part of the interaction time for most users. This is even more the case for users with access problems, and we have consequently paid special attention to navigation activities. The uni-directionality of signal connections makes it hard to implement semantic feedback. We have tried to overcome this problem by letting the so-called navigation connections be bi-directional. A navigation input point on a component gives the connected component access to a cursor in its data structure. A navigation protocol defines the messages that are allowed. These messages enable the connected component to move the cursor in an abstract tree structure, extract information about objects, ask for the set of possible operations and perform operations. Changes in the data structure lead to call-back events. All selection sets (e.g. keyboard emulation modules) and editors in the system implement this navigation protocol. Consequently, all operations in a system having to do with focus movement and item selection are dealt with in a uniform manner.

## 5. Implementing the Architecture

The architectural model does not map directly onto all existing software environments. The target environment has to provide a relatively fast asynchronous inter-process communication mechanism. Fortunately, such mechanisms are currently available on most of the target platforms (i.e. Apple Events in System 7, DDEs in Windows 3.0 and of course pipes in UNIX).

We have chosen a hybrid solution with modular applications capable of communicating with other applications through a well-defined communication protocol. The inter-application protocol at the operating system level is identical to the inter-component navigation protocol in the application. With this approach we hope to maintain the benefits of a simple architecture without introducing unnecessary computational overhead.

Applications that implements the inter-application protocol give alternate access systems direct access to their essential parts. This makes it possible to bypass the existing user interfaces in a structured way. For example, a drawing tool for children could automatically provide textual representations of its graphic objects such as: "A tiny red circle in the upper left corner". An alternate access system with a speech synthesiser and a scanning mechanism would in this case automatically offer a blind switch-using child meaningful access to this application.

In the final system, new COMSPEC components will be distributed as DLL/XCMD files that will automatically be integrated into the software environment. This feature makes it possible for third party developers to extend the available set of COMSPEC components without having to alter the systems software.

A pre-compiled version of the runtime kernel of COMSPEC makes it possible for developers to distribute COMSPEC applications as stand-alone programs.

## 6. Conclusion and future work

We have been encouraged by the positive comments made about the prototype system. Trained therapists have already used this design tool successfully to construct new applications from existing software components. We are convinced that a fully developed system will substantially improve the conditions for future production of a wide range of flexible, high quality communication and access aids for people with impairments of many kinds.

Experience from similar projects has taught us that it is very important for programmers to have available for inspection and modification all the source code for libraries and runtime modules. We therefore strongly recommend to put well-documented source code in the public domain both for the runtime kernel of COMSPEC and for the standard components. End products developed with the COMSPEC tool will not need to include the tool itself, and as long as the format of the COMSPEC application files are well documented, the developers will have full control over all parts of a distributed product.

## References

[1] A. Goldberg, Information Models, Views and Controllers: The key to reusability in Smalltalk-80 lies within MVC, Dr.Dobb's Journal of Software Tools, July 1990.

[2] J. P. Odor, Connecting External Systems to COMSPEC Aids, CALL Centre, Edinburgh, 1992.

[3] D. Olsen, A Browse/Edit Model for User Interface Management, Graphics Interface '88, June 1988.

[4] F. Shein et al., A Model for Alternate Access Systems, in Proceedings of 12th Annual RESNA Conference, New Orleans, 1989.

[5] D. Svanæs et al., The Specification of a Versatile Communication Aid and Writing Tool. To appear in ECKART'2 proceedings, Stockholm 1993.

[6] P. Wegner, Classification in Object-Oriented Systems, SIGPLAN Notices 21, 10, (October 1986), 173-182.

# Restoration of Gait in Paraplegics by Functional Electrical Stimulation and Orthoses (Hybrid Systems)

Peter H. Veltink, Bart F.J.M. Koopman, Hermie J. Hermens,
Henry M. Franken, Gert Baardman, Jacques Th.M.M. Cloostermans,
Jan A. van Alsté, Gerrit Zilvold, Henk J. Grootenboer and Herman B.K. Boom

*Centre for Rehabilitation Technology:*
*University of Twente, Biomedical Technological Institute,*
*P.O. Box 217, 7500 AE Enschede, the Netherlands.*
*and The Roessingh Rehabilitation Centre,*
*P.O. Box 310, 7500 AH Enschede, the Netherlands.*

**Abstract.** Gait restoration in paraplegics by means of electrical stimulation of paralysed muscles (FES) in combination with orthoses (hybrid systems) is being investigated at the Centre for Rehabilitation Technology (University of Twente and the Roessingh Rehabilitation Centre). The research is well embedded in concerted European efforts in this field. Research activities include electrical stimulation of paralysed muscles, orthosis design, automatic control systems, gait analysis, biomechanical modelling, and clinical application.

## 1. Introduction

Gait restoration in paraplegics by means of electrical stimulation of paralysed muscles (Functional Electrical Stimulation: FES) in combination with orthoses (hybrid systems) is a promising new technology in rehabilitation. The electrical stimulation of paralysed muscles can yield active generation of movement and the orthosis supplies adequate support and restricts the number of degrees of freedom of the movement. Transformation of the current technology in the areas of orthotics and muscle stimulation into a wide spread clinically accepted hybrid system for restoring paraplegic gait asks for an integrated design of the system [1].

The University of Twente and the Roessingh Rehabilitation Centre work together in the Centre for Rehabilitation Technology. They jointly undertake a substantial research effort in improving technology for gait restoration in paraplegics using hybrid systems (figure 1).

This research effort is well embedded in concerted European efforts in this area: the Centre of Rehabilitation Engineering takes part in the BIOMED1 concerted action RAFT, and previously in the preceeding concerted action MORE. Furthermore, joint efforts with industry are being undertaken in the Eureka project CALIES. M.Sc. and Ph.D. students,

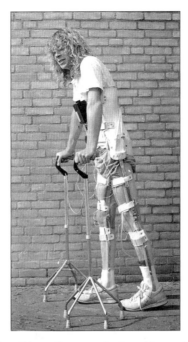

*Figure 1.* *Experimental walking of a paraplegic subject using a hybrid FES-orthosis system at the Twente Centre for Rehabilitation Technology.*

exchanged between European Universities in the ERASMUS student exchange program, contribute in the research efforts as part of their study. Furthermore, recently a Human Capital and Mobility proposal has been granted in the area of artificial neuromuscular sensing and control for a research network with exchange of post-doctoral fellows.

The goal of this paper is to give an overview of the current research activities of the Twente Centre for Rehabilitation Technology in the area of gait restoration in paraplegics using hybrid systems. Research areas encompass muscle stimulation, orthosis design, automatic control of hybrid systems, gait analysis, biomechanical modelling and clinical application.

## 2. Active generation of movement by electrical stimulation of paralysed muscles

In a hybrid system, a well defined set of degrees of freedom should be actively controlled by artificially stimulated paralysed muscles. The constitution of this set depends on the function to be restored. The other degrees of freedom should be restricted by the orthosis part of the system.

Muscles can be stimulated either by electrodes on the skin or by electrodes positioned within the body outside or inside nerves or muscles. Stimulation with electrodes in the body is potentially more selective and can lead to a better control of muscle contraction. It can be applied in combination with an implantable stimulator (CALIES project). However, it requires extensive surgery.

Electrical stimulation of paralysed muscles using skin electrodes inherently results in unphysiological muscle activation, characterised by synchronous activation and inverse recruitment of motor units of the muscle. However, stimulation by skin electrodes is a noninvasive method, acceptable in clinical practice, which will remain relevant as an alternative even if implantable stimulation systems become available.

In our centre the optimal activation of muscles for generation of functional movements is studied. The mechanical muscle response to stimulation of hip flexors, extensors and knee extensors by skin electrodes and its functional use are investigated [2], [3]. Also, the influence of stimulation parameters and movement parameters on muscle fatigue during electrical stimulation is an important research topic [4], [5], because muscle fatigue is one of the main limiting factors to the functional application of electrical stimulation. Muscle fatigue, defined in a relative sense, appeared not to depend on the recruitment level, and appeared to increase with increasing joint angular velocity and with increasing duty cycle.

## 3. Design of Orthoses for hybrid systems

The mechanical parts of hybrid systems for restoration of gait in paraplegics are based on the Reciprocating Gait Orthosis design [2]. An orthosis gives static support, which is not easily accomplished by electrical stimulation, because of muscle fatigue. It also limits the number of degrees of freedom to be controlled by active muscle contractions induced by electrical stimulation.

The Reciprocating Gait Orthosis used clinically to date only allows for hip movements in the sagittal plane. Hip extension in one leg is coupled with hip flexion in the other leg. These orthoses allow no knee flexion or ankle dorsi- or plantar flexion during walking, resulting in a rather unnatural walking pattern.

We investigate the integrated design of the orthosis - stimulation system, which should allow rather natural movements at lower energy cost and lower muscle fatigue. As for the orthosis part of the integrated design a new type of knee joint has been developed which allows for knee flexion during the swing phase of gait, and mechanically locks the knee during the stance phase. Furthermore, the ankle joint is being improved, allowing for limited dorsi- and plantar flexion.

## 4. Artificial control of motor tasks

Artificial control of a hybrid system is needed in order to perform the motor tasks desired by the user. The artificial control system should provide the user with maximal flexibility and a functional interface.

Artificial control of motor tasks like standing up [6], standing [7] and walking are important research topics at the Twente Centre of Rehabilitation Technology. Several control strategies have been designed and tested. For controlling cyclical tasks like walking, an adaptive optimal control strategy in combination with a high level finite state control strategy is being developed [8], [9].

## 5. Biomechanical modelling for individual optimisation of hybrid system design

The hybrid system can be viewed as a system with active and passive components: The active components are the artificially stimulated muscles which generate joint torques that may result in a movement and the passive components are orthotic components which stabilize the joints. To understand how these components interact and influence the walking movement, two computer models are being designed to simulate walking with a hybrid system.

The first model describes the 'external' biomechanics: The relation between the joint torques and the movement. It is based on the so-called direct dynamics method, in which the torques are prescribed and the resulting movement is predicted [10]. The influence of the orthosis is modelled as a set of constraints, placed upon the joints. This method is extended with the implementation of optimization techniques. In an optimal control scheme, only some end-conditions such as the step length and the average walking velocity are prescribed. By minimizing a certain criterion, such as the energy consumption, both the movement and the necessary joint moments of force can be predicted. The latter is important in determining how the muscles should be stimulated.

The second model describes the muscle dynamics: The relations between the joint torques and the muscle forces of the (artificially) stimulated muscles. These include effects such as the time-delay between stimulation and force production, force-length relations etc. At present, the model estimates the distribution of the muscle forces with given joint torques and movements but it may well be used the other way around. A detailed description of the anatomical structure of the muscles in the lower extremities is obtained with Magnetic Resonance Imaging Techniques for a better estimation of parameters such as muscle moment arms.

Both models depend on individual properties and abilities of the patient, such as body weight, dimensions and the maximal torques that can be generated at the joints. By combining the two models, the optimal configuration of the hybrid system for the individual can be determined to obtain a maximal walking performance. The information obtained can also be used to optimise the muscle training programme for the individual patient, in order to improve his walking ability.

## 6. Gait analysis for objective evaluation of task performance

Gait analysis is one of the tools to evaluate the performance of walking with a hybrid system. The walking movement is registered with a video-based measuring system by which markers, attached to the body of the subject, are tracked in space. An extensive software package has been developed to evaluate the measured data and to perform the gait analysis. The main part of this package is an inverse dynamics model to determine the biomechanical output at the joints (e.g. joint torques, joint powers) which was originally developed to analyse and predict normal and prosthetic gait [11]. This model is being extended to simulate the use of walking aids, which are essential in walking with a hybrid system, because it provides balance. Gait analysis can then be used to evaluate the effectiveness of how the  artificially stimulated muscles contribute to the forward propulsion and how this can be improved. At present, still the largest part of the energy needed for the propulsion is generated at the arm and shoulder joints.

## 7. Clinical application of hybrid systems for restoration of paraplegic gait

Hybrid systems for restoration of gait in paraplegics have been applied in a clinical program at the Roessingh Rehabilitation Centre now for over seven years, resulting in an extensive experience in this area.

In this clinical program newly developed technology is being tested [12], and if proven successful, incorporated in a modular clinical hybrid system.

## 8. Perspective

In the research effort described technological stimulation, orthosis and control strategy tools are being developed and their effects biomechanically analysed. Furthermore, the resulting motor task performance is evaluated by biomechanical and functional analysis procedures.

The goal of this joint effort is to develop procedures for optimal design of hybrid systems for each individual patient. An optimal system should be predicted on the basis of biomechanical analysis of the deficits in the motor performance of the individual and on the technological tools available. The patient should then be supplied and trained with the proposed optimal configuration. After this training phase, the motor performance is re-evaluated and compared with the predicted level of performance. On the basis of this procedure the prediction tools can be improved.

References
[1]   H.J. Hermens, A.J. Mulder, A. Schoute, G. Baardman, G. Zilvold, B.J. Andrews, C.A. Kirkwood, M.H. Granat and M. DeLargy, Development of Practical Hybrid FES Systems, *Proc. 3rd Vienna International Workshop on Functional Electrostimulation; Basics, Technology and Application*, September 1989, pp. 89-92.
[2]   G. Baardman, J.M. Vastenholt and H.J. Hermens, Assessment of Propulsive properties of Hip Muscle Stimulation Methods in Hybrid Systems, *Proc. 4th Vienna International Workshop on Functional Electrostimulation; Basics, Technology, Clinical Application*, September 1992, pp. 69-72.
[3]   P.H. Veltink, R. Tijsmans, H.M. Franken and H.B.K. Boom, Identification of Electrically Stimulated Quadriceps - Lower Leg Dynamics, *Proc. 14th Annual International Conference of the IEEE Engineering in Medicine and Biology Society*, Paris, November 1992, pp. 1339-1340.
[4]   H.B.K. Boom, A.J. Mulder and P.H. Veltink, Fatigue during Functional Neuromuscular Stimulation, *Progress in Brain Research*, accepted.
[5]   H.M. Franken, P.H. Veltink and H.B.K. Boom, Fatigue of Intermittently Stimulated Paralyzed Human Quadriceps during Imposed Cyclical Lower Leg Movements, *International Journal of Electromyography and Kinesiology*, accepted.
[6]   A.J. Mulder, P.H. Veltink and H.B.K. Boom, On/off Control in FES-induced Standing Up: a Model Study and Experiments, *Med. & Biol. Eng. & Comput.* 30 (1992) 205-212.
[7]   A.J. Mulder, P.H. Veltink, H.B.K. Boom and G. Zilvold, Low-level Finite State Control of Knee Joint in Paraplegic Standing, *J. Biomed. Eng.* 14 (1992) 3-8.
[8]   P.H. Veltink, Control of FES-induced Cyclical Movements of the Lower Leg, *Med. & Biol. Eng. & Comput.* 29 (1991) NS8-NS12.
[9]   P.H. Veltink, H.M. Franken, J.A. van Alsté and H.B.K. Boom, Modelling the Optimal Control of Cyclical Leg Movements induced by Functional Electrical Stimulation, *International Journal of Artificial Organs* 15 (1992) 746-755.
[10]  D. van de Belt, H.J. Grootenboer, H.F.J.M. Koopman, Simulation and Evaluation of FES-induced Walking, *Proc. 14th Annual International Conference of the IEEE Engineering in Medicine and Biology Society*, Paris, November 1992, pp. 1345-1346.
[11]  H.F.J.M. Koopman, The three-dimensional Analysis and Prediction of Human Walking, PhD-thesis, University of Twente, Enschede, 1989.
[12]  G. Baardman, A.G.M. Lissone and H.J. Hermens, Evaluation of the Functionality of Walking Systems, *Adv. in External Control of Human Extremities X*, D.B. Popovic (ed.), Dubrovnik 1989, pp. 381-386.

# Mobile Communications and Environment Control for Wheelchair Users

Barry REDMOND
*Dublin Institute of Technology, Kevin Street, Dublin 8, Ireland*

Robert ALLEN
*Central Remedial Clinic, Vernon Avenue, Dublin 3, Ireland*

Richard BULLOCK
*Quest Enabling Devices Ltd, Ability House, 242 Gosport Road, Fareham, Hampshire PO16 OSS, UK*

**Abstract.** This paper presents the results of the MECCS project run under the pilot phase of the TIDE programme. The objective of the project was to produce a prototype of a home control and communications system for wheelchair users. The paper gives brief descriptions of the system designed by the project, the problems encountered, and the conclusions reached.

## 1. Introduction

The objective of the MECCS project of the TIDE pilot programme was to produce a prototype of a home control and communications system for wheelchair users. The system is intended to allow a wheelchair user to have greater freedom within their home, and to function more independently for longer periods.

The project aimed to provide a user with a number of specific facilities directly from a powered or non-powered wheelchair as they move about within a normal domestic environment. The facilities to be provided included remote control of simple on/off electrical appliances, remote control and monitoring of the front door lock, remote channel selection and volume adjustment of a television, use of the telephone, a 2-way intercom link to the front door, and an emergency or alarm activation (Figure 1). The user would interact with the system via a single interface mounted on the wheelchair. The user's input to the interface would be by their choice of keyboard or alternative input switches. The system was to be modular in design so that it could easily be adapted to the initial and changing needs of a user, and so that further technical developments could be incorporated with a minimum of redesign. A major aim of the project was to provide these facilities in a cost-efficient system that could be brought to market quickly as a practical commercial product.

The project lasted 15 months, ending in March 1993, with a consortium consisting of just three partners, all of whom had existing working relationships before the project began.

## 2. MECCS System Overview

The project made use of existing commercial products wherever possible in order to take advantage of mass production cost savings. The X10 home control system was used to allow the system to control electrical appliances around the home.

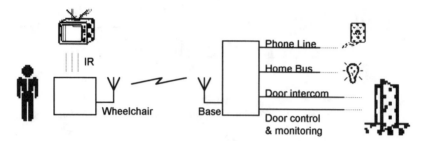

Figure 1.   System functions

An infra-red controller with a serial interface was used to provide television control;  A commercial cordless telephone was used to provide the voice communications;  A laptop PC was used for the user interface.

The system architecture is based on a number of modules with defined functions and interfaces.  The interfaces are almost all serial data links, using the MECCS Command Language (Figure 2).

### 3. User Needs

The original impetus for this project came from firsthand experience with wheelchair users in various settings.  The functions to be included in the system were selected by considering the activities and reported problems of some wheelchair users and the availability of technical devices which might be used to overcome them.  The underlying objective was to provide the means for a wheelchair user to function independently for significantly longer periods. The only requirement on the user is that he or she be able to operate the system via the keyboard or alternative switch input, and that they be able to read the information presented on the screen.

The consortium considered that although existing systems could provide the required functionality, no one system integrated all the control and communications functions. Typically, systems are assembled for each user from individual pieces of equipment from different manufacturers.  They tend to be expensive, difficult to adapt to changing needs, technically complex, and they can require intrusive equipment and cables around the home.

The project was begun without any formal research to support the need perceived by the partners in the consortium, but as part of the project a limited survey was carried out to determine users' needs more precisely.

### 4. User Interface

The user interface for the system is based on a laptop PC running Microsoft Windows with a specially designed software package.  A PC was used in order to reduce the development time, and to avoid duplication of equipment for users who may wish to use a PC for other purposes.  Microsoft Windows was selected because of its multi-tasking and task-switching capabilities.  The MECCS software on the PC was implemented as a user-oriented interface part and a system-oriented communications part.  The user interface was written using Microsoft Visual Basic and was optimised for a monochrome LCD screen.

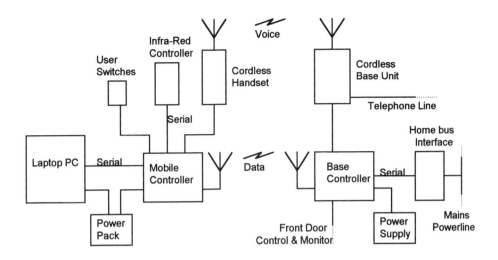

Figure 2.   System block diagram

The communications software was written as a Windows Dynamic Link Library (DLL) using Borland C.

The user interface software went through a number of iterations during the project, and a larger than expected proportion of the project resources was used in developing the user interface.   Since the system is intended to be usable by people who have no previous experience of computers, it is important that interaction with it be as intuitive as possible. To achieve this, the interface must be designed to act and react in ways that the user can easily anticipate.   This, in turn, is achieved by ensuring that the model of the user's environment presented on the screen matches the user's own model as closely as possible.

A graphical or map representation of the layout of the user's environment was rejected because it was felt that this is not how a person normally thinks of their surroundings, and because the relationship between the image on the screen and the real world would change as the wheelchair moved.   The representation chosen for the interface was to use the conventional Windows buttons and text boxes to present a list of rooms to the user, and then to present a selected room as a set of devices arranged in columns on the screen.   Each device is represented as an On and an Off button with a filled or empty box to report the device status.   More complex devices such as the telephone, television or front door are represented by appropriate sets of buttons and text boxes.

The user interface may be controlled by mouse, keyboard or alternative input switches. The mouse and keyboard control use the normal Windows functions.   Switch input may be either single or double switches connected to the MECCS Mobile Controller (Figure 2). Any operation of a switch causes a message to be sent to the user interface software in the PC.   Switch operation allows the user to scan rows and items to select a button or object on the screen.   In single switch mode, screen objects are automatically highlighted in sequence and operating the switch causes the highlighted object to be selected.   If the selected object requires text input then a keyboard simulation appears on the screen.

The user interface software has been designed to be highly configurable by the installer or end-user.   Rooms and devices may be added, descriptive text changed, individual configurations loaded and saved, and switch mode scanning delays adjusted.

## 5. Communications

Communication among the elements of the MECCS system uses a subset of the Esprit Home Systems (HS) command language. The command language defines the formats for exchanging commands and reports between the user interface software, the Mobile Controller and the Base Controller. By basing the MECCS command language on the HS definitions the consortium have ensured that the basis for future expansion of the system is in place. Connecting the MECCS system to the HS bus will not require complex protocol conversion software since the internal protocols are already a subset of the HS protocols and a single software task in the MECCS Base Controller handles messages to and from the home bus interface.

At present the use of the relatively limited X10 home bus means that a number of the functions implemented on the user interface and in the MECCS command language cannot actually be used because X10 does not support them.

Infra-red and radio were considered for the communications medium between the wheelchair and the fixed part of the system. Radio was selected for a number of reasons. Firstly it was decided by the consortium that an infra-red system to cover a number of rooms and areas in a house adequately would require a significant amount of extra wiring and transceivers. Secondly, radio technology has advanced rapidly in recent times and can now provide compact reliable and inexpensive low-power transceivers. Lastly, radio was judged to be appropriate given the objective of voice plus data communications, and the eventual possibility of using the Digital European Cordless Telephone (DECT) technology.

Initially it was hoped to use a standard voice plus data radio link but this proved impractical within the time scale and resources of the project. The DECT standard looks promising for applications such as this, but it is still relatively expensive. After considering a number of alternatives the consortium decided to use a combination of a specially designed radio link for data, and a separate commercial cordless telephone for voice. This gave the required functions using available technology and at a relatively low manufacturing cost.

At present there are no pan-European standards for radio frequencies to be used for short-range data, which means that different countries will require slightly different versions of the MECCS system.

## 6. Home Bus

The MECCS system was originally intended to use the Esprit Home Systems bus to control and monitor appliances around the home. When it became apparent that Home Systems components would not be available within the time scale of the MECCS project, other home bus systems were examined. X10 was selected because of its availability, low cost, and use of the power line for communications. These advantages were judged to outweigh the disadvantages of control only (no appliance status monitoring), and general lack of functions such as message acknowledgement and security. The X10 home bus system consists of a single controller unit and a number of small slave units at selected power outlets. The controller transmits a single unacknowledged message on the power line when it is required to turn one of the slave units on or off. The controller has no means of knowing whether the destination slave unit received the message correctly, or even if the slave unit exists.

The lack of feedback from controlled devices does not seriously limit the applications of the MECCS system. At worst, it may be an inconvenience for the user. The MECCS system does monitor the front door and the doorbell but these signals are not sent over the power line-based home bus in order that they will not be affected by a power cut.

The X10 home bus cannot be used to control the channel and volume of a television set. This was one of the specific objectives of the project, and therefore the MECCS system includes an infra-red remote control unit mounted on the wheelchair and controlled by the MECCS Mobile Controller.

The MECCS system has been designed to move to the Home Systems (HS) bus when it becomes commercially available. The modularity of the system design means that the MECCS system can be readily adapted by the manufacturers to use any home bus.


## 7. Power management

Power management is provided separately for the mobile and fixed equipment. On the wheelchair it is required that the equipment operate from batteries for as much as possible of a normal day. A period of 10 hours of average use was selected as giving reasonable freedom to the user. The MECCS equipment on the wheelchair operates from its own rechargeable batteries, independently of the motor batteries of a powered wheelchair. This is to minimise electrical interference between the motors and the MECCS electronics, to ensure that the MECCS system can still be used in the event that the motor batteries become discharged, and to allow the system to be fitted to non-powered wheelchairs.

The laptop PC used for the user interface is the biggest drain on the batteries on the wheelchair. Typical laptop computers have internal rechargeable batteries which give 2 to 3 hours of use. The MECCS system must therefore provide further battery capacity equivalent to about three times that contained within the laptop PC in order to run it for 10 hours. It is expected that current trends in power requirements for small computers will allow the battery capacity needed on the wheelchair to be significantly reduced in the near future.

The MECCS batteries on the wheelchair are recharged using a separate charger, typically overnight.

Under normal conditions the fixed MECCS equipment, at the base unit, is powered by the mains. However, for the safety and security of the user it is necessary for some of the facilities of the system to remain operational even if mains power should fail. Therefore a trickle-charged battery has been included to maintain power to the MECCS electronics, the telephone, and the front door monitoring and control functions. The battery provides 2 hours of operation after a mains failure.


## 8. Conclusions

The objectives of the project were met. The consortium intends to commercialise the prototype and to develop the system further. The project demonstrated the feasibility of the integrated modular approach and explored user interface requirements in this specialised area.

Future work will examine the user interface requirements in more detail, and will look at the possibility of incorporating emerging technology and standards such as DECT and HS. Integration of the MECCS system with other wheelchair mounted equipment will also be explored.

# The Information Prosthetic for Severely Physically Handicapped Children

E. Hoenkamp & R. Voort

*Psychological Laboratory, NICI, Postbus 9104, 6500 HE Nijmegen, Netherlands*
*LCN, Postbus 1408, 6501 BK Nijmegen, Netherlands*

**Abstract.** Physically handicapped children can derive exceptional benefits from computer applications. A careful evaluation of such applications is called for, however, to thwart unjustified hopes or claims. This paper describes the development and evaluation of a computer based environment, refered to as the 'information prosthetic'. It consists of pointing devices and a computer program. In a large scale pre-test post-test design, the information prosthetic was evaluated on its effects on attention and cognitive- and emotional development of physically handicapped children aged four to eight. The experimental group worked five months, twice a week, during 20 minutes with the computer. Teacher questionnaires confirmed previous research that immediate effects may be considerable. In contrast however, an analysis of variance (ANOVA) showed long term treatment effects to be negligible.

## 1. Introduction

The significance of evaluating the hard- and software presented here arises from three observations:

- A severe physical handicap not only prevents the child from manipulating objects at will, or explore its environment by itself, the lack of such experiences may delay the emotional and cognitive development of the child [1, 2, 3].
- A computer-based learning environment in which the child can be active independently may alleviate these problems [4, 5].
- Speculations in the literature for persistence of such benefits over time, have not been experimentally investigated.

The first two points more than justify exploring computer applications for children with special needs; the third point however calls for careful evaluation to avoid excessive hopes or claims. So, given the wide range of cognitive and motoric disabilities, we set out to develop a computer-based environment that could be easily tailored to each child's individual needs [6]. The design aimed at two goals. The first was to familiarize the child with the computer to make it less dependent, enabling it to play and act more on its own. The second goal was to assess the value of computer activities for the child's development. This article shows how we realized these goals. Section 2. introduces the computer-based environment ('information prosthetic'), and section 3. describes the evaluation research.

## 2. The 'Information Prosthetic'

The information prosthetic consists of pointing devices attached to a computer, and a program.

### 2.1. The Pointing Devices

We first used the following well-known devices: *single switches*, *mouse* and *joystick*. Since the single switch option pertained to only one program, and some children could not operate the mouse or the joystick correctly, several alternative input devices had to be developed.

The *button box* has four white buttons labeled with an arrow, one for each direction, and a red horizontal bar as the fire button. The cursor on the screen moves in the direction of the arrow as long as the button is held down. Besides motor problems some children had cognitive difficulties with the button box: As opposed to mouse and joystick, the movement of the cursor does not agree with the hand movement.

The *touch sensitive device* consists of five individual contact surfaces (analogous to the button box, but switching on contact). The contact surfaces can be varied in size and located freely, thus making it adaptable to individual (dis-)abilities.

The *scan system* has five lights, positioned around the screen: a green one on each side (for each direction), and a remaining red one in a corner as fire button. The computer turns the lights clockwise on and off. When a light is on, the user can respond by pressing a single switch. As long as the switch remains pressed, the cursor moves in the direction of the light. This device can even be used for very restricted motor skills: lifting a knee or nodding the head suffices. We found an unfortunate constraint on all pointing devices we tried: if it requires less motor skill, it requires more cognitive ability, and vice versa.

## 2.2. The Program

The program (published as 'Clowns' [7]) covers essential skills that young children must master, including: recognition of form, sort and classify by shape and color, determine sameness and difference among objects, develop one to one correspondence, and visual memory. The program works with pictograms, allowing children to work independently. There are nine games, varying from low to moderate complexity. Here are the games, together with their description and (sometimes obvious) purpose:

*Picture book:* when a single switch is pressed a new picture appears on the screen, so the child can browse through a book. It learns how its action evokes a reaction on the screen.

*Build a picture:* like the picture book, but with each key press a new part of a picture appears until the picture is complete.

*Guess a figure:* a figure is hidden by white squares. By moving the cursor to a square and pressing the fire button, a hidden part becomes visible. As more and more of the figure appears, the child can try to guess the completion. This game practices form recognition.

*Resemblance:* the child has to choose the pictures on the screen that resemble an example picture. This teaches shape and color discrimination.

*Drawing:* the child can select a color. Moving the pointing device leaves a track on the screen. Drawing stimulates the creativity of the child.

*Coloring book:* the child can select colors to fill the surfaces in the drawing.

*Mosaic:* a grid of squares appears. There are two modes: with or without an example. Reproducing the example teaches visual discrimination, visual analysis and visual synthesis. Without an example the child can make something by itself, stimulating creativity.

*One by One:* the child has to select two cards that belong to each other (i.e. same color, same form). This develops understanding one tot one correspondence.

*Memory:* the child has to select two identical cards that appear upside down on the screen. This teaches visual memory.

## 3. The Evaluation Research

Since the information prosthetic can be tailored to the individual without changing the (standardized) task, we started an evaluation of this instrument [8]. The evaluation research then, was conducted to answer the following questions:

- Does the information prosthetic have a significant effect on the cognitive and emotional development and the attention,
- What variables (i.e. diagnosis, severity of the handicap) determine how effective it is.

## 3.1. Method

### Subjects

Subjects were 138 physically handicapped children, enrolled in fourteen special schools for the physically handicapped. The sample represented circa 10% of the population in the

Netherlands. The 73 male and 65 female subjects ranged in age from 48 to 98 months (mean=74 months, SD=12).

To match experimental and a control group all children were classified by diagnosis: cerebral palsy (104), spina bifida (16) and motoric coordination dysfunction (14). Because we expected that diagnosis, severity of the handicap and intelligence could have an important influence the effect on the information prosthetic we classified the children also by these factors. Random block design assigned a child to the experimental or the control group [9]. This design tries to divide the population in blocks that are as homogeneous as possible for the variables under study. This resulted in 69 pairs of children who are comparable in diagnosis, severity of the handicap and intelligence score. Of each pair, one child was assigned to the experimental group and one to the control group. Each group contained 52 children with the diagnosis cerebral palsy, 8 children with a spina bifida and 9 children with a motoric co-ordination dysfunction. The experimental group closely resembled the control group on *sex* (experimental group 30 males and 30 females; control group 34 males and 35 females), *age* (mean age experimental group 74 months, control group 75 months), *intelligence* (SON-score experimental group 35,49 (SD=10,75), SON-score control group 43,51 (SD=11,96); Raven-score experimental group 7,77 (SD=4,68), Raven-score control group 7,69 (SD=5,75)) and *severity of hand movement disability* [8].

## Design

A pretest-posttest design was used. The children participated during one school year. At the start of the school year all children were given the pre-test that measured cognitive development, attention and emotional development. The same was measured at the end of the school year as post-test. A teacher questionnaire about the social validity of the information prosthetic was administered as post-test only. Attention during compture work was measured in an additional experiment.

## Procedure

Following the pre-test, forty-four teachers and six occupational therapists were instructed in working with the information prosthetic. Then the children in the experimental group were given microcomputer sessions during five months, twice a week, 20 minutes. The software used ('Clowns') was designed to enable the children to work independently and to teach them pre-school skills. Every child worked with the program at its own level. The control group did not work with the computer and received no alternative program. The rationale was that these children already receive much individual attention, and we didn't want to burden the teachers more than necessary.

## Measures

We measured the cognitive development with the SON 2,5-7 years and the Raven (using the sum of raw subtest-scores). The SON consists of five subtests: sort by color and form; mosaic; combine; visual memory; and drawing. The Raven tests reasoning by analogy. The child is asked to choose an alternative to complete a figure. We registered the right and wrong answers.

For measuring attention we developed an observation task. The children were observed in their class rooms during two tasks with pencil and paper. In the 'mosaic' task, the child has to copy an example consisting of a string of squares. In the 'coloring' task, the child has to color pictures in a small coloring book. The technique used was time-sampling. During ten minutes every ten seconds the behaviour of the child was recorded in one of six categories: (1) T= attention paid to the task; (2) TP= talk to someone about the tasks, while not looking at the task; (3) N= no attention paid to the task; (4) NT= paying no attention to, nor talking about the task; (5) L= stand up or walk away; (6) B= other factors like going to the toilet or sneezing. The inter-observer agreement was sufficient: ten out of twelve calculated scores reached al least 80%. For each child we counted the scored categories. For the mosaic task and the coloring task we computed the task attention score ($\%T=(T+TP)/(T+TP+N+NP+L+B)$) and the task not-attention score ($(\%N=(N+NP)/(T+TP+N+NP+L+B))$).

We measured the emotional development using the NCKS (Nijmegen California Kinder Sorteertechniek). The NCKS was designed and standardized by our department of developmental psychology, and helps the teacher to profile the independence of the child. The NCKS forces the rater to sort 100 cards containing sentences that refer to the child's behavioral characteristics. (This results in two scores: ego-flexibility and ego-control).

We assessed the social validity of the tests via a questionnaire [10]. The three parts of this questionnaire were: (1) the social significance of the goals (does the teacher want these goals?); (2) the social appropriateness of the procedures (does the teacher consider the treatment procedures acceptable?); (3) the social importance of the effects (is the teacher satisfied with the results?).

In an separate experiment we observed the attention of the children in the experimental group during work with the computer. The task was comparable to the observation of attention in the pre- and post-test. The children worked ten minutes with a mosaic task and ten minutes on a coloring task on the computer. The observation categories used are the same as in the pre- and post-test. We calculated for both tasks the task attention score ($\%T=(T+TP)/(T+TP+N+NP+L+B)$) and the task not-attention score (($\%N=(N+NP)/(T+TP+N+NP+L+B)$). The scores for working with the computer are compared with the scores during for with pencil and paper.

## 3.2. Results

### Pre- and Post-test
The mean scores and standard deviations for the experimental and control group on the pre- and post-test are summarized in Table 1.

None of the differences (except one) between experimental and control group were significant ($p<.05$). There was only a significant difference at the post-test on the ego-control score (ego-control: $F(1,128)=5,12$; $p=0,03$). Since there was also a difference (though not significant) at the pre-test on the ego-control score, the difference score of experimental and control group on ego control was compared. This difference was not significant ($F (1,128)=3,06$; $p=0,08$).

The scores offer no evidence that working with the information prosthetic has a positive effect on attention, cognitive data, or emotional data. Nor does regression analysis demonstrate an effect of diagnosis, severity of the handicap in the hands, or age on the progress scores of the different tests.

### Teacher questionnaire
Analysis of the first part of the questionnaire (the social significance of the goals) revealed that teachers judged the goal 'the child obtains a tool to take initiatives on its own' as most significant. The answers in the second part, concerning the treatment procedures, were acceptable. The third part showed that teachers were undecided about the social importance of the effects. Some remarks are: "it is too early to see a clear result" and "hard to say, there are more factors involved". Some specific remarks were "the child became more self confident", "the child gets a higher self esteem by working with the computer" and "clear improvement of concentration". More than 83% of the teachers said they took pleasure from supporting the children, mainly because the children enjoyed it. Given the same age group, 91,7% of the teachers would use the information prosthetic in their class room again.

### Attention during work with the computer

Table 1. Mean scores and standard deviations of the experimental and control group on the pre- and post-test

| | Pre-test | | Post-test | |
| | Control | Experimental | Control | Experimental |
| Tests | Mean (SD) | Mean (SD) | Mean (SD) | Mean (SD) |
|---|---|---|---|---|
| *Cognitive data* | | | | |
| SON | 35.5 (10.8) | 34.5 (12) | 40.7 (11) | 38.8 (11.8) |
| Raven | 7.8 (4.7) | 7.7 (5.8) | 9.6 (6) | 9.6 (6.6) |
| *Attention* | | | | |
| % T mosaic-task | 74.8 (14.2) | 74.8 (14.7) | 76.4 (12.8) | 72.8 (18.7) |
| % N mosaic-task | 23.5 (14.0) | 23.4 (14.2) | 21.8 (12.0) | 25.6 (18.2) |
| % T color-task | 75.1 (13.5) | 71.7 (16.7) | 74.2 (14.0) | 73.4 (14.0) |
| % N color-task | 22.7 (14.3) | 24.1 (14.0) | 24.0 (14.5) | 23.6 (11.9) |
| *Emotional data* | | | | |
| Ego-flexibility | 0.12 (0.3) | 0.19 (0.3) | 0.15 (0.4) | 0.17 (0.4) |
| Ego-control | 0.06 (0.2) | 0.02 (0.2) | 0.06 (0.2) | -0.03 (0.3) |

The difference between attention scores on the mosaic task per computer and the mosaic task with pencil and paper is significant (F1,134)=50,32; p=0,0001). At the coloring task the difference between the computer and the pen and paper version is also significant (F(1,124)=90,71; p=0,0001). So for comparable tasks, children paid significantly more attention to the task during work with the computer than during work with paper and pencil.

## 3.3. Discussion

Many publications about the use of computers by young children emphasize the pleasure they may derive from it. In this paper we desribed the special hard- and software we developed to let even severely disabled children share this experience. We found however, that the literature lacks objective information about the effects of the technology other than immediate satisfaction [11]. We set out to carefully examine this issue experimentally and highlighted the difference between immediate effects and long term efficacy. The study comfirms the immediate effects so often alluded to. Yet, the results showed no positive effects of the information prosthetic on the cognitive development, the attention and the emotional development. Although we conducted a large-scale experiment over a moderate interval (a normal school year) the negative results merit some discussion. Lahm [12] mentioned that physically handicapped children are characteristically slow learners, so the intervention period may have been to short. A second factor is the variability of the population. Although we used the method of random block design, the group is extremely heterogeneous in severity of the handicap and intelligence. May be the nature of the variability of the population may indicate the more appropriate use of single case experimental designs rather than group designs to ensure changes that may be clinically significant are detected [12,13]. Third, it may be that we cannot expect an effect on general measures as intelligence and emotional tests.

We would like to conclude with advice to educators concerning computers in the classroom, particularly for the severely handicapped: High hopes for longer term effects are thus far unsubstantiated. The immediate effects of working with the information prosthetic fall into two catogories:

For the children:
• A positive influence on concentration and attention span during work with the computer,
• Satisfaction on tasks that are otherwise difficult to perform.

For the educator:
• An informal asssessment by teachers that several children made progress,
• Satisfaction about the information prosthetic as a tool for learning.

## References

[1]   P. Campbell and G. Fein, Young children and micro-computers. Prentice-Hall, Englewood Cliffs, 1986.
[2]   L. Fisher and J. McDonald, Fixed effects analysis of variance. Academic Press, New York, 1978.
[3]   P. Goldenberg, Special technology for special children. University Park Press, Baltimore, 1979.
[4]   D. Hagen, Microcomputer resource book for special education. Prentice-Hal, Reston (VA), 1984.
[5]   E.A. Lahm, Technology with low incidende populations: promoting access to education and learning. Center for special education technology, Reston (VA), 1989.
[6]   M. Pagen, R. Voort, E. Hoenkamp and W. Hulstijn, De computer als informatieprothese voor jonge, ernstig motorisch gehandicapte kinderen. KUN (Intern Rapport 88 NICI 07), Nijmegen, 1988.
[7]   R. Voort, R. Liauw and E. Hoenkamp, Handleiding Clowns. Malmberg b.v., Den Bosch, 1990.
[8]   R. Voort and E. Hoenkamp, Een evaluatieonderzoek naar het gebruik van de informatieprothese in het byzonder voor tertiaire preventie. KUN (Technical Report 92-03), Nijmegen, 1991.
[9]   S. Weir, Cultivating minds. A Logo-casebook. Harper & Row, New York, 1987.
[10]  S. Weir, Logo as an information prosthesis for the handicapped. MIT (Working paper MIT, WP-9), Cambridge, 1981.
[11]  P.B. Waldrop, Computer use with young children: present perspectives and future possibilities, *Early child development and care*, **32**, (1988) 59-68.
[12]  M.M. Wolf, Social validity: the case for subjective measurement or how applied behavior analysis is finding its heart, *Journal of applied behavior analysis*, **11**, (1978) 203-214.

# A SAFE AND EASY TO USE INTEGRATED CONTROL AND COMMUNICATION METHOD, M3S

J.A. van Woerden; TPD-TNO-TU Delft
on behalf of the partners in M3S
FST, Neuchatel, Swiss; Indes BV, Hengelo, Netherlands; Exact Dynamics, Zevenaar, Netherlands; IPA, Stuttgart, Germany, Penny & Giles Technology Ltd, Dorset, UK; Permobil, Åkersberga, Sweden; IRV, Hoensbroek, Netherlands; Imperial College, London, UK; Cambridge University, Cambridge, UK; Keep Able Foundation, Brentford Middlesex, UK; Creati, Parthenay, France; Meyra, Vlatho, Germany.

## ABSTRACT
Integrated Control Systems allow disabled and elderly people access to multiple functions from a single input device (for example a joystick with a switch). Multiple handicapped users are thereby able to switch efficiently between wheelchair control, manipulator control, control of their environment, computer access and communication without help. The control of integrated systems is a safe and easy to use possibility with the general purpose interface M3S.

## USER NEEDS FOR INTEGRATED AND STANDARDIZED SYSTEMS
Technical aids for motor handicapped people, young as well as elderly, may generally be divided in the following groups:
- mobility with (electrically powered) wheelchairs
- autonomy by control of the environment and by use of manipulators
- communication of mute people, especially by means of synthetic speech output
- adaptations of the work place, at school, at home or in the professional environment by means of special keyboards for computers

About a decade ago, the use of a technical aids was generally restricted to one system out of the groups mentioned above. This situation has considerably been changed. As en example, in Switzerland, about 50% of the users have technical aids in more than one application field and this trend will keep on growing.

Since there is no "standard" for communication between devices sofar, it has not yet been possible for designers of technical aids to rationalize their work. Until now the technical aids were developed in a number of products not compatible with each other. In order to form a set of functions necessary for the autonomy, the disabled person is forced to buy a number of products each with its own user interface and possibility overlapping functionality. It resulted in a vertical concept of a series of products where the needs in various domains automatically involve the cumulation of specific and/or separate apparatus to satisfy the needs of a physical handicapped person.

The main disadvantages of this vertical approach are:

- Users (and their direct environment) cannot sufficiently use their experience in applying a product when an additional technical aid is required.
- Professionals in re-education have to learn the use of a too large range of products which makes it impossible to have sufficient knowledge of all the necessary products.
- Agents and consultants in the field responsible for promotion and training of the products have difficulties to sufficiently master the totality of products and their selection.
- Technicians are confronted with a diversity of technologies obstructing rationalisation of production and after-sales service, and sometimes these engineers have to develop all the elements for every product.

While, as indicated, users need often more than one end-effector nowadays an integrated control system is needed to allow a user to access various end-effectors from a single input device. A flexible and open interface method is needed for this horizontal approach and standardisation seems to be needed.

## INTRODUCTION TO M3S
The aim of M3S is both to design a general purpose interface method and a safe, easy to operate and simple to configure integrated control system.

Therefore the M3S project specified and developed a new flexible and open interface method for systems to be used by disabled and elderly people to control their mobility and their environment. The M3S Multiple-Master-Multiple-Slave intelligent interface is meant to be used as a 'standardised' communication method.

In the M3S system different types of input devices are able to interface to different types of end-effectors. Manufacturers of input and end-effector devices are able to adapt their devices to meet these specifications which ensure compatibility in the field.

The M3S specification aims to be cost-effective both for high tech environments (powered wheelchair with features) and for low tech applications (synthetic speech output with scanner).

## STANDARDS
The M3S communication method has the ISO 7176-17 "serial interface for wheelchair controllers" as a background. Part of the M3S project was to investigate standard communication protocols (as available on silicon) for their applicability. The CAN (Controller-Area-Network) protocol with add-ons for safety (DMS and keyline) was selected. The M3S bussystem is upwards compatible with CAN and fits in the ISO-OSI specification for communication. Communication to homesystems was investigated in the project, and will be made available in the future.

## M3S SPECIFICATION
The M3S general purpose interface is specified in:

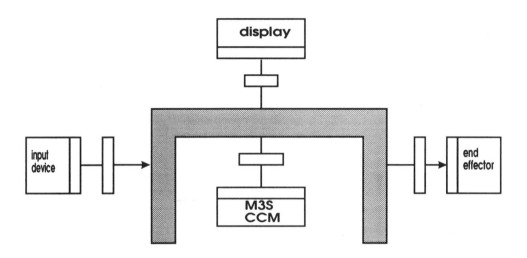

* a basic hardware architecture
* a bus communication system
* a configurable method

The 7 wires bus has 2 power lines, 2 CAN lines, 2 safety lines, 1 shield, and 1 special support line (harness number).

The M3S interface with integrated control can be configured in a flexible way. Human interface support is available for ease of use.

The bus is described as intelligent because it will allow the system to be optimally configured to the user's needs. The intelligence in the system exists in the controllers of the individual end-effectors and also in the control and configuration module (CCM) which forms part of every implementation of the M3S bus. The intelligence in the M3S CCM deals with the processing necessary to configure the system and the ongoing need to monitor the safety of the system while it is in use. The CCM is linked to a simple display which allows the user to select and operate each effector. The CCM processor itself contains the master menu used to select individual effectors.

While the main purpose of the bus is to simplify the use of multiple end-effectors, it opens the possibility for the user to access a wide range of devices via a wireless link, using infra-red or radio, to a home bus. In this way, a wheelchair user has control over any system which can be controlled via a home bus.

## MAN-MACHINE-INTERFACE

The Man-Machine-Interface in M3S assists the user in operating a system of output actions, with the goal of making the operations as easy, fast and reliable as possible.

At the simplest level, the Man-Machine-Interface is the point of contact between the human operator and the machine. At the highest level, the Man-Machine-Interface is the strategy to allow the user to control a system with a mismatched number of input and output actions.

Requirements to set up a multiple master multiple slave system with bus communication are analyzed and a three mode operation is defined: initialisation, configuring a system, operating a system.

Device generalisation, which includes user-specific information, is part of the MMI concept. The generalisation takes into account the fact that the function of individual input actions are interdependent and that these interdependencies are user specific in a rehabilitation environment.

A major effort in the design work on the user interface has the aim of reducing the cognitive load on the user and on the rehabilitation professional involved.

## SAFETY ISSUES IN CONTROL

One of the problems for moving devices in the environment of persons is that safety issues are unclear. A manipulator is generally functioning as a replacement for a human helper. The benefits that accrue are therefore as a result of the cost saving of the helper and the convenience of the disabled person having a measure of independence with all the psychological and physical benefits. Since these benefits are not 'life-critical' but are based on cost and convenience, the safety measures needed and how much they can be justified in terms of cost and complexity are less clear. What is needed, is for the medical manipulator community to make recommendations of a level of safety which is acceptable, with the various implications discussed so that the users, helpers, relatives, and public at large can come to a consensus of what is an agreed standard. The same holds for the safety of the mobility function.

The safety of the communication of signals is 'guaranteed' through the addition of two safety lines, a DMS line (Dead-Man-Switch) and a keyline plus a safety monitor.

In conclusion safety is reached through (apart from the functioning of the CAN bus):
*   self check of the system at start up
*   safety monitor on the bus
*   extra hardware to:
    - stop movements (DMS)
    - switch on-off of systems (keyline)

## STATUS AND RESULTS
The result of the M3S project will be a specification available in the public domain describing
○ A basic hardware architecture with a:
- CAN bus system
- Power distribution system
- Safety system
- Standard connector
- Device identification system
○ A bus communication protocol

○ A configuration method
- with MMI support
- with a M3S configuration editor

Products with M3S interface are owned by partners.

## DESIGN EVALUATIONS
The M3S specification will be implemented and evaluated in two demonstrator platforms early 1993.

- A Permobil wheelchair with a M3S interface made by Permobil.
- A MANUS manipulator with a M3S interface made by Exact Dynamics.
- A Rencom environmental controller with a M3S interface made by Keep Able Foundation.
- A joystick with a M3S interface made by Penny & Giles.
- A chincontroller with a M3S interface made by Penny & Giles.
- A M3S CCM with LCD display, text to speech synthesizer safety monitor and a M3S bus interface designed and realised by FST.

optional:
- An optical headpointer with a M3S interface made by FST.


- A Huka MAKS wheelchair with a M3S interface made by Indes.
- A MANUS manipulator with a M3S interface made by Exact Dynamics.
- A Rencom environmental controller with a M3S interface made by Keep Able Foundation.
- A Zofcom tongue controller with a M3S interface realised by Keep Able Foundation.
- A headrest sensor with a M3S interface made by IRV.
- A joystick with a M3S interface from Penny & Giles.
- A M3S CCM with LCD display, safety monitor and a M3S bus interface designed and realised by TPD.

## ACKNOWLEDGEMENTS

M3S is a project in the European Community research programme TIDE (Technology for the Integration of Disabled and Elderly people). Tide pilot action number 128.

J.A. van Woerden
TNO Institute of Applied Physics
(TPD-TNO-TU Delft)
Stieltjesweg 1, 2628 CK  Delft
P.O.Box 155, 2600 AD  Delft
The Netherlands

# Innovative Concept for Teaching Elderly CAD - The TECAD Project

Michael Collet
Universität Bremen-BIK, Badgasteiner Str. 1, D-2800 Bremen 33

## Abstract

Technological change imposes special training needs on the elderly. We introduce a concept for flexible, self-directed learning in the workplace. Standard workstations without additional multimedia-hardware running CAD-software in a Unix-environment with the X-Window system are basis for our development. In this way the people with training needs can access the trainig-modules in their actual environment, out of real-world problem situations which they encounter. This will enhance their capabilities and provide guidance especially to those elderly workers in the construction-office without prior computer knowledge.

## 1 Introduction

Most work in CBT research is carried out on standard PC-type devices. Most serious CAD-applications run on workstations with operating systems other than DOS. The TECAD project is intended for use in the workplace (in this case: small and medium sized construction offices), so we had to do scale up. We decided to design a CBT system from bottom up to gain flexibility and adaptability. TECAD is both: a generic CBT framework, which can be filled with contents of completely different learning topics, and an example contents tailored to the CAD-application program of one major vendor in the market of software for mechanical design.

As well as we can fill the framework with different topics, we can prepare the same topic in a different way to meet the expectations of different user communities.

### 1.1 Elderly People and Technological Change

The technological change imposes special training needs on the elderly. Elderly people in general have lower formal qualifications and to a greater degree incomplete vocational education. They have to compete in the workplace with young and highly skilled workers. An increasing number of workplaces especially in the engineering departments will be equipped with data-processing facilities in the near future. The elderly have to keep pace with this challenging development.

## 1.2   Multidisciplinary Approach

In TECAD we use a multidisciplinary approach. The BREMER INSTITUT FÜR KON-STRUKTIONSTECHNIK – BIK works in tight cooperation with colleagues in the social siences and with several small and medium sized enterprises on developing courseware for CAD-education with special consideration of the needs of elderly people.

## 1.3   Aims and Scope

In TECAD we are realizing a concept utilizing computer assisted learning (CAL) in the working place. We provide a SECURITY CELL SOFTWARE for elderly workers in the construction-office which will guide them through the process of acquiring initial and advanced CAD knowledge in an exploratory and self-directed way without beeing obliged to ask for help each time they are exposed to system related trouble. Our focus is on exploring the cognitive gaps of elderly people with no or small computer experience and how to bridge this gap using online accesssible teachware modules. The TECAD-software will be built using object oriented programming on Unix-based workstations with OSF-Motif user-interface. Programming techniques considered to provide maximum flexibility and ease of use in the user-interface are hypertextlike organization of the training modules, adaptability to the specific needs of the individual elderly user and direct access to training modules out of the running application.

# 2   The TECAD Framework

The basic concept exploited in this approach is a learning graph. We can see a small example of a learning context with twelve vertices in figure 1. The knowledge of some application area, which shall be communicated to the users, is partitioned into small entities contained in each vertex. In TECAD each vertex contains one entitity composed of some text and graphic. Conceptionally, it is possible to integrate sound and video output into this framework to achieve multimedia capabilities. Actually, there is no possibility of viewing video output at the workstations out in the offices without supplying additional hardware. Sound output would impose unwanted noise onto colleagues of users of the TECAD training modules, who mostly share their rooms with several persons.

## 2.1   Design Guidelines

In the following, we will discuss some guidelines in the approach we used. A major principle was the fostering of self-directed learning by supplying maximum flexibility in the user-interface.

### 2.1.1   Fostering of Self-directed Learning

Traditional CBT-programs force learners to follow a predefined path through the material provided by the author of the training modules. Learners have little or no chance to structure the provided knowledge according to their very needs. Using this software, learners can follow a predefined path, which might be of great importance for novel learners. More skilled learners can define a path of their own to gather the knowledge they want to obtain. This all happens in the workplace, where the need for education is obvious and motivation is strong.

### 2.1.2 Ease-Of-Use

We provide four main windows in standard layout. A learning software should not impose unnecessary complexity of its own onto possible users. During each session, the windows appear in turn:

- The first window (figure 2, topleft corner) is the start-window. Learners can access it by selecting a menu-choice of the running CAD-application. Actually, it is not possible to catch the context of the learners task performed before accessing the training modules.

- the second window (figure 2, topright corner) shows a table of contents. Learners can select between courses in the scrollable lists. A text-window just below the lists provides an abstract of a selected module.

- The third window provides the entire learning screen. The upper pane just below the menubar displays graphics, the other pane shows text. The lower part of this window is crowded by some control buttons which allow to proceed, to raise a help facility and so on.

- The fourth window in the bottomright corner of figure 2 displays the notepad. Here learners can make textual and graphical annotations. These notes are tied to the module they are actually working on. An author-mode allows it, to save a note as personalized learning module which can be inserted into a learning path. Everybody can enhance his lessons!

## 2.2 Tracking of User-Behaviour

We track user behaviour for research purposes. The user in TECAD is modelled as a person taking some path through the learning graph of figure 1. Each entering of a vertex, the time spent here and the way taken to the next node is logged in a protocol-file. This will allow to improve weaknesses in the initial modules and/or learning-paths provided.

# 3 Tutorial Concept

Courseware alone will not do the job. In addition we develop an educational concept which will provide for the organizational framework in the enterprises. This includes a tutorial concept (with human tutors). Additionally, the TECAD project will investigate the feasibility of the above mentioned electronic tutor, a facilitiy to send notes including graphics and text to a skilled colleague or system expert who returns his advice in the same way.

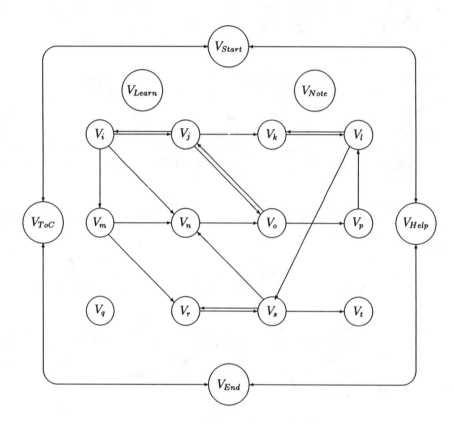

Fig.1: Example TECAD learning-graph

# 4 Outlook and future work

Actually we are evaluating a prototype of the TECAD-software in a field test in some construction-offices in northern Germany. The results of this first user-testing will be taken into account and a possibly redesigned version of TECAD which incorporates the feedback of initial users will be evaluated during summer 93.

Furthermore we would like to enhance the TECAD environment to catch the actual context of the task users are performing with their CAD-application. This would enhance greatly our abilities in providing electronic advice and guidance.

In BIK we are also discussing the implications of providing a tele-tutor service, a concept of mailing TECAD notes to some expert in a remote location who provides assistance in a hotline manner.

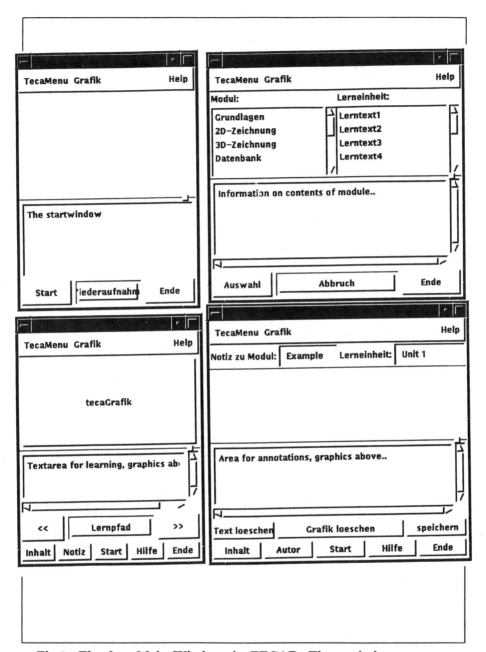

**Fig.2:** The four Main Windows in TECAD. These windows correspond with the vertices of the learning-graph on the previous page. The upper-left window belongs to $V_{Start}$ , upper-right is the table of contents with $V_{ToC}$, bottom-left is the actual learning-window $V_{Learn}$ and bottom-right the notepad-window which is represented by $V_{Note}$.

# Videotelephony: Support for Elderly People

*T. Erkert, S. Robinson*

**Abstract:**

The contribution describes the opportunities for providing support to elderly persons in their homes using videotelephony. Such services were tested in Frankfurt am Main as part of the Project, "Application Pilot for People with Special Needs (APPSN)" in the CEC RACE Programme.

Videotelephony offers opportunities to provide services to the home, encouraging and supporting an independent way of life and thereby reducing elderly people´s need to recourse to institutional care. It is shown that services which can be provided using videotelephony in a local care scheme can potentially help maintain social competence, motivating and enabling continued participation in social activities, thereby helping to prevent decline into dependence. Other opportunities to provide help centre on informing the elderly about activities and events, providing refresher exercises between regular therapy sessions, and general assistance in coping with problems of everyday living.

Data from logging files were used to analyse the usage levels of the new services. An overview of frequency, duration and patterns of calls is given. Besides these automatically generated data, information was gathered in several surveys with participants and staff of the pilot project. The surveys were carried out as part of the evaluation of the videotelephony-based support services.

It can be shown that the implementation of a videotelephony-based social support service has a potential to assist professional carers in their difficult tasks and a potential to improve the quality of life of the elderly with special needs.

## 1. Introduction

The main objective of the RACE Project Application Pilot for People with Special Needs is to develop and demonstrate the types of support services within the care sector which will be commercially viable using video-telephony. In the EC, the population of elderly people will total 50 million in the year 2000 and the disabled 36 to 48 million [1]. Through the provision of Integrated Broadband Communication (IBC) services to homes using bi-directional transmission of video signals these groups can be given regular support services, which up until now have required by daily visits or, for 4-5% (for the german elderly) [2], transfer to a residential place of care.

In the pilot service set up in Frankfurt am Main 17 elderly persons in 15 households are connected via specially developed videophones to a service centre located in a residental care centre. The pilot clients are connected to the service centre using cable-tv network. This network was modified to support reverse channels to carry audio and video signals from the client to the service centre [3]. A number of servives were developed and implemented during the pilot phase.

The services, named "Haus-Tele-Dienst", are run by the Frankfurter Verband für Alten- und Behindertenhilfe e.V.(FV), the care organisation providing the majority of sheltered housing, old peoples homes and day care facilities in the city of Frankfurt am Main. In addition, the FV provides alarm telephone services to over a thousand clients in the area.

## 2. The service concept

The services on trial in Frankfurt have the overall aim of promoting the ability of the elderly and mobility-impaired to live independently and to reduce the load on social service resources required to do this. Investigation of current service provision and consultation with providers of care services led to a number of service "components" as follows:

Remote care on demand
The user group benefiting from this service is mainly family members who care for elderly and disabled relatives in their home. In many cases even short periods of absence are hardly possible or involve great difficulties, reliance on others or stress and risk. Since carers are often unable to ask someone else to come to their home, the remote care can give carers some relief from their 24 hour job.

Information and assistance service
The aim of this service is to provide support to continued competence in mastering every-day life under the changes aging brings to people´s situation and needs. Clients can be helped in filling out official forms, in understanding complex bills, or for a whole range of organisational tasks; including for instance in arranging special senior citizen vacations.

Active information and care
This service component was expected to be most useful for those elderly living alone and who are, therefore, prone to depression and withdrawal. As this group is also cut of from normal levels of contact with people outside the home, the regular contact with service centre personnel can help as a minimum by acting as a vital safety valve.

Remote response to emergency, "alarm service"
Clients who know or fear that they might be in a dangerous situation can call the service centre and receive reassurance and help. This service component is an advancement on traditional phone-based emergency intercom systems, providing the opportunity of a visual assessment of clients needs and situation.

Remote access to expertise, "counselling service"
The counselling service is designed to give clients opportunities to put questions to experts on specific topics, helping them gain access to information relevant to their needs. Appropriate experts are those in fields which regular service staff cannot be expected to gain detailed knowledge of, such as law, specific rights to state benefits, or detailed dietary plans.

Training and exercise service
This service component covers a large range of types of training, including communication training, memory training or physical exercises. Those receiving some forms of therapy, can be given short refresher sessions of exercise in the intervals between full sessions. These services can partly also be offered using videotapes.

Support for carers

The system enables service staff to provide support to nonprofessional carers having to carry out tasks such as bathing, or changing clothes. Correct care techniques are often unknown by family carers with no training. Remote advice can enable them to fulfill even more difficult tasks.

Although the service concept consists of different service components, it is necessary to note that these components are based on regular and close contacts between the service providers and the pilot clients. Based on these relationships, needs could be identified which would otherwise not have been discovered by regular staff. Personalised help could be offered, creating a feeling of security and integration.

## 3. Evaluation results

Evaluation efforts in this project are based on several surveys [4] and automatically gathered data from software supported call logging. First a general overview of usage based on the logging file data will be given.

### 3.1 General service usage patterns

The period of time for which calls were logged amounted to 315 days lasting from the 24th of January to the 31st of December. Altogether 4239 calls were registered in this time.

Figure 1: Frequency of calls by month

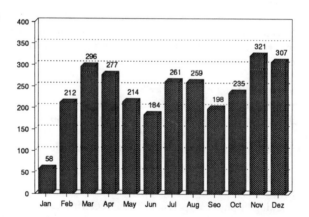

Looking at the trend of calls over time, a remarkable increase in calls can be seen up until March 1991. This and a second peak in November can be partly explained by the fact that in these months, new clients joined the service. The irregularities can be explained by differences regarding the days in which the system actually was in use. Taking the number of all days on which the system was in use and calls were registered, the average was, at the beginning of the year, 10 calls per day. Towards the end of the year the average rose to 11 calls per day.

For an analysis of the feasability of the overall service concept, the duration of calls is also of great importance:

Figure 2: Duration of calls

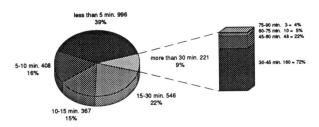

A sizeable minority of calls (39%) lasted less than five minutes. 16% of the calls lasted between 5 and 10 minutes and 22% between 15 and 30 minutes. In 9% of all cases, contact between client and service centre was established for longer than half an hour, some of them were up to an hour and a quarter in length. A trend towards an increase of conversation time was observed.

Figure 3: Frequency and duration of calls per month (absolute numbers and trend)

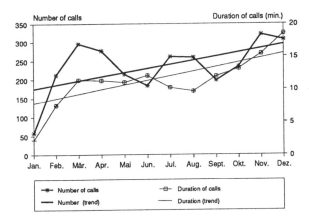

Analysing the development of the number of calls in comparison with the overall length of contact reveals that the length of calls increased relatively fast in the beginning. The high level was reached early, and since then the figures have changed only slightly. The client's need for contact is enormous. The average duration of all calls is over 11 minutes. On the basis of experience it seems that one can rely on an average of 10 to 15 minutes for a contact between client and service centre.

Given that intensive human relationships are involved in the pilot service, one main concern in the research was to find out if there is any evidence of discrimination for or against individual clients.

Figure 4: Number and average duration of calls per client

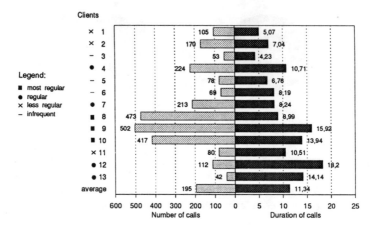

With the exception of 3 participants, all pilot clients can be regarded as frequent users. They differ only in the regularity of their calls. Some call twice or three times a day. This consumes three fifth of the total speaking time of the service providers. Others call very regular once a day. The average connection time of this group is 12.3 minutes, only half a minute shorter than the group described before. A third group of frequent users calls on average every second day. The group of infrequent users contains a total of 3 users. As expected, the calls of these infrequent users are less extensive than calls by frequent users. The shortest average connection time was 4.23 minutes. It is worth pointing out that a trend towards increasing call length was observed not only for those clients who frequently call the service centre but also for those who could be described as infrequent users.

Interview data revealed no evidence of any significant discrimination of specific users. Those who used the service little did so of their own accord. The duration of calls can be regarded as an indicator for the intensity of the conversation and also for the quality of all contacts. In both respects the results are very positive and promising for a future regular service.

## 3.2 Service provision experience

The service components described at the beginning of this chapter were the subject of an additional qualitative assessment. Here, the reflection of the three service provider staff on their experience is given.

The picture component of the integrated **alarm service** enables the service provider to assess the emergency situation better. Such a videobased emergency system is better than a regular telephone-based emergency intercom system. In an emergency situation it helps create a feeling of security while emergency services are on the way.

The **remote care on demand** service has probably the highest potential of all service elements. This service component offers a real and direct help to the relatives. It allows them to continue a 'normal' way of living by offering a secure way of caring via videophone. This element also enables relatives to get advice e.g. with specific care techniques.

Although the **counselling** service is very time consuming in preparation, it is a useful source of help for elderly people, enabling them to get in touch with expertise which they would not be able to travel to. It reduces the fear of asking experts, because the well-known service provider can lower inhibitions by mediation between the experts and the elderly.

Most of the calls made could be associated with the **active information and care** service component. The ongoing and regular possibility to ask the service provider whenever there is a need to, seems to be especially important to the elderly. The service providers believe that this service element is the most important one to the pilot clients. Many senior citizens obviously just need someone to talk to when they feel isolated and/or lonely.

The **training and exercise** lessons were frequently joined by several of the pilot clients. Remarkable improvements could be observed in the case of a lady who frequently joined memory training exercises. The physical fitness training motivated people to do some additional exercises at a senior citizens' club.

The service provider staff and the service provider organisation summarised their experiences with the new sevice as follows: The video-based Haus-Tele-Dienst fills into a gap in social services. Fast and effective help is possible. One of the biggest advantages of the new system is to reduce unnecessary travel time. During the regular service hours an opportunity for communication exists. This ongoing connection leads to a close relationship to the clients, enabling the service providers to activate and motivate the elderly. A feeling of security can be given. The close and regular contacts lead to a recognisable improvement in personal health and well-being. A wide range of services is thinkable, supporting the work of regular carers in the field. This example emphasises at the same time the most important limitation of the new service. The Haus-Tele-Dienst was not designed to replace but to augment direct personal contacts.

Issues of acceptability of cameras in the home were much less important than researchers and especially the service provider organisation expected. After a relative short time the personnel at the service centre felt comfortable using the new technology. Even when technical problems occured during the first months they could handle the system. This issue was also of little importance for the elderly.

*3.3 Service use experience*

Due in large measure to a special simple remote control device, most of the elderly users had no problems at all with the usage of the equipment. A more important problem was the fact that the system at the beginning of the pilot was not completely reliable. Technical problems at the beginning of the project led to critisism by some users, stating that technical improvements were necessary. At the end of the pilot project the system was much more reliable, so that none of the clients had complaints about the technical system.

In general the "Haus-Tele-Dienst" was rated very positively by users. Suggestions for improvements concerned additional personnel and longer service hours, if possible 24 hours a day. The most valuable service component was the active care and information service, although it has to be make clear that most users saw the Haus-Tele-Dienst-services as a general service, not a set of different service elements. 10 of the users pointed out that the opportunity to get in contact with someone when they want is most important for them. The second most important advantage of the service is the possibility to immediately get direct help if needed. Almost all of the users emphasised the very personal and close relationship to the staff. The new service has had quite an impact on their lives. Five of them believe that the service directly changed their life. Statements range from "I don't feel lonely anymore" to "I have a more regular daily routines, I've regular meals again" or "I have more joy in my life".

To summarise the pilot client's impression, it can be said that all of them think that the new service is appropriate for all senior citizens, with a emphasis on people with special needs. All of the clients asked for an extension of the services.


## 4. Summary

The contribution describes the opportunities for providing services to elderly people in their homes using picture telecommunication. It could be shown that videotelephony offers opportunities to provide support services to the home, encouraging and supporting an independent way of life and thereby reducing elderly people´s need for institutional care. Services which can be provided using videotelephony can potentially help to maintain social competence, motivating and enabling continued participation in social activities, thereby helping to prevent isolation, loneliness and dependence. Other opportunities to offer help centre on informing the elderly about activities and events, providing refreshment exercises between regular therapy sessions, and general assistance in coping with problems of everday living.

The results of the Application Pilot for People with Special Needs in Frankfurt am Main were seen by all concerned as very positive and motivating. A continuation and a expansion of the research effort is possible within RACE project "TeleCommunity", which runs from 1992 to 1994. In this project, opportunities for extending support services to various forms of sheltered accomodation are being explored for an extension of the field trial in Frankfurt am Main.

### References

[1]Organisation for Economic Co-Operation and Development. Aging Populations: The Social Policy Implications. OECD, Paris, 1988.
[2]W. Krug, Pflegebedürftige in Heimen, Studie im Auftrag des Bundesministeriums für Familie und Senioren. ISBN 3 17 012178 2 . Kohlhammer, Stuttgart, 1992.
[3]S. Robinson, Support for Elderly People using Videotelephony. In: H. Bouma, J. Graafmans (Ed.), Gerontechnology. ISBN 90 5199 072 3. IOS Press, Amsterdam, 1992, pp. 305-316.
[4]T. Erkert, Elderly Persons and Communications. In H. Bouma, J. Graafmans (Ed.), Gerontechnology. ISBN 90 5199 072 3. IOS Press, Amsterdam, 1992, pp. 293-303.

# Open Control Architecture for an Intelligent Omni-Directional Wheelchair

Helmut HOYER and Ralf HOELPER

*FernUniversität Hagen, Chair of Process Control, Hagen, Germany*

**Abstract.** This paper presents an open control architecture for a smart omni-directional wheelchair allowing a flexible configuration of user required functionality, which is essential for an individual adaptation to the special needs of severely physically disabled and mentally handicapped people. The demand for a large functionality with high flexibility, leads to a modular structured control system, composed of different smart units. Each unit is provided with local intelligence to yield a high independence from other modules as well as to get an open control system.

## 1 Introduction

The use of power wheelchairs is one of the great steps towards the integration of severely physically disabled and mentally handicapped people, enableing them self-controlled mobility without external help. However, many of them, especially those with restricted psycho-mental capabilities, are not able to operate conventional wheelchairs.

There are two reasons why those systems can not address these people: their limited mobility and the restricted functionality. Normal domestic environments (e.g. bathrooms) are often complex structured and therefore require a high manoeuvrability. Because of their kinematic constraints, conventional wheelchairs are hardly suitable to move within packed rooms. In this context complex manoeuvres often overcharge the user. An increase of the mobility could be reached by the use of omni-directional driving concepts e.g. based on Mecanum wheels, which give an all-around freedom of motion, so that any combination of forward, sideways, and rotational movement is possible (movement with three degrees of freedom in a plane).

To offer the people with restricted capabilities a higher degree of independence, the wheelchair also has to be provided with an expanded functionality and the possibility to control it on different levels of abstraction. This requires a control structure, that allows not only acting on a low-level (e.g. direct control by using a joystick) but completes the line up to executing task-oriented commands (such as "wash hands"), which generate an automatic, sensor supported navigation to a predefined position. Therefore, the control system has to integrate intelligent components to ensure navigational accuracy and occupant safety through the use of collision sensors in order to enable the wheelchair to compensate specific handicaps.

## 2   Omni-directional wheelchair

To satisfy the demand of a higher mobility, new driving concepts have to be taken in consideration. Therfore a study [1] of the suitability of vehicles with omni-directional steering capability for the use in the rehabilitation was conducted.

Wheeled mobile robots (WMR) with such driving features are wellknown in the field of robotics, e.g. Muir [2] has proved that WMRs using four omni-directional, actuated and sensed wheels provide three degree-of-freedom (DOF) locomotion.

Within the scope of the study, experiments with such an omni-directional wheel-driven vehicle have shown that its performance is almost equal to those based on conventional wheels, with respect to various kinds of floor (stone, PVC, carpet) under several conditions (dry, wet, slippery) and on different gradients (flat to 25%) [1], [3].

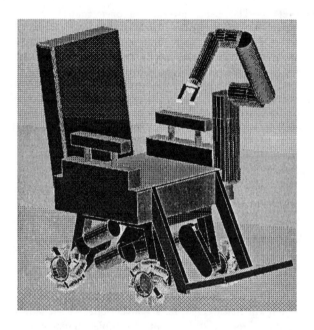

Figure 1: Simulation of the omni-directional wheelchair

Moreover, simulations (fig. 1) have illustrated the increase of mobility that can be yield by the use of such omni-directional driving concepts, which allow to move even within packed indoor environments because of a non-restricted positioning capability.

As a result, a prototype wheelchair equiped with four so-called Mecanum wheels has been developed, able to move with three DOF in a plane, so that in spite of its floor constraints, the wheelchair almost has the movability of a hovercraft.

The omni-directional wheelchair not only overcomes the kinematic constraints of conventional ones and provides the user with a higher manoeuvrability, but also allows to simulate other wheelchairs with steering axes, which makes it useful for an individual training [4].

## 3   System Architecture

The demand for a large functionality with high flexibility, leads to a modular structured control system, composed of different smart units. Each unit is provided with local intelligence to yield a high independence from other modules as well as to get an open control system. This enables a flexible reaction and increases the reliability because of a mutual verification of the transferred data. Figure 2.a shows the system architecture as well as the hardware design. From the viewpoint of the level of abstraction, the system can be devided in a low-level control including the motion unit, a sensor module and a robot manipulator, and a high-level functionality, which encompasses a path-planning module as well as a task-planner to execute task-oriented commands (such as "wash hands"). Several functions of the low-level control, e.g. the servo-controller (motion unit), require real-time processing. Therefore modules, which use hardware resources, are realized on a VME bus based system using pSOS$^+$, which is an operating system kernel providing multi-tasking and multi-processor features. The high-level functionality is located on a PC/Laptop running under Unix operating system. The link between the high-level sytem and the low-level control can be either infrared in the case of remote control or a RS-232 interface.

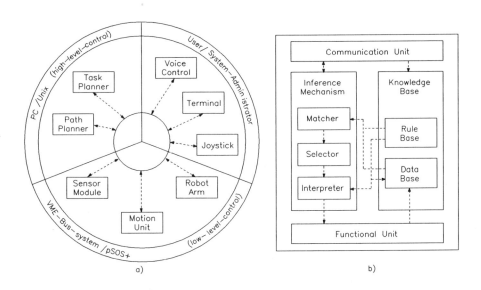

Figure 2: a) System architecture; b) Module structure [4]

The different modules, realized in C$^{++}$ programming language, share an identical underlying structure, which is illustrated in fig. 2.b.

### 3.1   Module Structure

The main components of the module structure are the local knowledge base, the inferernce mechanism, the communication unit and the functional unit (see fig. 2.b).

### 3.1.1 Communication Unit

The module communication is established during the module initialization phase and supported by a message-passing-mechanism. First, the module creates a message queue and enters its identification number ($Q_{id}$) in a so called module connection list. In a second step, the module sends its interface requirements (i.e. what kind of data it can process) to each of the modules whose $Q_{id}$ is already stored in the list. Those modules who are able to communicate with the transmitter because of their compatibility to its interface, enter the transmitter's identification number in a communication link list. Using the exchanged interface information, a fault tolerant module interprocessing can be established, trying to reorganize the communication if an error occurs. For example, within an initial state the terminal informs the other modules that it is able to process user input/output data. In case of a terminal error, those modules, which try to communicate with the user via this device, look within their communication link list whether there is another module accepting input/output data in order to reorganize the interaction with the user.

### 3.1.2 Local knowledge base

The module knowledge is represented in a hybrid knowledge base [5]. On the one hand the declarative knowledge, including specific information about the current module status (e.g. init, ready) as well as facts about the functionality and the links to other modules, is stored in the data base. On the other hand the rule base, which contains the procedural knowledge about how to act in dependence on the available data (e.g. it holds the information how to establish the communication with the other modules and how to react in case of an error or the absence of a module).

### 3.1.3 Inference Mechanism

The processing of the declarative and procedural knowledge by the inference mechanism runs through three phases: (1) Accessing the local knowledge base, the matcher identifies all applicable rules by comparing the current module data with the rule premise. All rules, whose conditions match the facts and module data (e.g. status) stored in the data base, are passed to the rule selector. (2) From amongst the set of applicable rules, the selector has to determine that rule which should be executed. This is done by evaluating the priorities attached to each rule. (3) Finally, the interpreter executes the conclusion of the selected rule. The effectuation of the rule conclusion can delete, modify or create new facts in the data base or cause elementary actions. The inference mechanism is event controlled, i.e. it is invoked by receiving a message from other modules or by a changing of the internal module status (e.g. in case of a module error).

### 3.1.4 Functional Unit

The functional unit consists of a set of functions, which operate the specific module hardware/software resources. For example, the functional unit of the motion module includes algorithms to control the wheelchair position, while the sensor module can execute task as e.g. obstacle localization to avoid collisions. The functions are activated by the interpreter and may change the module status.

# 4 Conclusion

In this paper an open control architecture for a smart omni-directional wheelchair is introduced, allowing a flexible configuration of an individually adaptable functionality. The system architecture consists of different intelligent modules, which are able to organize their interaction by themselves. The communication is event controlled and established by sending messages, which contain only the information that is essential for the addressed units ('information hiding', 'client-server model'). Because of the self-organizing feature of the module communication mechanism and the modular architecture, the system is open and its functionality can easily be expanded, so that the integration of high-level processing, such as task-oriented programming, path-planning etc., requires no system modification. The distributed intelligence allows the design of a fault tolerant system, that means, using the local knowledge base the system is provided with the capability of continuing to operate with reduced functionality in case of the absence of a module from the system (every unit knows how to react if one failures).

The presented control architecture makes it feasible to act on different levels of abstraction and supports the user with several modes of operation, e.g. movement with sensoric, back-tracing, play-back, etc. Because of the modular structure, special features of the omni-directional driving concept, e.g. the simulation of other wheelchairs with steering axes, can easily be realized for an individual training.

Furthermore, the open architecture of the control system is able to integrate technically modified and/or additional devices, e.g. a robotic service arm or special user interfaces. This allows to compensate specific handicaps and gives an adjusted and matched system to the individual.

## Acknowledgment

This work was done in cooperation with the *Forschungsinstitut Technologie – Behindertenhilfe (FTB), Volmarstein* and supported by the *Ministerium für Wissenschaft und Forschung (MWF) des Landes Nordrhein - Westfalen.*

## References

[1] FTB : Elektrorollstuhl mit hoher Manövrierfähigkeit. Internal Study B92-2, Forschungsinstitut Technologie – Behindertenhilfe (FTB), Volmarstein, 1992.

[2] Muir, P.F. and Neuman, P. : Kinematic Modelling for Feedback Control of an Omnidirectional Wheeled Mobile Robot. IEEE International Conference on Robotics and Automation, pp. 1772–1778, 1987.

[3] Bühler, C. and Humann, W. : Smart Wheelchair with high Manoeuvrability. European Conference on the Advancement of Rehabilitation Technology (ECART II), Stockholm, 1993.

[4] Hoelper, R. : Konzept für ein flexibel konfigurierbares, modular strukturiertes Robotersteuerungssystem. Internal Report RH/92-I, Chair of Process Control, FernUniversität Hagen, Hagen, 1992.

[5] Rzevski, G. [Ed.] : Applications of Artificial Intelligence in Engineering V. ISBN: 0-945824-67-X, Computational Mechanics Publications, Boston, USA, 1990.

# THE MARCUS INTELLIGENT HAND PROSTHESIS

P Kyberd, R Tregidgo
Oxford Orthopaedic Engineering Centre, University of Oxford, UK
R Sachetti, H Schmidl
Centro Prosthetico, INAIL, Bologna, Italy
M Snaith, O Holland
Technology Applications Group, Alnwick, Northumberland, UK
S Marchese, M Bergamasco
Scienzia Machinale, Pisa, Italy
P Bagwell, P Chappell
Electrical Engineering Dept., University of Southampton, UK

**Abstract** The application of mechatronics principles to artificial hands has lagged a long way behind other areas of medical technology. Current provision uses simple open loop grippers that require concentration to be controlled successfully, and can only perform a limited range of tasks. By adding sensors and a microprocessor it is possible to control a more complex and functional hand with simpler instructions.

## 1. Introduction

Many artificial hands are driven through direct mechanical links to the operator. They are successful in use, but have only a single motion and are visually unattractive. To some members of the limb deficient population appearance is very important, and these individuals therefore opt for hands that are more natural in appearance but have little or no function. The active cosmetic hands have only one degree of freedom, with all the digits opening and closing together, this limits their functional range. To add more function necessitates the addition of further independent degrees of freedom at the gripper. Received wisdom asserts that for each independent degree of freedom there must be an independent control channel but it is difficult to co-ordinate independent inputs. However, successful control of such a device requires careful choice of control methodology.

### 1.1 Control methods for artificial hands

The type and form of control adopted for an upper limb prosthesis dictates the success with which it can be used. If the user interface and feedback loops are poor or difficult to maintain, then the operator will under-use or completely reject the device. The key issue in the control is that of the *appropriate* form of the control input.

Human control of natural limbs is hierarchical, Figure 1. The high level conscious instructions from the Central Nervous System, (CNS) are simple. The person simply wishes to grasp an object and it is achieved. The simple instructions feed down to a layer that co-ordinates finger and limb motion (posture) with the force required to hold the object stable without tiring the person. At the lowest level these instructions are implemented by the individual joints. Conventional prostheses are controlled at this lowest level by the conscious part of the operator's mind, which makes the control slow and tiring. Users must consciously instruct the hand to open and close, controlling the grip force and size using only visual cues.

## 1.2 Extended Physiological Proprioception

Extended Physiological Proprioception (EPP) [1,2], is an important example of an appropriate control method. It utilises the basic mechanisms of limb control; force demand and position feedback. The method's virtue is that, because its form is similar to the control the operator uses for other bodily motions this control is easily learned and tasks such as tracking can be performed precisely [3,4]. The control is serial, it manages several joints down the length of the arm. This control then allows the low levels of the user's central nervous system to attend to the task rather than requiring conscious decisions. EPP is less successful at controlling parallel actions, such as grasping objects with a multi-degree of freedom hand. For this more information would be needed, and so more channels would have to be used. The consequence of this would be to overload the operator and degrade the performance.

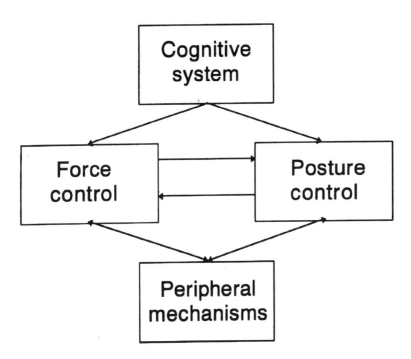

Figure 1 The hierarchical control of the human Central Nervous System

## 1.3 Hierarchical Control

The alternative is to divorce the low level control of the hand to a computer, mimicking the manner which the natural hand is controlled. This is a control method that employs only very simple user commands to open, close, hold, squeeze, or release the target object [5], Figure 2. The detailed task of hand shape or grip tension is devolved to a computer. When an object is touched the hand automatically adopts one of a set of generic shapes which is then adapted to maximise the contact area between the hand and object as well as to minimise the grip force. If the object slips this is then detected and the force is increased until the sliding stops. The advantage of this form of autonomous control is that the operator needs only to issue supervisory commands, and so is free to perform the strategic task planning similar to the natural grasping process.

The user commands can be of any one of a number of forms, the computer only needs the command to be converted to digital voltage changes. In addition the precise details of the control scheme can be altered easily to suit the user. The most common form of input for any commercial electric hand is a two electrode electromyographic system: Electrodes on the surface of the arm are placed over two antagonistic muscles. Small voltages are generated when the muscle contracts, these are amplified and used to form two user input channels. Tension in one muscle opens the hand and tension in the other closes it. For hierarchical control the two channels are used differently. The control of the device is then much more like that of a natural hand. The degree of hand flexion is made proportional to the extensor tension of the command channel, thus the hand opens progressively, and closes automatically (POSITION), Figure 2, there is no additional user input. The second channel, (flexor muscle) can then be used for command input. In addition the threshold to open the hand when it is grasping an object can be made different to when it is empty, thus the grip is more secure and the operation less tiring.

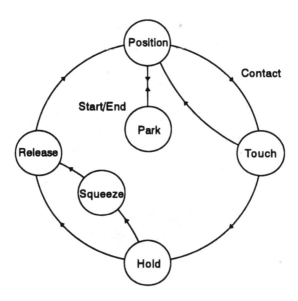

Figure 2 Control diagram for the MARCUS artificial hand

When the hand closes on an object the sensors detect this and it causes the controller to maintain the lightest touch force (TOUCH). If this force changes, the hand responds to return it to the original value, closing the hand further or opening it up. Thus the grip can be adjusted by the user, before the controller is instructed to hold the object. Once in HOLD mode, the controller monitors the sensors in the hand to detect when an object slips within the grasp. If this occurs the grip force is increased until the slide is arrested. The user can also override the grip reflex and apply a force in proportion to the commanding muscle tension (SQUEEZE), or they can open than hand completely and RELEASE the object.

Finally co-contraction of both muscles causes the hand to be disabled, and the system is then shut down to conserve power (PARK).

The computer system can thus be used to minimise the power consumption so that the duration of the hand on a single charge is over eight hours, which has been identified as the average time individuals use the hand in a day. In addition the computer can maintain a check on the rest of the hand systems, it measures the rate of change of the sensors' output so that any sensor failure is detected and the hand is safely powered down.

This procedure has been applied to a number of mechanisms, first in the laboratory and more recently in the field, [5,6,7]. Users have found it easy to learn and use.

## 2. The MARCUS hand

The MARCUS hand uses the hierarchical control scheme on a two degree of freedom anthropomorphic prosthesis [8]. The hand has two degrees of freedom, these are; finger flexion and thumb flexion. This configuration allows differential flexion speeds for the fingers and thumb, which is supported by the work of Wing [9] (who showed that the thumb does not move during grasping but is held as a strut onto which the fingers close). So powerful is this tendency that individuals with standard prostheses (where the flexion speed is equal for both) correct the deviation by using shoulder rotation to fix the thumb in space relative to the target [10]. Two major clinical research centres in Italy and England will test the hand mechanism.

The MARCUS hand mechanism is more anthropomorphic in geometry than conventional prostheses, Figure 3. The thumb partly adducts as it flexes, the fingers also curl progressively with flexion. The hand can therefore open wider than other prostheses and so pick up larger objects and those with irregular profiles more securely.

The separated degrees of freedom also allow the hand to adopt both of the standard grip types that a human can employ; *precision* grip when the thumb opposes the tips of the other digits, and *power* grip, where the thumb wraps around the rear of the fingers.

A survey of the user population, [11], showed that one of the principle problems with conventional external cosmetic gloves is that they are not durable and are hard to clean. For the MARCUS hand a silicone glove of superior construction and cosmesis was chosen. It is produced by the bio-engineering unit at Princess Margaret Rose hospital, in Edinburgh, Scotland.

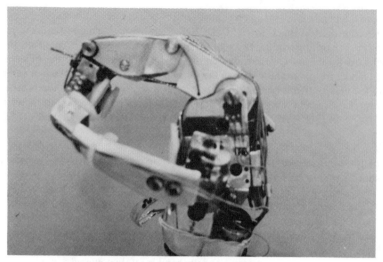

Figure 3 Prototype MARCUS artificial hand

Trials of the new hand system are designed to compare the new control with conventional schemes and thus assess the ease of operation and the functional range of the hand.

### References

[1] D.J Gow, T.D Dick, et al (1983), *The physiologically appropriate control of an electrically powered hand prosthesis.* International Society of Prosthetics and Orthotics, 4th World Congress, London, September 1983.

[2] D. C. SIMPSON, G. KENWORTHY (1973), *The design of a complete arm prosthesis.* Biomedical engineering, February 1973.

[3] D. T. GIBBONS, M. D. O. RAIN and J. S. PHILLIPE-AUGUSTE (1988), *A multi-functional prosthesis employing extended physiological proprioception and programmed linkages.* First workshop on medical robotics. Ottawa 1988.

[4] J. A. DOUBLER and D. S. CHILDRESS (1984), *An analysis of extended physiological proprioception as a prosthesis control technique.* Journal of rehabilitation research and development. **21** no.1 BPR 10 - 39 pp 5 - 18.

[5] P.H Chappell, P.J Kyberd (1991) *The Prehensile control of a hand prosthesis by a microcontroller.* J. Biomed. Eng. **13**, September 1991. pp 363 - 369.

[6] D. Moore (1980), *Development of multifunctional adaptive hand prosthesis.* PhD thesis, University of Southampton.

[7] P.J Kyberd, N. Mustapha F. Carnegie and P.H Chappell (1993) *Clinical experience with a hierarchically controlled myoelectric hand prosthesis with vibro-tactile feedback.* Journal of International Society of Prosthetics and Orthotics, *In press.*

[8] P.J Kyberd et al. (1992) *Development and use of an intelligent myoelectic prosthesis.* International Society of Prosthetics and Orthotics, World Congress, Chicago 27th June - 3rd July 1992.

[9] A. Wing and C. FRASER (1987), et al. (1986), *The contribution of the thumb to reaching movements.* Quarterly journal of experimental psychology. 1987, **35A**, pp 297 - 30.

[10] A. M. WING, and C. FRASER (1988), *Artificial hand use in grasp and release phase of reaching.* International symposium on teleoperation and control. Bristol, July 1988.

[11] P.J Kyberd, D.J. Beard, D. Morrison, J. Davey, (1993) *Survey of the population of upper limb users in the Oxfordshire region* International Society of Prosthetics and Orthotics, UK meeting, Swansea 28th March - 3rd April 1993.

# A Soft Assistant Arm for Tetraplegics

Alícia CASALS, Ricard VILLÀ, Daniel CASALS
*Dep. of Automatic Control. Universitat Politècnica de Catalunya*
*Pau Gargallo nº5  08028 BARCELONA  (SPAIN)*

**Abstract.** *Tou* is a robotic arm conceived to provide tetraplegic people with some autonomy in their daily life. The main characteristic of *Tou* is to be intrinsically safe due to its soft structure. This, together with the fact that the user's orders are imprecise, implies the need to develop special control algorithms. *Tou* is not aimed to substitute an human assistant but to avoid the need of continuous dependance on others of the severely disabled in tasks such as picking up light objects, scratching or to turn the pages of a book.

## 1. Introduction

A large number of projects on assistant robot arms have been developed or are in course of development with the aim to provide disabled people with some degree of autonomy either in their home life [1], [2] or at work [3] [4] .

The first prototypes developed already in the seventies were mainly prosthetic and orthetic devices [5]. Further effort has been done in the adaptation of existing robots for assistance use [6], [7], [8] or in the development of specific arms for this purpose [9], [10]. Also, much progress have been done in the development of workstations based on a robotic arm for the integration of disabled people [11], [12]. Nevertheless, the real commercialisation of this equipment and the user's acceptance is not easy to attain. Often, the real user's requirements are not known sufficiently and the interface may lead to a too tedious a control. That's the reason why many projects have not lead to a final commercial prototype and have rested unfinished.

Fortunately, a great effort is being done now to join together the work, experience and resources of researchers to drive the developments toward the market needs. Also, the general aspects as social implication, market and safety are being studied [13], as well as the legal issues.

The main goal of *Tou* is to become a friendly arm, intrinsically safe, able to obey very simple orders given by a severely disabled user, a tetraplegic. An additional condition is its low cost in order to be available not only to big clinical centers, but fot domestic use. The functions to be realised by *Tou* are not too ambitious, but it is expected to provide wheelchair confined or bedridden users with a certain level of autonomy in their daily life to avoid the continuous assistance of an human in simple tasks such as: to pick and approach objects, to read, to rearange the bedding or to appart an insect.

The orders given by the user differ substantially from those used for industrial robots. They are mainly simple movement and grasping commands that can be provided orally if the user can talk or by means of his residual mobility. These orders are imprecise and can not be defined numerically. Nevertheless, the lack of quantification of the operation to perform is corrected by the user himself, which closes the loop of the control system.

## 2. General Structure

The robotic system consists basically on the arm, a PC to control it and the communication interface with the user. The arm is built from foam-rubber cylindrical modules each of which can bend in two orthogonal directions with respect to the previous one. The movement of the arm is produced by the adequate deformation of each module through wires. When the wires are pulled by the motors located on the robot base they compress the modules in the x or y direction. The number and size of these modules have been defined to obtain the desired accessibility at the user´s environment. With the aim of reaching all the bed width, the length of the arm is 1,6 m (Fig. 1).

Since tetraplegic people, as happens in most types of disabilities, have different communication capabilities, three different interfaces have been used and tested: a speech recognition system, a joystick and a specific keyboard. According to the user's needs the three interfaces are interchangeable.

The use of a PC as the arm control unit has allowed a low cost system but has forced the development of specific and simplified algorithms to control the arm at a reasonable speed. The low precision attainable due both to the soft and flexible structure and to the imprecise orders given by the user doesn't become a real problem, because the user can correct the positioning errors by additional corrective orders or by his own limited mobility. Fig. 2 shows the assistant arm *Tou* at work.

## 3. User's interface.

The basic commands to control the arm position and trajectory are those corresponding to the elemental movements: up-down, approach-go and right-left. With these commands the hand of *Tou* can reach any object on the user's environment or a part of his body. The additional orders: open-close and stop, complete a set of generic commands which allow the user to order the arm to do many elemental operations required repeatedly in his daily life. Nevertheless, many operations may become tedious, that's why the system is able to learn more specific orders and to execute them automatically. For example, the order scratch, already executes repeatedly a sequence of movements up-down or left-right in the zone selected by the user without the need to explicit them. The way the user gives these orders depends on the interface, selected according to his abilities. Fig 3.

### 3.1. Oral communication.

The first interface utilised has been a speech recognition system based on a commercial PC board. Thus, only an adaptation to the system has been necessary. The interface is configured as to be user's independent. In order to increase its discrimination capability in the first prototype the catalan words chosen for each order are chosen to be very different. Anyway, the user can substitute new words for the same orders according to his preferences. If the user has speech difficulties some differentiated sounds could also be used as the programmed commands. Besides the user's possibility to change the words for each order, the system is open to add additional orders to increase the arm performance.

## 3.2. Manual communication.

Initially to solve the problem to make the arm available to users that are not able to speak, an interface to connect a joystick was developed. The first problems found were that only a restricted number of orders could be given. The stick allows to control the movement of the arm only in two dimensions. By coding the signals generated with the two buttons of the joystick, the orders corresponding to the movement in the third dimension and to the control of the grasping movement are given. After a short experimentation period, the joystick has shown to be a device difficult to control by tretraplegics with only some residual mobility in the hand.

Afterwards, a specific keyboard has been designed and built. To avoid the lack of control the user's have in positioning their fingers and the pressure to apply to the keys, the keys are substituted by a material sensible to the touch and are slightly sunk with respect to the keyboard surface. Fig. 4.

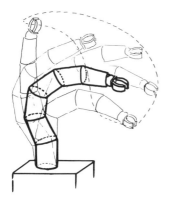

Fig. 1 The structure of *Tou*

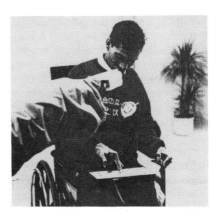

Fig. 2 Tou, the assistant arm in operation

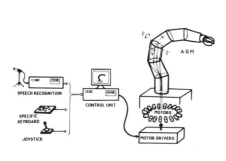

Fig. 3 Man machine communication options

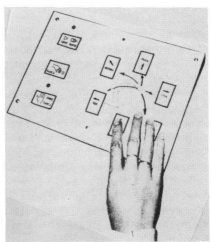

Fig. 4 Specific interface for the manual control of the arm

## 4. Sensing capabilities

The sensing requirements depend on the operations the arm is expected to do and their performance. As internal or positioning sensors, *Tou* uses potentiometers placed over the pulleys that move the wires. Although their precision is low the control unit is able to obey the imprecise orders of movement given by the user. But, due to the hysteresis of the arm material the precise final positioning of the hand results hard to attain.

*Tou* is provided with an additional internal sensor to assure the right orientation of the hand when it carries an object in horizontal or vertical position. This sensor consists on a small pendular device in the wrist.

Since the arm is directly controlled by means of the orders given by the user, who continually closes the control loop by visual tracking of the arm movements and the supervision of its hand final position, the environment sensing requirements are low. In spite of this, to increase the arm performance some sensors are specially useful for some operations. External sensors can also help the user in the control of the arm. This is the case of reading.

In order to turn the pages of a book the hand is provided with an adhesive strip that helps to pull a page when they get in touch. A proximity sensor in the outer part of the hand indicates when contact with an object is near.

The control of grasping objects by the user can be difficult if his visual point of view is not adequate. Vision provides an additional aid in the operation of grasping objects. The approach to an object can be done automatically with a vision system able to locate the different objects on the user's environment. Thus, the user only has to approach the hand to the object. The vision system will guide the arm towards the object that appears nearest to the hand. In case the objects were not the desired, the user's orders would correct the trajectory towards the selected object. The final positioning will be done by the vision system. (Fig. 5). This not only aids to make the control of the approaching and grasping operation less tedious but is useful in some cases when the arm itself can occlude the object and then impede the user's control.

## 5. Results

After an experimentation period in the laboratory the arm was brought to the "Centre Hospitalari del Parc Taulí" in Sabadell (near Barcelona). *Tou* has been tested by two kinds of tetraplegics, a spastic and a flaccid. In the first experimental phase the tasks done by *Tou* have been very simple. the arm has not been seen as a useful tool for daily use but as an exercise for learning, experimentation and as an ocupational work. *Tou* has been generally very welcome. Nevertheless, other kind of help must be sought for those who have strong feelings against all kinds of technological aid.

The tasks previously foreseen have been proved to be useful to the users and now we are working on the development of a more efficient hand able to, handle safely different objects as for instance a cigarette. The inability to smoke has been reported to be very frustrating when the disability has been produced suddenly by an accident. We are also working on the integration of the vision system that will increase the arm performance and thus the degree of utilisation by the users.

With respect to the communication interface, the voice is clearly the must comfortable one but unfortunately many tetraplegic people, mainly if the disability is due to a disease, not an accident, are not able to talk. With respect to the manual communication the spastic user can control the arm with difficulty by means of the joystic while it was really hard for the flaccid, who only controled the stick not the buttons. The specific keyboard has proved to be useful and easy for both.

**Acknowledgements.** This project has been developed with the support of CICYT (Comisión Interministerial de Ciencia y Tecnología). We wish to specially thank the contribution of the personnel of the Residencia Albada (Centre Hospitalari del Parc Taulí) in Sabadell for their interest in the project and their contribution to provide the means of testing the arm effectiveness and to assess on the user's main requirements. We also wish to mention and thank the contribution of the group of people in our department that has cooperated in some part of the project.

**References**

[1] S. Landau et al, A Low-Cost Robotic Manipulator Feeding Device. Proc. $2^{on}$ Int. Conf. on Rehabilitation Engineering, Otawa, 1984.

[2] J.M. Detriché et al, The Domestical Robot Master for the disabled. Cardiotism 88, 6th. Int. Congress, Monaco, 1988.

[3] M.F. Machiel Van der Loos et al, Assessing the Impact of Robotic Devices for the Severely Physically Disabled. Int. Advanced Robotics Programme, Canada, 1988.

[4] Holloway et al, Vocational applications of a Robotic Aid. $2^{on}$ Int. Conference on Rehabilitation Engineering.

[5] $3^{rd}$ Int. Symposium on Theory and Practice of Robot and Manipulators. Elsewier Scientific Pub. Company, 1978.

[6] RTX robot arm. PCW. December, 1978.

[7] Dario et al, Advanced Rehabilitative Robots. Proc. Int. Symposium and Exp. on Robots, Sydney, 1988.

[8] Journal or Rehabilitation Research and Development. R&D Progress Report. Department of Veterans Affairs (Periodic).

[9] A. Casals et al, TOU, Assistant Robot Arm. Design Considerations. $2^{on}$ National Congress of AER, Spanish, 1991.

[10]"Undergoing research subjects in Japan relating to disability". Welfare equipment Development Center of Japan, 1991.

[11]M.R. Hillman et al, A Robot Workstation for the Disabled. 1st. Int. Workshop on Robotic Applications in Medical and Health Care, Otawa, 1986.

[12]J.M. Detriche, The Robotized System Master for Helping the Disabled Persons. 1st Workshop on Domestic Robots and 2on Work on Medical and Healthcare Robotics, Newcastle, 1989.

[13]Safety issues. Specific session on $2^{on}$ Cambridge Workshop on Rehabilitation Robotics. April, 1991.

# RAID Robotic end-effector developments

Gunnar Bolmsjö

*Dept. of Production and Materials Engineering, Lund University*

Håkan Eftring

*CERTEC, Center for Rehabilitation Engineering, Lund University*

**Abstract.** This paper presents recent developments in end-effector design for a robotised workstation for disabled people. The workstation is intended for use at computerised office work places and the robot tasks will primarily be within the area of paper and book handling including page turning. Additional tasks, such as loading diskettes and serving refreshments are included as well. During initial tests the end-effcetors have shown excellent results with respect to expected functionality and reliability. Future developments will be concentrated on integrating more sensors to the end-effectors and the robot controller in order to produce more autonomous and flexible robot tasks in a less structured environment.

## 1  Introduction

The RAID project (Robot for Assisting the Integration of the Disabled) is concerned with the development of a robotised computerised office environment. The aim of the project is to demonstrate a prototype robotic workstation for use by disabled people. The project is part of the European Community TIDE programme.

The partners in the RAID project are: Armstrong Projects Ltd, UK; Cambridge University, UK; Oxford Intelligent Machines Ltd, UK; Papworth Group, UK; UMI Group, UK; CEA/DTA/UR, France; Equal Design, France; HADAR, Sweden and Lund University, Sweden.

The robotised system is intended primarily for vocational use in an office environment. The selected application for demonstration in March 1993 is CAD (Computer Aided Design), which is an application full of handling tasks for the robot. If the demonstration shows a satisfactorily result, a number of other applications can be extracted from the CAD application such as graphics layout, desk top publishing NC programming etc.

During the initial work of the end-effectors it was evident that we should design the end-effectors with as high degree of flexibility as possible in order to minimise tool changing operations. The technical solution is based on two end-effectors, called "book gripper" and "page turner".

## 2 End-effector design

The two end-effectors are outlined in Figs. 1 and 2.

The book gripper is designed to handle books catalogues, manuals and ring bound files with varying thickness and geometrical size (max. 2 kg, max. width 75 mm) between the book shelf and the reader board.

The book gripper is based on a pneumatic clamping device. The movements of the gripper's "thumb" are controlled by a double acting pneumatic cylinder (dia. 16 mm). The gripper will hold a book with a force of 30 N, if the air pressure is set to 0,6 MPa (6 bar). The grasped book is supported by a small shelf to reduce the maximum clamping force needed. The approximate friction coefficient of the surface of the "thumb" is 1 and the weight of the book gripper is 0,8 kg.

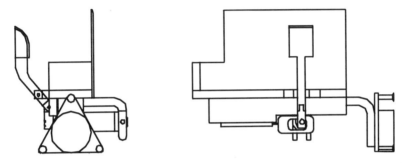

Fig. 1. The book gripper from the top view (left) and from the side view (right).

The design of the book gripper resulted mainly from the user requirements saying that the books should be stored in a normal upright position and that the book shelf should look as normal as possible. These requirements are met with the exception that the books must be stored in separate locations in the book shelf. The width of these locations must be at least 100 mm, which is the width of the book gripper when it is open. A photo electric switch detects if a book is in the gripper.

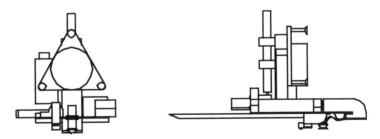

Fig. 2. The page turner from the top view (left) and from side view (right).

The page turner is designed to open books at any point and page turn forwards or backwards from that point. The page turner can also grasp papers of varying sizes and move them between the printer, the reader board, the scanner, the storage racks and the input and output trays. The page turner is also designed to handle disks and drinks served on a specially designed tray.

The three main parts of the page turner are a "knife", a suction cup and a clamping device placed close to the suction cup. The "knife" is a plastic plate with the size of a human hand. It is used for opening books and for turning multiple pages simultaneously. The suction cup and the clamping device are used for single page turning. The bellow type suction cup lifts a single page when it reaches the page surface. A push button is mounted next to the suction cup and detects when the suction cup has reached the page surface. The activated push button stops the approaching movement of the robot arm. The page is then lifted and grasped with the clamping device, which is connected to a double acting pneumatic cylinder.

Some arrangements has been made at the reader board, to prevent small books from moving when they are opened and prevent unwanted page movements when pages are turned in small books with stiff pages. A big suction cup, placed in a hole in the reader board, will prevent small books from moving. A "finger" has been added to the lower part of the reader board, to press down the pages and prevent unwanted page movements. The "finger" is connected to a double acting pneumatic cylinder, which is controlled by the robot. The "finger" is removed for a short time during the page turning process.

The "knife" is also used when handling papers (up to approx. 50 pages), handling disks and serving drinks. The clamping force is produced by a single acting pneumatic cylinder (dia 6 mm). The clamping device is activated towards the "knife", which is used as a supporting surface for the papers, the disks and the drink tray. A force of 15 N will hold the objects, if the air pressure is set to 0,6 MPa (6 bar). The approximate friction coefficient of the surface of the clamping device is 1 and the weight of the page turner is 0,7 kg. A photo electric switch detects if an object is in the gripper.

The end-effectors are mounted on a robot tool changer, which makes it possible for the robot to change end-effectors automatically. The tool changer also increases the flexibility of the RAID workstation. New handling tasks, which perhaps would require a separate gripper, could then be added more easily. The possibility to adapt RAID to individual needs is an important user requirement.

The tool changer SOMMER WW 50 has been selected, mainly because of safety reasons but also because of the small dimensions. The gripper mounted on the tool changer will not fall off, neither in the event of electric power failure nor air supply failure. Additionally, grasped objects won't be dropped, because of the introduction of non-return valves and the choise of the grasped mode as the non-activated mode.

## 3   Tests, results and problems

The development of the end-effectors has been an iterative process, where tests continually have been done during the RAID project. From the beginning prototypes have been developed and tested, not only to evaluate the technical functionality but also to be able to incorporate as much as possible of the users' point of view. Therefore, the development has been done in close contact with a reference group [2]. The end-effector prototypes have subsequently been modified several times.

The final tests of the RAID demonstrator with users in action will take place at HADAR in Malmö, Sweden between March and April 1993. Not until then we have the possibility to test the end- effectors' real performance in the specified environment. At present, January 1993, the system integration phase of the RAID project is in its final stage and the different sub-systems like the modified RT100 robot, end-effectors, latest version of the MASTER control language, reader board etc. will all be integrated into the RAID work station demonstrator.

A specific problem in the development of the end-effectors have been the demand for high degree of flexibility in functionality. As an example, we try to adapt the environment (book shelves etc) as little as possible. This has also caused a lot of modifications during the project in order to meet all demands and changes of the peripheral equipment and layout of the system.

Initial tests have been made with the end-effectors mounted on a standard instead of the modified RT100 robot, that is used in the RAID demonstrator. Simple prototype versions of the book shelf, paper storage racks and reader board have been constructed for these initial tests. The results during these tests are described below.

## 3.1 Book gripper

The time to move a book from the book shelf to the reader board is 60 s. With the modified RT100 robot the time should be reduced to 20-30 s. Grasping a book from the shelf has not caused any problem. When positioning soft catalogues at the reader board, the robot has to make some extra movements to prevent the pages from being folded. In addition, to grasp a book from the reader board has caused some problems with varying positions of the book in the gripper. However, this does not cause any problems when returning the book to the shelf again except for catalogues that have a tendency to fold.

## 3.2 Page turner

When opening a book it is only possible to reach an accuracy of $\pm 20$ pages. To reach a specific page the user then has to turn one page at a time. The cycle time for turning one page is 15 s. This is expected to be reduced to 5-10 s in the demonstrator. In order to test the performance of the page turner at higher speed, the page turner was mounted and tested on an ABB IRb1000 industrial robot. The cycle time obtained with full functionality of the page turner was 3 s and approx. 100 pages could be turned without errors. Furthermore, in case of an error, the robot could still proceed the operation by turning backwards and forwards. The errors during page turning was (1) missed to lift and turn a page, (2) turned two or more pages at one time or (3) made an uncompleted page turn. In all cases, a subsequent page turn without human interaction corrected any problems caused by the error. At this stage it is not possible to have one task program for all books. Our approach is to make one program for each book with respect to their size. Furthermore, the tilt angle of the reader board have to be specified. It is anticipated that the angle can be a parameter in the program. Page turning at the beginning and at the end of books cause some problems, because the corners are not in the same position. Some user interaction may be needed during robot execution. Stiff pages get slightly folded in their upper corners due to a clamping device on the page turner. Some noise is produced by a vacuum ejector and pneumatic valves during operation. An electric vacuum pump was tested but was rejected by the reference group.

The only problem observed in paper handling is positioning paper sheets of size A3 on the reader board. It is only possible to grasp them at the short side from the printer or storage.

Disk handling tasks has proven successful with a high reliability. Straight line interpolation and good robot repeatability is needed during this operation. However, the page turner is not ideal for this task due to geometrical constraints.

A special tray is adapted to the page turner in order to serve refreshments. No problems have occurred.

### 3.3 Future work

In order to fulfil user requirements and increase the flexibility and reliability of the end-effectors, the following parts should be developed further: (1) Redesign the end-effectors emphasising on the appearance to the end user and reduce the geometrical size. (2) Improve the book gripper to make it able to get books from a normal shelf. (3) Increase use of sensors in order to develop control functions in the task and a higher degree of flexibility and autonomy in a less structured environment. (4) Develop process models in the control system for different tasks that can produce a "generic" task, for example grasp a book and turn up page 153 for different types of books.

## 4  Conclusions

Two end-effector prototypes for use in the RAID demonstrator have been constructed and a test programme is defined and will cover both technical and user requirements. Initial technical tests have shown a good performance both with respect to cycle time, reliability and functionality. However, this kind of end-effectors need pre-programmed procedures and a structured environment that is known beforehand. In order to increase the flexibility of the system, we are aiming towards more autonomous functions for the specified tasks. This will be taken care of in two ways: increase the functionality of the robot and hence the robot controller, and increase the functionality of the end-effectors by introducing sensors which, integrated to the controller, can greatly improve the robot performance in less structured environment that is likely to occur in human operated work stations. It must also be pointed out that improved autonomy through better robot controller and integrated sensors have in this context a specific value; It is simply more important to increase the reliability, functionality and autonomy of the robot when applying robot technology for disabled people since an error during execution may just not be acceptable. Enhanced autonomy of the end-effectors will also increase the possibility to use the robot for certain tasks in manual or semi-manual mode that today in most cases can be quite time consuming.

### References

[1] J.L. Dallaway and R.D. Jackson, RAID — A Vocational Robotic Workstation. In: *Proceeding of ICORR 92*, 1992.

[2] G. Bolmsjö and L. Holmberg, User Requirements and Test Results. In: *Proceeding of the 1st TIDE Congress*, Brussels, April 1993. To be published.

# Speech Processing for the Profoundly Hearing Impaired

Arjan J. Bosman and Guido F. Smoorenburg
Laboratory of Experimental Audiology, Department of Otorhinolaryngology
University Hospital Utrecht, Heidelberglaan 100, NL-3584 CX Utrecht
The Netherlands

**Abstract.** Many profoundly hearing impaired listeners experience not only an increase in auditory threshold but also a severe loss in hearing differences among sounds at any level above their threshold. We studied audio-visual perception of natural speech versus synthesized speech based on voice fundamental frequency and on one or two vowel formants. Intelligibility scores of four profoundly hearing impaired subjects showed an interdependency between the type of speech processing scheme and the type of residual hearing. This project was performed within the project 'STRIDE' of the TIDE program.

## 1. Introduction

Hearing impaired listeners with a hearing loss greater than 90 dB, the profoundly hearing impaired, often derive little benefit from conventional hearing aids. Their residual hearing capacities are so small that even with optimum amplification they cannot extract sufficient information to understand speech. The small range of levels between just-detectable sounds and uncomfortably loud sounds, the so-called dynamic range, is one of the limiting factors. Also, residual hearing is often only present at frequencies below 1 or 2 kHz. This causes a severe low-pass filtering of speech which obscures contrasts between some phonemes (e.g., /u/ versus /i/, /f/ versus /s/). Apart from the reductions in dynamic range and frequency range, the frequency resolving power of the impaired ear is often also reduced. Consequently, spectral contrasts are perceived less well by the hearing impaired than by normal-hearing listeners [1]. Since the receptive ability of the impaired ear is limited in several ways, one might improve their speech reception by reducing the information contained in the acoustic speech signal, so that it better matches the limited auditory capacity.

For the profoundly hearing impaired lipreading is the most important means of communication with the normal-hearing world; amplified speech may provide, at best, additional information to lipreading. So, when providing acoustic signals to the listener, attention should be focussed on features that give optimal support for lipreading. The presentation of these features must be adapted as closely as possible to the residual hearing.

Both the analysis of features and the presentation thereof can be readily achieved by digital signal processing. An example of a digital speech processing hearing aid is the SiVo (Sinusoidal Voicing) aid developed by Fourcin and his co-workers [1]. The SiVo extracts the fundamental frequency from the speech signal and presents it as a pure tone to the listener. Speech perception based on the presentation of vowel formants (i.e. maxima in the envelope of vowel spectra) has been studied by Breeuwer and Plomp [2], but only with normal-hearing listeners.

In this study we will compare intelligibility scores in four profoundly deaf subjects for (1) unprocessed speech and for speech representations based on: (2) voice fundamental frequency (SiVo-like), (3) one vowel formant, and (4) two vowel formants. All conditions were presented audio-visually.

## 2. Speech Analysis and Synthesis

Speech can be analyzed on the basis of the following model. Voiced sounds (vowels and voiced consonants) originate from quasi-periodic vibration of the vocal chords, whereas unvoiced sounds (consonants) originate from turbulent air passing some narrow constriction in the vocal tract. The vocal tract acts as an acoustic filter and the resonances of the vocal tract introduce maxima in the envelope of the speech spectrum (formants). As both the excitation sources and the shape of the vocal tract behave relatively independently and vary only slowly with time, speech parameters can be accurately estimated with Linear Predictive Coding (LPC) [3]. The LPC-parameters are: fundamental frequency, voiced/unvoiced classification, waveform amplitude and filter coefficients. The formant values follow directly from the poles of the filter transfer function.

In the perception of speech, voice fundamental frequency, $f_0$, carries prosodic information like intonation and stress, whereas formants provide information about speech elements. Vowels and voiced consonants can be identified on the basis of their formants and formant transitions.

In our $f_0$-synthesis we represented $f_0$ as a pure tone during voiced speech; white noise was used during unvoiced speech. In the waveforms representing one ($F_1$) or two ($F_1$ and $F_2$) formants during voiced speech two adjacent harmonics of $f_0$ were used for each formant to indicate formant frequency. During unvoiced speech, white noise was used.

Finally, in all cases the time-envelope of the synthesized waveform was set as closely as possible to the envelope of the original waveform. The advantage of providing two harmonics of $f_0$ per formant is that both formants can be more easily interpreted as belonging to one sound source; secondly, due to the phenomenon of residue pitch [4] the pitch corresponding to $f_0$ is implicitly encoded by time-domain information (the beats correspond to the difference frequency $f_0$).

The procedure of synthesizing formants is illustrated in Fig. 1. The left-hand panel of Fig. 1 shows a spectrum of the vowel /o/ (as in "low") and its envelope estimated with LPC-analysis; the right-hand panel shows the synthesized spectrum for the same vowel with two harmonics for both $F_1$ and $F_2$.

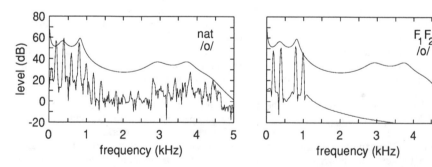

Fig. 1. Left panel: FFT-spectrum of the vowel /o/ (as in "low") excised from running speech. The spectral envelope was estimated with a 12th order LPC-analysis. Right panel: FFT-spectrum of the $F_1F_2$ synthesized signal consisting of two harmonics of $f_0$ per formant. Due to the low $F_1$ the lowest harmonic coincides with $f_0$; for higher values of $F_1$ only true harmonics of $f_0$ are present.

## 3. Methods

Four subjects (age: 14 to 18 years) from a school for the hard of hearing participated in the experiments. They all wore hearing aids. Detection thresholds for pure tones were measured at octave frequencies from 125 Hz up to 2 kHz. Both detection thresholds (THR), most comfortable levels (MCL) and levels of discomfort (UCL) are shown in Fig. 2.

The speech material consisted of sentences of 8 or 9 syllables, representative of everyday Dutch [5]. The video-taped material was read out by a female speaker. LPC-analysis of the speech signal was carried out off-line with Entropics software running on a SUN workstation. In a few cases hand-correction of LPC-parameters was carried out.

The speech stimuli consisted of 1) natural speech (nat); 2) voice fundamental frequency coded as a pure tone for voiced fragments and white noise for unvoiced fragments ($f_0$); 3) first formant coded by two adjacent harmonics of $f_0$ ($F_1$); 4) first and second formant coded by two harmonics of $f_0$ each ($F_1F_2$). The spectra of all signals were shaped according to the MCL curves in Fig. 2 using a 1/3 octave equalizer (Boss GE131). Before the experiment 5 minutes training was given to acquaint the listener to the coded stimuli.

The four speech stimuli were presented at each listener's most comfortable level. Subject's responses were written down by the observer and the percentage of correctly identified syllables in sentences (syllable score) was scored.

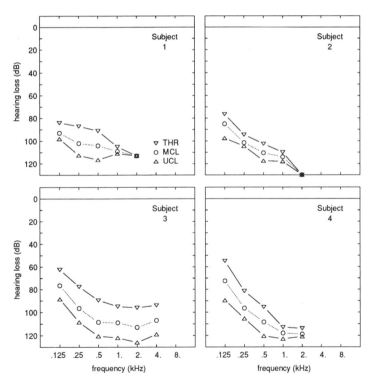

Fig. 2. Tone audiogram with detection thresholds (THR), most comfortable levels (MCL) and uncomfortable levels (UCL) for pure tones. All levels are relative to the average detection thresholds for normal-hearing listeners. Data are given for each subject individually.

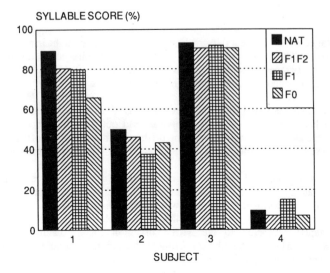

Fig. 3. The percentages correctly identified syllables (syllable scores) for the four encoding strategies. The sentences were presented audiovisually. NAT: natural, unprocessed speech; $f_0$: fundamental frequency only; $F_1$: first formant encoded by two harmonics of $f_0$; $F_1F_2$: both $F_1$ and $F_2$ encoded by two harmonics of $f_0$. Data are given for each subject individually. In lipreading alone, the average syllable score for this material is 18 % with an interindividual standard deviation of 16 % [7].

## 4. Results

The syllable scores for the four speech conditions are shown in Fig. 3. As scores can be modeled as a binomial variable, standard deviations are largest for scores around 50 %. For this material, scores near 50 % have standard deviations of about 5 % [6]. For three subjects the highest scores are found with the natural speech condition. Subject 4 shows highest scores with $F_1$-encoded speech.
For the coded speech conditions subject 1 has higher scores for both $F_1$ and $F_1F_2$ encoding than for $f_0$ encoding. Subject 2 has higher scores for the $f_0$ and $F_1F_2$ condition than for the $F_1$ condition. Subject 3 shows no clear difference scores among coding strategies. Subject 4 comes to the highest score with $F_1$-encoding, with $f_0$ en $F_1F_2$-encoding about equal. For comparison, in lipreading alone the average syllable score for this material is 18 % with an interindividual standard deviation of 16 % [7].

## 5. Discussion

The lower scores for three of the four subjects in the coded conditions may be due to a lack of experience with these new types of speech coding.
More interestingly, subject 1 has about equal scores for $F_1$ and $F_1F_2$-encoding, while scores for $f_0$-encoding are lower. Apparently, this subject makes use of spectral information in the region up to about 1 kHz. For this subject the high-frequency information of the second formant in the $F_1F_2$-encoding falls beyond his hearing range. So, when spectral resolution is relatively intact, $F_1$-encoding seems best for subjects with residual hearing limited to 1 kHz.
Subject 2 shows about the same scores for $f_0$ and $F_1F_2$-encoding. The dynamic range for this subject is smallest. This suggests that in cases with marginal residual hearing and little spectral resolution $f_0$-encoding may be best. The score for natural speech

was higher than for $f_0$-encoded speech, suggesting that training is necessary to exploit the full potential of this new speech code.

Scores were highest in subject 3. Subject 3 is a good lipreader and thus, ceiling effects may have obscured differences in scores due to the encoding. The large dynamic range in this subject and his relatively good hearing thresholds up to 4 kHz suggest that $F_1F_2$-encoding would be the best choice.

The scores for subject 4 were lower than for the other subjects. This may be due to his relatively poor lipreading abilities. Also, in this case $F_1$-encoding provides the highest scores.

So, the choice of an optimum encoding strategy depends on the individual's residual hearing. More research is needed into the (psychophysical) parameters that predict the optimum encoding strategy.

## Acknowledgments

We thank our subjects for their cooperation throughout the experiments. We also thank Marjan Bruins of the Alfonsi Corti school for her help in selecting the subjects. This project was performed within the project 'STRIDE' of the TIDE program.

## References

[1] Faulkner, A., Ball, V., Rosen, S., Moore, B.C.J. and Fourcin, A., Speech pattern hearing aids for the profoundly hearing impaired: Speech perception and auditory abilities, J. Acoust. Soc. Am. **91** (1992) 2136-2155.

[2] Breeuwer, M. and Plomp, R., Speech reading supplemented with formant-frequency information from voiced speech, J. Acoust. Soc. Am. **77** (1985) 314-317.

[3] Rabiner, L.R. and Schafer, R.W., Digital processing of speech signals. Prentice-Hall, London, 1978.

[4] Moore, B.C.J., An Introduction to the psychology of hearing. Academic Press, London, 1982.

[5] Plomp, R. and Mimpen, A.M., Improving the reliability of testing the speech reception threshold for sentences, Audiology **18** (1979) 43-52.

[6] Bosman, A.J. Speech perception by the hearing impaired. Doctoral Dissertation, University of Utrecht, 1989.

[7] Huiskamp, T.M.I. Twee onderzoeken op het gebied van liplezen. Master's thesis, Laboratory of Experimental Audiology, University of Utrecht, 1992.

118

# Multi-modality Aids for People with Impaired Communication (MAPIC)

*P A Cudd, Department of Electronic & Electrical Engineering, University of Sheffield, Mappin Street, Sheffield S1 3JD UK*

*M S Hawley, Department of Medical Physics & Clinical Engineering, Barnsley District General Hospital, Gawber Road, Barnsley S75 2EP UK*

*P Dalsgaard, Speech Technology Centre, Institute of Electronic Systems, 7 Fredrik Bajers Vej, DK 9220 Aalborg, Denmark*

*L Azevedo, Centro Analise Processamento Sinais (CAPS), CAPS/Complexo I, Avenida Rovisco Pais, 1096 Lisbon, Portugal*

*S Aguilera, ETSI Telecommunicacion (UPM), Ciudad Universitaria s/n, 28040 Madrid, Spain*

*B Granstrom, Department of Speech Communication and Music Acoustics, KTH, PO Box 70014, S-100 44 Stockholm, Sweden*

**Abstract :** The paper gives an overview of a research project submitted to the CEC Human Capital & Mobility programme. The aim of the project is to initiate research to improve communication for the communication impaired using a single hardware and software platform. The project will build on current state-of-the-art techniques in multi-lingual "normal" speech recognition, processing and synthesis but will use clinical assessment and analysis to fundamentally re-appraise speech processing parameters. Novel techniques will be brought to the graphical interfacing for visual communication, which will start from the use of symbolic language systems. If successful, the speech recognition and speech synthesis work will have benefits for general applications as well as for speakers with disability.

## 1. Introduction

Due to the relatively low incidence of severe physical disability in the general population, the cost of development and provision of aids for communication and mobility tends to be relatively high. The research described below has developed from a recognition that by combining expertise and technologies in a modular approach, opportunities exist to develop and extend the applications of widely available and relatively inexpensive computer systems to a large range of different levels and types of disability, including those who have short-term disability.

The planned research aims to establish a software and computer peripheral base which will enhance a portable personal computer so that it can be used to augment human-machine and human-human communication. The resulting modular aid will aim to optimize communication and control for people with a range of communication and motor disabilities.

The research programme has on-going clinical assessment as an essential provider of feedback to the technical investigations. People with moderately severe to severe cerebral palsy will form the main subject group for the clinical facets of the research, although speakers who are severely dysarthric as a result of CVA (stroke), head injury or degenerative neurological conditions (such as motor neurone disease) may also be included. The exploitation of speech recognition techniques, including those used for multi-lingual recognizers, will be used to identify parameters characterizing voice and speech quality for this group of patients as an aid to later synthesis of speech designed to be perceived as appropriate to the individual, and, to improve automatic impaired-speech recognition.

In the following sections an indication is given of the authors' research programme in the MAPIC proposal. Whether or not it succeeds in being supported by the CEC, the authors felt that it was worth airing our proposed research at the TIDE Congress. Furthermore the authors recognize that even with the 30 man-years of work requested in their proposal, a high performance solution is unlikely, not least for the automatic impaired-speech recognition, since the research is at an early stage. The MAPIC proposal fits the requirements of the Human Capital & Mobility programme well, because it will train post-doctoral researchers in a multi-disciplinary way, who will then return to their countries to hopefully continue working on related research.

## 2. Speech Recognition

The aim of the Sheffield group is to investigate the feasibility of oral communication aids which will translate an individual's vocalizations into clearly enunciated appropriate speech. In order to assess this it will first of all be necessary to carry out a substantial amount of fundamental scientific investigation into the two main aspects of the translator; impaired-speech recognition and high quality speech synthesis.

The research will work towards the automatic, or semi-automatic, estimation of appropriate parameters to represent any individual's speech. Firstly though, exploratory work will be conducted to characterize the acoustic features of vocalization patterns produced by individuals with different degrees of communicative disability. There is also a need to establish the limits of repeatability of the vocal patterns produced by individuals within each group of speech-impaired patients. This will be investigated jointly with the Aalborg team using stochastic signal processing techniques (such as principal components analysis), clustering algorithms (k-means etc) and/or self-organising (Kohonen) artificial neural networks, as appropriate.

The research at Aalborg will work on refinements and robustness of the signal processing, as opposed to signal analysis techniques normally used in connection with speech recognition. The latter will be used in clinical tests being carried out to assist in and improve the ability of deaf children in their lip-reading.

The Madrid team has wide experience in developing automatic speech recognition systems. At present, they are adjusting an inexpensive large vocabulary, isolated word, adaptive speaker speech recognition system based on a verification paradigm and a bottom-up strategy. The system contains three main modules:

* A front-end module (feature extractor) to parameterize the speech input.

* An acoustic module based on a connected speech algorithm (One-pass of Ney) working with an allophones library (context and word independent allophones, 25-40 allophones in Spanish) using Discrete Hidden Markov models.

\* An optimal access lexical module based on a Dynamic Programming algorithm with the possibility of dealing with these errors using a confusion matrix and other kinds of information (allophone duration, phonological rules, ....).

Initial studies of data collected at Lisbon and at Madrid, using the Spanish speech recognizer, will be used to indicate the sort of changes that may be required in any re-parameterization and to indicate what sort of speech data should be collected. To allow multi-language comparison of any new recognizer to be made the protocol for speech data collection will be adapted from that decided on at Sheffield. Investigations to re-parameterize the Aalborg recognizer to encompass the Romanic language impaired-speech will then commence.

## 3. Speech Synthesis

In the development of the synthetic speech output, concerted efforts will be made to achieve a high level of naturalness and acceptability to the subjects in the study, and to others with impaired speech. This is necessary because patients often reject the currently available speech communication aids due to the inappropriate voice (ie. typically robot-like and/or sounding North American). In order to achieve this, a preliminary investigation into the speaker and voice types preferred by the patients will be necessary. This will include consideration of local accent features and intonation patterns, for example. Once the preferred speaker and speech parameters have been identified they can be modelled in the synthetic speech output.

The research on speech synthesis will be the major contribution of the Madrid team and will be pursued in three ways. Firstly, to enhance the current synthesizer and secondly to investigate a Diphone synthesizer, the point of this being to compare the performance of these synthesizers. The adaptations and novel modelling in the synthesizers will be investigated from the basis of adapting the normal automatic speech recognition to pathological speech. Speaker adaptation will also be considered in the latter analysis. Collaboration with the Sheffield group on looking for multi-lingual parameters for the impaired-speech of cerebral palsy people is planned.

Novel techniques for customizing speech synthesis will be investigated. This includes both configuring different voices and switching speaking styles. Ways of expressing attitudes and emotions in an artificial voice is an important sub-project. In this the Madrid team want to include both the basic speech production development and the man-machine interface giving the disabled person access to these facilities. This is expected to call for new solutions since the attitudes and emotions are by nature different from the strictly linguistic content of an utterance.

In the speech synthesis area, the Madrid team will try to enhance the segmental quality of their formant-based (Klatt) speech synthesizer. The necessary changes will be investigated by consideration of the results of intelligibility tests to be performed as a first step in the project schedule. All the modifications needed to improve this quality (other than the rules of the synthesizer) will be studied and, if possible, implemented.

Another avenue to be investigated is the use of waveform concatenation methods for synthesis. These methods are known to perform better than the methods involving strong quantization of speech. Pitch-synchronous overlap-add was chosen because of its superior modification capability. Yet, another task in synthesis is the capability of changing the type of voice to be synthesized. The user should be able to select a type of voice in the installation procedure or, in the case of the Klatt synthesizer, change the voice by including a code in the text.

## 4. Human-Computer Interface

The Lisbon team want to develop graphical user interfaces for the multi-modality (MAPIC) system. These graphical interfaces will use both symbolic language systems currently in use (BLISS, PIC, SPC, etc), as well as new techniques for visual communication methods. These graphical interfaces will be particularly helpful for severely physically disabled or elderly people, but will also have application for people with cognitive impairment. A graphical user interface environment will be developed which will allow graphical symbols used by people with impaired speech to be transduced into linguistic concepts.

## 5. Tactile Communication

The Aalborg group are currently working on a tactile support for lipreading, in face to face situations, for post-lingually deaf persons. Optimizing this communication mode calls for efficient evaluation techniques and we are working on the development of a computer assisted speech tracking procedure. This will allow the system to be standardized so that intra-laboratory as well as inter-laboratory comparisons of results can be made.

Speech analysis parameters for this task will in a first assessment set-up be presented to the deaf children via three tactile vibrators positioned at individual finger tips, while the deaf children will also get some speech information by simultaneously using a behind the ear hearing aid, which is specially designed to amplify the speech signal frequencies up to 500Hz. Later on in the project the speech signal analysis parameters may be presented, for example visually instead of via the tactile vibrators. In the first experiments, the parameters are a set of acoustic phonetic features. These are: frontness versus backness and two manner-of-articulation features (closed versus open) for the vowels, and two place-of-articulation features (velar versus alveolar) for the consonants. However, an optimal form of presentation of a relevant set of features will be identified within the task of the project.

## 6. Control of Assistive Devices

There are a large number of people with congential or acquired neurological disorders who only have very limited controllable movement but have a greater range of vocalization. For these people, speech activation would be much quicker than switch input, allowing them to use their limited vocal ability as an aid to independent action. Control will be achieved via an integrated control system with a friendly user interface based on the standard computer system to be used by each of the laboratories. The aim is to allow severely disabled people to control a large number of essential functions, for example mobility (powered wheelchairs), environment, communication, all from the same source and means of input. Research will be carried out into optimum control strategies and into the best means of feedback to the user via the visual display and audible means.

Interfacing of the computer system to existing equipment controllers produced in Barnsley and Sheffield and those being developed in other European projects (eg. the Modular environmental control and communications system project running under TIDE) will be explored. In parallel with this, algorithms from recognition of impaired voices will be investigated in conjunction with the Aalborg, Sheffield and Madrid teams, with emphasis on accurate recognition of a relatively small vocabulary. Particular prominence will be given to ensuring the safety of control systems. User trials will take place in the final year of the project.

## 7. Clinical Involvement

The whole programme has on-going clinical assessment as an essential provider of feedback to the technical investigations.

The Sheffield group can provide their own clinical input to the speech characterization and the Barnsley group will assist in data collection. The Lisbon group will provide clinical input for the Madrid team on the speech research. They will collect impaired-speech data in Portuguese according to a modified version of the Sheffield protocol and will work closely with the Madrid team on the assessment process for speech synthesis and recognition. The Lisbon group are well placed to provide clinical assessment of their visual interfacing.

The teachers of Aalborg School of Deaf Children will carry out clinical assessments related to the lip-reading task of the project, and will give feedback to the STC researchers on improvements and modifications needed and being identified during the real-life assessment.

## 8. Conclusions

The successful development of aids such as those proposed here should enable people with severe long-term disabilities to participate and interact more readily with others within their own and other communities. There is clearly a potential for such a system to be used across the EC and it has clear economic and social implications for the communication impaired, not least in terms of increased choice and participation in education and employment.

The proposed research is a necessary precursor to the arrival of affordable systems and will help to ensure that there is a European alternative to the currently pervasive English language based American aids. By emphasising the multi-lingual approach, the future applicability of the prototype system developed should lead to all EC countries enjoying the benefits. The modular approach being adopted will allow only those features required to be provided, while the use of IBM compatibles will ensure a continuing availability of platform.

The work programme strikes a balance between clinical assessment of techniques and equipment and engineering design and implementation. This multi-disciplinary approach is the best way of carrying out this type of cross-discipline research and will give the highest possibility of success. It will also provide a broad-based training for researchers, providing the human resources for the EC to compete in this increasingly competitive field.

## 9. Acknowledgements

The authors would like to thank all their colleagues who helped to put together the research proposal and this paper, especially Ms. M. Freeman and Dr. S. Whiteside from the Speech Science Unit of the University of Sheffield.

# A New Communication Device
# for Handicapped Persons:
# The Brain-Computer Interface[1]

Gert PFURTSCHELLER, Joachim KALCHER, Doris FLOTZINGER
*Institute of Biomedical Engineering, Department of Medical Informatics, and
Ludwig Boltzmann Institute of Medical Informatics and Neuroinformatics,
Brockmanngasse 41, A-8010 Graz, University of Technology, Austria*

**Abstract.** For patients who are unable to perform normal movements or normally communicate with others it is important to search for a new communication device, which allows the patient to perform simple movements either by functional stimulation or by a robotic device, or to give answers to simple questions without a verbal response. The prerequisites for such a communication is mental activity (thoughts), represented in a specific spatio-temporal EEG pattern, that can be classified on-line.

This paper reports on prerequisites to classify mental activity and on a simple self-learning EEG-based Brain-Computer Interface (BCI) which consists of EEG amplifiers, an analog/digital converter and a PC. This BCI transforms the EEG pattern into a code to control the movement of a cursor on a monitor. With the PC, features are extracted from the EEG which are then classified by an artificial neural network. With classification of EEG segments recorded during mental activity ("thinking"), the cursor can be moved either to the left or right into the indicated target on the monitor. After 3 days of training about 85% correct movements could be obtained.

## 1. Introduction

Patients with hemiplegia or quadriplegia cannot perform normal movements with their limbs; signals from the motor cortex that do not reach the muscles because of a lesion in the cervical spine are the reason for this. Patients with a locked-in syndrom are not able to make any conscious movement including speech although they are fully conscious. This means patients with a locked-in syndrom cannot respond or communicate with others. A Brain-Computer Interface (BCI), a system which can transform their thoughts into action, would enable such patients to lead a much more normal life.

The first EEG-based BCI was reported by Wolpaw et al [6]. This BCI uses one EEG recording and induces the movement of up or down of a cursor on a monitor by "thinking" only. Their work showed for the first time that a BCI is in principle possible and that "thoughts" can be decoded. For control they used the amplitude of the central mu rhythm: several amplitude ranges were defined to map the measured amplitude into a command for

[1] Supported by grants of the Austrian Ministry of Science and Research (GZ 45,167 13-278 91), the Lorenz Böhler Foundation (project 7/92), and the Austrian Science Foundation (project P9043).

the cursor. The disadvantage of that approach is, however, that the patients had to learn to change their mu rhythm amplitude by biofeedback, which took several months until a reasonable performance. It would be more efficient to adapt the system, i.e., to train the system to detect some predefined EEG patterns. This can be achieved by building a self-learning system which is trained on a set of examples and can be used to classify new patterns. First results on such a BCI, which allows cursor movements by mental activity alone, was reported by Pfurtscheller et al [7]. They showed that the classifier can be adapted to reliably identify various states of the brain within a few days.

This paper shortly reviews the principles of a Brain-Computer Interface and presents first results of the Graz BCI.

## 2. Mental Activity and Event-Related Desynchronization

Different mental activities are associated with different patterns of neural activity and are reflected in the potential distribution which can be measured with scalp electrodes. The event-related desynchronization (ERD) of alpha rhythms is a well-known electro-physiological correlate of planning or preparation of movement ([4], [5], and [8]) For quantification of the ERD, the averaging technique must be used; i.e., events (special "thoughts") have to be repeated at least about 30 times in intervals of some seconds before a series of ERD maps can be computed. Figure 1 shows ERD maps for planning of left and right hand movement and for actual movement along with the experimental paradigm.

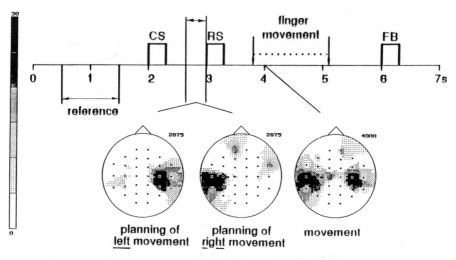

Fig.1: Experimental paradigm and ERD maps for planning of left and right hand movement and actual movement. CS represents the cue for 'left' or 'right', RS the request to start the movement.

## 3. Experimental Paradigm for Classification of ERD in Single Trials

For the construction of a BCI, spatio-temporal ERD patterns have to be classified without averaging techniques, i.e., on a single-trial basis. This is possible by using a neural network-based classifier. To prove that such a classifier can be used for classification of single-trial data, a movement experiment was designed in which the subject was asked to press a microswitch with the index finger, whereby 'left' or 'right' was indicated by a cue (CS). The experimental paradigm is displayed in Figure 1. The time window used for classification to predict which hand will be moved lies between the two cues CS and RS and represents the movement planning phase ("preparatory state"). The recorded data were divided into a training and a testing set: using the training set a classifier was created and its performance was then verified on the testing set.

Classification results obtained in 3 subjects were presented in [8]: the side of index finger movement could be predicted from multi-channel EEG data recorded prior to movement with an accuracy of 70-85% (performance on the testing set). These results show that planning or preparation of right or left finger movement can be differentiated by analyzing single-trial ERD patterns.

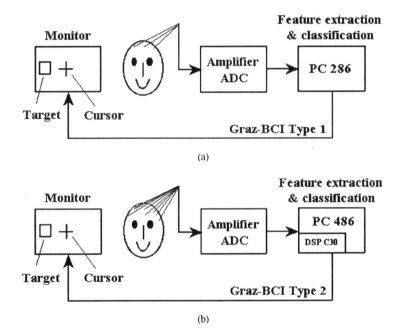

(a)

(b)

Fig. 2: BCI setups. (a) Graz BCI 1, (b) Graz BCI 2.

## 4. Graz BCI

### 4.1. Experimental Setup

The first one-dimensional BCI developed in Graz (Graz BCI 1) includes an EEG amplifier and a PC 286 with a 12 bit analog-digital converter (see Fig. 2, upper part). The next generation (Graz BCI 2), currently under development, is based on a PC 486 and additionally uses a digital signal processing board (see Fig. 2, lower part).

Since the classifier has to be trained for each user individually, to distinguish between two kinds of patterns, here the planning of left and right finger movements, a seperate recording has to be performed with a paradigm similar to the one described in chapter 3. The EEG recorded during the preparation of movement is used to create a classifier which stores the characteristics for planning of left and right finger movements for this specific user (Figure 3a). After this, the user can control a cursor by merely going through the planning phase of either left or right finger movement without actual motor output (Figure 3b).

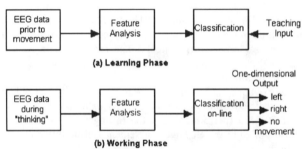

Fig. 3: Outline of the Graz BCI for one-dimensional movements.

## 4.2. Feature extraction and Classification

The Graz BCI 1 uses no digital signal processing (DSP) board and the limited processing speed of the PC 286 allows only the analysis of 2 EEG signals. The features used for classification are 9 power estimates calculated from the two electrode positions C3 and C4 (international 10-20 system). The experimental paradigm can be summarized as follows (see Fig. 4): the target (square) to be moved is placed either on the left or right half of the monitor in front of the subject. The subject has the instruction to move the cursor (cross), which appears one second after the presentation of the target, either to the left or right into the indicated target. The time interval which is used for classification is shown in Figure 4. It starts with the presentation of the target and ends at the presentation the cursor (cue) whose movement is determined by the decision rule stated below and is shown to the user via feedback after 2 seconds.

By shifting a sliding window of size 5 over these 9 timepoints, 5 feature vectors were created in each trial and were classified either to 'left' or 'right' ([2]). These 5 classifications were combined to one final decision, which moved the cursor on the screen, by majority voting. This classification method has the advantage over classifying all 9 timepoints in one step that it does not suppose that the reaction to the external stimulus (presentation of the target) always starts at exactly the same timepoint. It therefore incorporates a form of shift-tolerance of the starting point of the ERD.

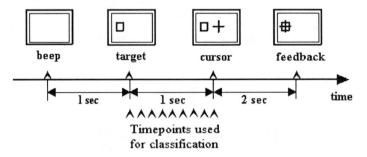

Fig. 4: Working-phase of the Graz-BCI

## 4.3. Classifier

The classifier used in the Graz BCI 1 is the Learning Vector Quantizer (LVQ), a machine learning method developed by Kohonen ([3]). This classification method is related to vector quantization methods in which the (usually higher-dimensional) input space is divided into a number of regions, where each region has a reference vector and a class label attached. In the recognition stage, an unknown input vector is classified to the class label of the reference vector that is closest to that input vector. Kohonen presents several versions of the learning algorithm, which finds near-optimal placements for the reference vectors. Here, version LVQ3 was used.

## 4.4. Results

The results obtained in one subject in 4 sessions (on different days) are summarized in Table 1. After the first session a performance of 70% correct movements was reached; in the 4th session the performance increased to 86%. This means that by presenting a target either on the left or right half of the monitor, the subject was able to move a cursor into the target by "thoughts" alone. In two other subjects the classification performance obtained after 4 and 6 sessions, respectively, was close to 70%.

Table 1: Results of four on-line cursor control sessions in one subject.

|  | No. of left movements | No. of right movements | Overall performance |
|---|---|---|---|
| 1st on-line session | 18 out of 40 | 40 out of 43 | 70% |
| 2nd on-line session | 48 out of 53 | 36 out of 61 | 73% |
| 3rd on-line session | 68 out of 74 | 30 out of 40 | 86% |
| 4th on-line session | 31 out of 35 | 36 out of 43 | 86% |

## 5. Conclusion

It was shown that it is possible to create an EEG-based BCI which can be trained by preclassified spatiotemporal EEG patterns. The Graz BCI 1 is only a first minor step but shows, after the pioneer work of Wolpaw et al. [6], that a BCI can be realized within a few days when artificial neural networks are used. Next important steps are the increase of dimensionality and the performance of the BCI. For this it is important to use EEG signals from multiple electrodes whereby the following parameters have to be optimized: location and number of electrodes, location and size of the time window used for classification, type and number of EEG parameters, type and parameters of the classifier, and the experimental paradigms for the learning and the working phase. For selecting the proper electrode locations, experiments with a great number of electrodes have to be performed. Concerning EEG parameters, the best filter range in the alpha and/or beta range has to be specified.

## References

[1] D. Flotzinger, Neural Network-based classification of spatiotemporal EEG-data, MSc Thesis, Graz University of Technology, Austria, 1991.
[2] D. Flotzinger, J. Kalcher, and G. Pfurtscheller, EEG Classification by Learning Vector Quantization, *Biomed. Technik*, 37: 303-309, 1992.
[3] T. Kohonen, *Self-organization and associative memory*, 3rd ed., Springer, Berlin 1988.
[4] G. Pfurtscheller and A. Aranibar, Evaluation of event-related desynchronization (ERD) preceding and following voluntary self-paced movement, *Electroenceph. clin. Neurophysiol.*, 46:138-146, 1979.
[5] G. Pfurtscheller and A. Berghold, Patterns of cortical activation during planning of voluntary movement, *Electroenceph. clin. Neurophysiol.*, 72:250-258, 1989.
[6] J.R. Wolpaw, D. McFarland, G.W. Neat, and C.A. Forneris, An EEG-based brain-computer interface for cursor control, *Electroenceph. clin. Neurophysiol.*, 78:252-259, 1991.
[7] G. Pfurtscheller, D. Flotzinger, and J. Kalcher, Brain-Compter Interface - a new communication device for handicapped persons, Computers for Handicapped Persons, Zagler W. (Eds.), R. Oldenbourg Wien München, 409-415, 1992.
[8] G. Pfurtscheller, D. Flotzinger, W. Mohl, and M. Peltoranta, Prediction of the side of hand movements from single-trial multi-channel EEG data using neural networks, *Electroenceph. clin. Neurophysiol.*, 82:313-315, 1992.

# Speech Analytic Hearing Aids for the Profoundly Deaf: STRIDE[12]

*A. Fourcin*

**Abstract**

This project is concerned with the structured development of a new approach to the design and prescription of hearing aids within the European Community. These new instruments for hearing are based on the use of speech pattern-seeking algorithms which extract specially important speech components from the complete speech signal and which can operate in normal conditions of noise and reverberation. Field trials using wearable aids produced for the project are in progress in the Dutch, English, French and Swedish languages. Deafness is perhaps the most widespread single disability in Europe; it affects about 5% of the population. For the majority of these handicapped people, conventional amplifying hearing aids are of great value and are adequate to ensure integration within normal family and working life. However, some 160,000 adults within the Community as a whole are so profoundly hearing impaired that they are not able to make adequate use of amplifying aids. Here, the use of lip-reading presents the only real basis for interaction with the normally communicating world. The use of a structured approach to the implementation of the new speech pattern element aids makes it feasible to address the needs of these people by the clear auditory provision of those components of speech which are most needed to complement the visual information available from lip-reading. In our work, each patient is provided with a wearable speech pattern processing hearing aid which gives an output matched to the individual's hearing characteristics. Controlled assessments of the value of the approach compared with the use of conventional aids are based on the use of carefully designed, common standard, fitting, training and evaluation procedures in each of the four present language environments. This concerted activity can be briefly summarised:

- a basic set of speech pattern element priorities in the auditory supplementation of lipreading has been defined. Robust means of analysis have been developed and applied to the provision of these speech pattern elements; voice pitch/larynx frequency; loudness/intensity of the speech signal; frication/aperiodicity. The first work has been directed towards English but the special requirements of Dutch, French and Swedish can be catered for.
- a specially designed signal processing wearable hearing aid has been developed and made in first prototype quantities for the present four-country trials
- comprehensive common psycho-acoustic and speech assessment tools have been defined; standard cross comparable phonetic structures and evaluation and training methods are in use for all four languages

## 1 Project objectives

The STRIDE project has been designed to provide crucial rehabilitation assistance to an important group of "difficult-to-help people" who do not get sufficient help in lipreading from even the best conventional prostheses. We now have the possibility of providing a highly cost effective solution to many of the problems of this group, by the design and initial prototype development of a new speech technology-based pattern element-processing hearing aid - **SiVo**. Our work is supported by the parallel development of standard speech-based assessment and training in the different languages of the project as well as by the use of common psychoacoustic methods of evaluation.

Within Europe at least 5% of the population are handicapped to a greater or lesser degree, by hearing impairment, and for those over 60 years of age, this proportion rises to 30% [1]. Although persons with a moderate hearing loss derive very significant benefit from current hearing aids, this is not the case for the profound loss population [2]. Those who suffer profound hearing impairment - of the type associated with a four frequency (0.5, 1, 2 and 4 kHz) average loss of 107 dB HL or more - are unable to gain adequate benefit in speech communication from conventional hearing aids even in the support of lipreading. This group represents about 0.05% of the population, an approximate total of 160,000 adults within the Community as a whole. A rather larger sector, about 2% of the population, that is, about 8 M in Europe, have average hearing losses of 90 dB or more [2], and are generally unable to gain useful speech information from hearing aids without the assistance of lipreading [3]. Hearing impairments, including profound losses, are particularly prevalent in the elderly [4], and, given expected demographic changes, more and more people are likely to suffer from this handicap. Most hearing impairments are of sensorineural origin, and they are not amenable to medical or surgical cure, nor is there any indication that such intervention is possible in the foreseeable future. Management of the impairment is therefore confined to rehabilitation, predominantly by hearing aids and other technical devices.

The essential contribution of our work has been both to provide speech analysis within the aid itself and to match its output to the residual hearing ability of the listener so as to ease the task of the impaired ear. Although some consider that the most effective potential source of help for these profoundly deaf people comes from the provision of electro-cochlear implants, this is often inappropriate when factors of patient choice, cost, and likely damage to residual auditory function are considered. In patients with residual hearing, for whom both an implant and the SiVo might be considered, SiVo has an approximate ten-to-one cost advantage, and it may be more acceptable to many since it involves no surgical intervention, and unlike an implant, cannot damage residual hearing. Although our first research and development activity has been concerned with the provision of a lipreading aid, the work as a whole is designed to provide a longer term contribution to the more widespread improvement of hearing aid design and construction with the aim of enhancing speech contrastive clarity so as to permit, for some users, improved speech comprehension without the assistance of lipreading.

## 2 Speech pattern element hearing aids

Work carried out over the last 15 years has produced an initial definition of the potential of speech pattern element hearing aids [5,6], and has led to the practical realization of the SiVo aid [7]; the first acoustic speech pattern element hearing aid. The SiVo aid provides voice fundamental frequency information as a frequency-controlled sinusoid, and has proved to be an effective lipreading aid in a number of profoundly hearing impaired subjects who were quite unable to use amplifying hearing aids [7,8]. The potency of voice fundamental frequency information in aiding lipreading arises because it conveys important speech contrasts based on voicing and intonation, both of which are invisible to the lipreader.

### 2.1 Receptive abilities of the profoundly hearing impaired

The success of the simplification used in the SiVo aid is due to the very limited auditory processing capacity of the profoundly hearing impaired. One major limitation is that auditory frequency analysis, which is so important in speech perception [9], is either absent, or very markedly impaired in this population [10]. Other major limitations arise from the severe restriction of the auditory receptive range [11]; the frequency range is often no more than 1 kHz, and the intensity range between threshold and discomfort is often less than 10 dB above 500 Hz. Despite these gross impairments, these people can usually perform auditory discriminations on the basis of temporal factors such as gross amplitude, the contrast between periodic and aperiodic stimulation, and changes in frequency of periodic stimulation [11]. Furthermore, even the limited frequency resolution seen in many listeners has a potential for the encoding of simple aspects of the speech spectrum [10, 12].

### 2.2 Optimal selection of speech pattern elements to aid lipreading

Those aspects of speech which are largely invisible to the lipreader, yet which bear a substantial communicative load, include voicing, intonation, manner of articulation and some aspects of vowel quality [13, 14]. Given a limited auditory receptive capacity, an aid designed to supplement lipreading should, therefore, provide speech pattern elements related to these factors. The relative priorities of these factors may differ between languages but is likely that in the European languages, the ordering above is appropriate [14].

*Signal Processing*

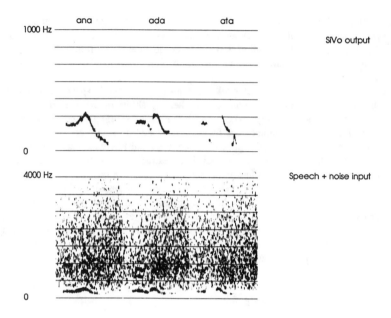

Fig 1. Spectrographs of speech+noise input and SiVo aid output. The voicing pattern is clearly preserved in the output and contrasts the voiceless [t] from the voiced [d] and [n], and also the distinguishes the nasal [n] from the plosive [d]

## 2.3 Matching speech information to the profoundly hearing impaired

The residual abilities of the profoundly hearing impaired offer significant scope for the encoding of important speech pattern contrasts, provided that information can be matched to the hearing impaired person's receptive abilities and communicative needs. Provided that the acoustic patterns used to encode speech contrasts preserve basic auditory relationships with the patterns of speech itself, matching can make use of the cognitive process of normalization. For example, the SiVo aid allows fundamental frequency information to be matched to the patient's regions of better hearing through transformations known as MAPITCH [15], whereby the fundamental frequency pattern is lowered so that the high-pitched voice of a child or woman is brought into a frequency region where the auditory resolution of frequency change is relatively superior, and at the same time, the range of fundamental frequency variation is expanded to compensate for the impaired resolution of frequency change. Similarly, the high-frequency aperiodic content of voiceless speech sounds can be mapped on to the hearing impaired person's auditory area by the use of a lower frequency noise [8]. Additionally, amplitude patterning based upon both low and high frequency speech components can be presented as an amplitude modulation of the fundamental frequency and voiceless pattern elements. By a combination of mappings in frequency and intensity, important speech components can be made comfortably audible in ways impossible to achieve with amplifying aids. The SiVo family of hearing aids incorporates provision for the assessment of the individual listener's hearing ability by means of the aid itself. In this way both comfortable sound levels and mapping adjustments can be made with exact self-calibration, and free from errors which could arise from the use of different acoustic transducers in assessment.

## 3 Benefits to users

The clarifying potential of the SiVo approach is illustrated in fig 1, which shows the output of the aid with an input of speech in speech-spectrum shaped noise at a 10 dB speech-to-noise ratio. At these noise levels, which are common in everyday life, the profoundly hearing impaired have considerable difficulty in extracting useful speech information with amplifying hearing aids [16]. However, the SiVo aid extracts very effectively the voicing pattern information required to distinguish the sounds shown here, which look very similar to the lipreader. With only modest amounts of training, profoundly hearing impaired users can become well able to make use of this simplified acoustic information, and we are beginning to see corresponding benefit in their overall ability to receive speech information. Examples of user results are shown in fig 2; here the advantages seen for the SiVo approach are based on speech in quiet; in noise, even greater advantage is likely.

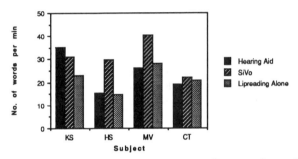

Fig 2. Performance of four users in a connected discourse tracking task. Better speech reception is found with the SiVo aid than with a conventional aid in the three users who show lower levels of residual hearing.

## 4 Achievements of Project

- The SiVo aid has been produced as a wearable programmable device using state of the art codec and microprocessor chips. We now have the basis for solving the practical problems associated with the auditory matching of the output of speech technology-based processing to the needs of this important deaf population.
- Neural net algorithms for the robust extraction of essential speech features have been developed [17, 18]. The development of this type of speech processing will continue, and will be compared with other speech technology-based approaches, in systematic work with patients, in order to ensure that the most efficient algorithms are available.
- Common cross-comparable assessment and training methods are being achieved by the use of standard procedures and protocols, and common clinical facilities. The resulting EURAUD (EURopean AUDiological) workstation will be made commercially available in complement with the PCLX speech training and assessment system.
- Other rehabilitation "spin-offs" are potentially possible - the SiVo aid can, additionally, be programmed flexibly to operate not only as an acoustic but also as tactile and as electro-cochlear prostheses - and these extensions will be actively pursued.
- The project brings together a substantial concentration of European research expertise. The results will be of interest to other European workers and should lead to applications for other non-European language communities. The fundamental developments have broad implications in many speech and hearing related areas and will not be without value for the education and management of the hearing impaired child.

• Much larger markets can be served on the basis of the work - for example Chinese profoundly deaf tone language speakers can benefit from the basic SiVo. The addition of further speech elements can lead in the longer term to important new prostheses for another group, those with severe-to-profound hearing losses for whom conventional aids allow only minimal speech reception in the absence of lipreading.

## 5 References

1. Martin MC (1990) "Amplification for hearing-impaired people" Proceedings of 2nd European Conference on policy related to Telematics and Disability, COST 219, pp 110-117.
2. Thornton A. R. D. (1986), "Estimation of the number of patients who might be suitable for cochlear implant and similar procedures", Br. J. Audiol. **20**, 221-230.
3. Boothroyd A (1990) "Signal processing for the profoundly deaf" Acta Otolaryngol. (Stockh.), **Suppl. 469**, 166-171
4. McEwan J (1990) "RACE Projects: TUDOR and APPSN" Proceedings of 2nd European Conference on policy related to Telematics and Disability, COST 219, pp 41-51.
5. Fourcin, A. J. (1977). "English speech patterns with special reference to artificial auditory stimulation," in *A review of artificial auditory stimulation: Medical Research Council Working Group Report*, edited by A. R. D. Thornton (Inst. Sound and Vib. Res., University of Southampton), pp. 42-44.
6. Fourcin A. J., Rosen S. M., Moore B. C. J. et al., (1979), "External electrical stimulation of the cochlea: Clinical, psychophysical, speech-perceptual and histological findings", Br. J. Audiol. **13**, 85-107.
7. Rosen, S., Walliker, J. R., Fourcin, A. J., and Ball, V. (1987) "A microprocessor-based acoustic hearing aid for the profoundly impaired listener". J Rehab Res Devt, **24**, 239-260.
8. Faulkner, A., Ball, V., Rosen, S. R., Moore, B. C. J., and Fourcin A. J. (1992) "Speech pattern hearing aids for the profoundly hearing-impaired: Speech perception and auditory abilities". Journal of the Acoustical Society of America, 91, 2136-2155.
9. Rosen S. and Fourcin A. J. (1986) "Frequency selectivity and the perception of speech", in Frequency Selectivity in Hearing, edited by B. C. J. Moore (Academic Press, London), pp 373-487.
10. Faulkner, A., Rosen, S., and Moore, B. C. J. (1990). "Residual frequency selectivity in the profoundly hearing-impaired listener," Br. J. Audiol. **24**, 381-392.
11. Rosen S, Faulkner A, and Smith DAJ (1990) "The psychoacoustics of profound hearing impairment" Acta Oto-laryngologica (Stockh), **Suppl. 469**, pp 16-22.
12. van Son, N., Bosman, A. J., Lamoré, P. J. J., and Smoorenburg, G. F. (1991) "Auditory pattern perception in the profoundly hearing impaired and speech reading" Proc 2nd Int Workshop on Hearing Impairment and Signal-Processing Hearing Aids, London, 1991.
13. Summerfield, Q (1985) "Speech-processing alternatives for electrical auditory stimulation" In Cochlear Implants, RA Schindler and MM Merzenich (Eds), Raven Press, New York, pp 195-222.
14. Fourcin, A. J. (1990) "Prospects for speech pattern element aids". Acta Oto-laryngologica (Stockh), **Suppl. 469**, pp 257-267.
15. Fourcin A. J., Douek E. E., Moore B. C. J., et al. (1984), "Speech pattern element stimulation in electrical hearing", Arch. Otolaryngol. **110**, 145-153.
16. Faulkner A., Vickers, D. A., and Fourcin A. J. (1992) "The STRIDE project: Background to the project and first patient results from a prototype multi-layer perceptron based speech pattern extracting hearing aid" Proceedings 2nd International Conference on Tactile Aids, Hearing Aids, and Cochlear Implants. KTH, Stockholm, in press.
17. Howard, I. (1991) *Speech fundamental period estimation using pattern classification*, Ph.D thesis, Dept. of Phonetics & Linguistics, University College London.
18. Walliker JR and Howard I (1990) "Real-time portable multi-layer perceptron voice fundamental-period extractor for hearing aids and cochlear implants". Speech Communication, **9**, pp 63-71.

1. The STRIDE consortium comprises: Department of Phonetics and Linguistics, University College London, and Laryngograph Ltd, UK; Oticon AS, Denmark; CCA Wagram, Paris, France; CNRS Parole et Langage, Aix-en-Provence, France; Department of Experimental Audiology, University Hospital Utrecht, Netherlands; Instituut voor Doven, St Michielsgestel, Netherlands; Department of Speech Communication and Music Acoustics, KTH, Stockholm, Sweden.

2. Contact address: Professor AJ Fourcin, Department of Phonetics and Linguistics, University College London, Wolfson House, 4 Stephenson Way, LONDON NW1 2HE, UK.

# Session 2:

## Market and Service Delivery

# Copyright problems for rehabilitation: new technological solutions

Graham P Cornish
Copyright Officer
British Library, Boston Spa, Wetherby, West Yorkshire, LS23 7BQ, UK

**Abstract:** A crucial element in any programme of rehabilitation is access to published material in a form appropriate to the needs of the user. Transcription of print into audio, braille or computer formats cannot be done without the permission of the copyright owner. Seeking permission is administratively expensive and can lead to refusals or just silence, leading to frustration.

The increasing use of digital technology for the production of text, visual images and sound has enabled the development of the CITED (Copyright in Transmitted Electronic Documents) generic model which allows access to digital materials whilst enabling the copyright owner to monitor use, control distribution and receive royalties if necessary. The project is a joint venture between manufacturers, publishers and libraries and is funded by the EC ESPRIT Programme.

## 1. Introduction

One of the most important challenges facing a person with any kind of print-handicap is the fact that the majority of the world's intellectual output is in the form of print on paper. This is true whether the need is for high-level academic research material, recreational reading, current news or the routines of daily life. Although some publishers, information providers and manufacturers are now aware of this problem, economics often prevent the necessary action being taken in all areas.

## 2. Copyright

Most of the textual information that is required for any aspect of life is, in fact, the intellectual property of someone else, either the author or the publisher. This aspect of intellectual property, called copyright, enables the owner to exercise exclusive rights over the copying, publication, disruption or performance of the work. As this right lasts for at least 50 years after the author dies, and in some countries, longer, very little published information can be used by other people without the owner's consent.

The need that the print-handicapped have to change works from print to other appropriate formats necessarily involves copying the work and often distributing it in the new format. But these are rights exercised exclusively by the owners and these actions cannot be undertaken without permission. Obtaining permission is often administratively slow and expensive and there are no guarantees that permission will be granted. Few countries have any legislation which permits transferring material from one format to another and those which do often limit this to making sound recordings of published books.

## 3. The digital environment

The widespread use of electronic technology to produce, store, manipulate and distribute information of all kinds is one of the great achievements of the information explosion. The arrival of digital technologies for text, sound and visual images has made the possibilities almost limitless. Not only can material be manipulated within its own form but multimedia packages can be created, information from different sources downloaded, copied, edited and repackaged to suit the user or generate completely new products which can be made available on the open information market.

It is already obvious that some information providers are reluctant to make their products available in digital form simply because of the threat that copyright infringement poses. But history shows that new technical developments are never prevented by such problems. In the end the question surrounding copyright materials is not so much "How shall we prevent access and use?" as "How shall we monitor access and use?" The real issue is to link monitoring, control and compensation. The ideal is a system which can undertake several different tasks, preferably all at the same time. The first task is to monitor use. Creators and owners are unwilling to lose control over how their intellectual property is used, regardless of the economics of that use. Not everyone wants their music used to promote motor cars or their writings used in political campaigns! In addition, the way in which intellectual property is used, in terms of quality, quantity and purpose is valuable marketing information for any publisher. So there is also a need to be able to limit the use to which material is put. It may be acceptable to allow the making of paper copies but not download electronic versions of a text or playing of a sound recording may be allowed but not copying of it. In addition there may be a requirement to allow different uses to different people. For example, access to a whole database may be allowed to a senior professor but only a small part may be available to a student. Similarly, copying the whole of a work may be prohibited generally but allowed for some groups such as the print-handicapped. Or changing format might be allowed for one group but not for another. Having managed to negotiate who uses what, and how, there is still a need to provide a mechanism to pay the owner for the use of the copyright material. Again, payment levels may vary according to use. It is to be hoped that an industrial company using material in digital format for carrying out research into a high-revenue process would pay more to use the materials than someone who needed to convert the material into an appropriate format because of a handicap.

Ideally all these different tasks could be carried out by one system. Such a system may sound more like a dream than a reality but it has been said that "when one man dreams, it is a dream; when several men dream the same thing it is the beginning of a reality."

Of course, not all the materials we need to use are in digital formats. Although digital technology is used increasingly for typesetting and printing the digital formats for many documents remains exclusively in the hands of the printer or publisher and is not publicly accessible. Where it is used to generate publicly-available databases this is certainly a major plus. Similarly, many publications are still produced by non-digital means so there is a vast corpus of material in printed form to which access is denied to the print-handicapped. However, with the introduction of various character recognition systems using digital signals it will at least be possible to negotiate that transferring printed material to electronic digital formats with publishers using appropriate protection mechanisms. It is these mechanisms with which the CITED Project is concerned.

## 4. The CITED solution

It was said earlier that any system which could carry out all the functions needed by both users and owners was nothing but a dream. Fortunately several men and women had the same dream and joined together to form a consortium which they called CITED (Copyright in Transmitted Electronic Documents). The group made a bid under the 6th Call for ESPRIT II under a Workpackage entitled "Electronic Copyright" which was accepted. The partners in the project are from France, Netherlands, Germany, Spain, United Kingdom and Belgium and include electronic publishers, a computer manufacturer, a library, a barrister, security and software specialists and experts in databases and networking. In addition to the obvious skills partners also bring considerable experience of the sound recording industry through both the Computer Industry Research Unit and the British Library National Sound Archive.

The basic philosophy of the CITED project is that, when we are dealing with information that is stored and, more particularly, processed digitally, it is therefore possible, in the digital environment, to control the processes which are an inevitable part of digital technology and, in consequence, control the copying of copyright material. In the present context it is immaterial what information is represented by the digital signal in any given case; what is now possible is the development of a generic model of copyright protection of digital information (the CITED model) together with corresponding guidelines and toolkit to enable the model to be implemented in specified domains. The generic nature of the CITED model means that it can be relatively easily applied in any legal background, both now and in the future regardless of technological developments. It is also capable of acting as a standard against which to test systems developed by other information providers in the information industry. CITED compliance with the model can be established to a range of standards, and via a number of different technical strategies. The level of protection can be defined, depending on the nature of the information to be protected, and the rights of various CITED users can be specified. These rights will be specified according to the user, but the effective right to gain access to a particular piece of information will, in practice, depend on the protection level of that information. The CITED model is primarily concerned with the relationship between "events" (ie those actions which users may wish to undertake) and "rights" (ie those legal rights which owners, distributors and end-users enjoy, either through legislation or by contract. The CITED model is concerned to record the actions undertaken by users and the response to these actions will depend on the rights which users of the appropriate information have acquired by legislation, purchase or agreement. Although the primary method of acquiring rights is to purchase these, there is no reason why a CITED facility should not permit free access if the owner so wishes or legislation requires. What CITED would permit is the monitoring of the free use which would in itself be a valuable piece of data. Naturally a critical area is the detection of actions which are not permitted, either generally or to a particular user. Of course, CITED can be used as a countermeasure to such threats but it can also be used as a marketing tool. Attempts at unauthorised use may bring not just a negative response but information as to how the event which has been refused could be executed. The CITED environment is therefore dynamic and can respond to a range of possibilities.

Naturally some of the technical tools used in the CITED project are adopted from the repertoire developed for the security industry. However, within the CITED project these are viewed as placing a protective guard around the copyright information in a manner which, while preventing unauthorised copying, never the less permits convenient access for authorised use. In fact CITED is a sort of tool kit which provides a variety of implements which may be needed in some, but not all, environments.

## 5. The needs of the print-handicapped

It hardly needs saying that the needs of the print-handicapped are many and various. Even so, it can reasonably be said that the alternatives to standard methods of publishing are enlarged print, braille (or Moon), audio and tactile computer displays with the occasional need for electronic text for those with physical, but not visual, impairments.

Once material is in digital format nearly all of these can be achieved easily. Where a publisher produces material in digital format initially there should, in theory, be no serious problem. However, the market for special format materials is small compared to the standard methods of production so there may be little incentive to generate output in different formats. However, if the electronic format of a publication can be made available publicly and the output determined by the final user, either directly or through an appropriate organisation, this could change publishers' attitudes. Their fear in this situation is that the electronic format will be abused by unauthorised copying, downloading and distribution. The CITED Model offers a way of ensuring this does not take place and could unlock many electronically stored texts for wider use among communities to whom they are denied at present.

Where material is not available in digital form the CITED Model still has an important role to play. Printed material can still be converted to digital format with the consent of the copyright owner and an agreement to protect the digital text which results from this using a CITED Model. There is, of necessity, an element of trust between the owner and the user in this situation as the owner would have to rely on the honesty of the person permitted to make the electronic copy to ensure that protection was built into the system. But the exploitation of all intellectual property relies, in part at least, on the concept of trust. When a publisher sells a book or journal, a record company distributes a disc or a computer firm sells some software there is always the chance that it will be copied either once or even many times for commercial gain. The law can prohibit such acts but only a combination of technology and trust can prohibit them.

Some would argue that such copying should be permitted under the law or that publishers should not be permitted to prohibit such copying as it meets the needs of a group of disadvantaged persons. It is often argued that those with print-handicaps would not buy printed materials so there is no loss to the publisher if a sound recording or braille version is made. This argument has always had one serious fault and the coming of the digital age has now given it a second one. Firstly, just because people have a handicap it does not mean that they wish to be given exceptional privileges. They should, and do, expect to be treated in the same way as everyone else. This should mean that access to information (in its widest) sense should cost the print-handicapped person the same as other people but no more. The second argument, that the publisher is not losing anything is confounded by digital technology because this enables a publisher to obtain some payment for use of copyright material by any person, regardless of the precise use to which it is put. Thus it is quite possible for a publisher, who cannot generate braille or sound recordings of work, to permit this to be done under controlled conditions by others licensed to do so and in return for appropriate payment. Therefore the argument of no lost revenue now falls down, probably to the benefit of the print-handicapped community as they will gain wider access to materials in the future.

## 6. The future

On the basis of their wide experience across a whole range of the information industry, the partners of the CITED project have been able to design a coherent model for the protection of all kinds of copyright information in digital form. They have shown how the model can form a consistent basis for a repertoire of technological guidelines and tools for the protection of copyright in digital materials in various fields in the information industry. Two demonstrators and test scenarios have been developed and are being used to validate the model and to develop the guidelines and tools by which the problem of copyright protection in this area can be mastered.

The CITED Consortium is also addressing the question of legal and technical standards in relation to the CITED approach. These concern the relationship of the CITED model to the legal framework, particularly as it is developing as a result of EC Directives on such matters as computer software, database protection, reprography and even data protection and personal privacy. The lack of any Directive in the pipeline making provision for the needs of the print-handicapped is a major source of regret but the CITED model could play an important role in developing such legislation if there were the political will to do so. Attention is particularly directed to the international developments which WIPO (the World Intellectual Property Organisation) are sponsoring. At a technical level, the question of standardisation of CITED rights, the monitoring of acts of copying and recording of the rights which are either owned or have been acquired is still being addressed. Eventually it is possible to envisage a Pan-European CITED clearance centre to provide the necessary infrastructure for a comprehensive system of copyright protection.

Implementing new information technology

A review of problems and possibilities
*H. Michels*

The Centre for Talking Magazines in Holland is one of five
libraries for the blind and partially sighted in our country. We
are specialized in producing talking magazines. At this moment we
publish over 275 magazines on audio-cassettes, covering such
areas as national and local newspapers, weekly magazines, professional and scientific journals and all sorts of special interest
magazines. It is our goal to give blind and partially sighted
people access to as wide a variety of newspapers and magazines as
possible. We try to accomplish this goal by using technology as a
means to our end. The adoption of audio-tape and later on the
technology of compact cassette production, made it possible to
produce talking magazines for the visually handicapped. The
recent developments in computer-technology have given us the
opportunity to advance in our efforts to give visually handicapped people a more equal opportunity to participate in the process
of information-gathering. I would like to tell you about the
possibilities and problems one encounters when trying to introduce a new technology in such a field as the library-services for
blind or partially sighted people.

Innovation is an expression often used as some kind of magic
trick that will take care of all your problems. Our civilisation
is build on the idea of constant technological development
leading towards a situation in which several problems of today
will be solved thanks to new technology. In the field of service
for the handicapped you will encounter this kind of thinking over
and over again. We often look upon a physical handicap as something that has to be "corrected" by some artificial device that
will take over the functions of that part of the body that does
not do what it is supposed to do. This kind of thinking has lead
us to amazing results. People have regained the possibility to
walk because of new prosthesises. Technical aides enable people
with hearing problems to at least hear something. All these
technical inventions have certainly improved the quality of life
of handicapped people. Innovations of information technology have
similar effect on the possibilities of blind people to read. To
invest in the development of these new technologies is therefore
an important aspect of trying to improve the living-conditions of
people with disabilities.

One of the most recent developments in the field of visually
handicapped is the appearance of electronic newspapers. As a
result of innovations in more than one area, it is today possible
to give blind or partially sighted people access to daily newspapers. In Holland we have started a newspaper-project with the
daily national newspaper Trouw. Over a period of two years, fifty
blind or partially sighted people have read the newspaper via
their personal computer with braille- or speech-output. The

newspaper was delivered every day by means of radio-transmission.
The radio-signal consisted of digitalized information, allowing
us to distribute the entire newspaper within 10 minutes. The
technology used in our project was developed in Sweden by Textalk
AB. In 1985 the first experiments with an electronic daily
newspaper for the visually handicapped started in Gothenburg,
Sweden. The cooperation with Textalk has developed over the years
and at this moment we are investigating ways of improving electronic publishing for the visually handicapped. Textalk has a.o.
participated in the CAPS-project, funded by TIDE.

During our project the focus was not so much on the technological
development. We knew from the experience of our Swedish partners
that the technology worked, although improvements are always
possible and desirable. The main focus of our project however was
to discover the ways in which the electronic newspaper could be
introduced in our country so that in the near future a reasonable
amount of people with a visual handicap could profit from it. In
doing so we discovered that the problems of introducing a new
technology had not so much to do with the technology as such, but
more with the social structure in which services for the handicapped are rooted. In brief, three different levels can be
distinguished:

* First level: the development and improvement of technology for
people with handicaps;
* Second level: the implementation of the technology in practical
service;
* Third level: the acceptance of the technology as a means to an
end by the community of handicapped people.

With regard to all these fields one can localize several problems, concerning:

1. Who is responsible for doing the job?
2. Who is going to determine what has to be done?
3. Who is going to pay for it?

I will consider these problems one by one for every level.

**The first level: developing and improving technology**

The development of new technology often takes place at universities or research-laboratories. Since the handicapped community is
not a rich one, universities are a very important source for new
developments. In several fields of science there are interesting
possibilities. We should some how focus on these possibilities
and try to put them into use for the people with a handicap.
Since the handicapped community is not an interesting commercial
market, I don't think that commercial research-laboratories will
be very interested in doing some work in this area.
So our first problem seems to be solved: universities should be
doing research and development on several handicaps. The Massachusetts Institute of Technology in the USA and the Institute of

Perception Research in Holland are examples of university-insti-
tutions involved in r & d for the handicapped. The technology of
the electronic newspaper was originally developed at Chalmers
University of Technology in Gothenburg, Sweden.
Now let's look at our second problem, being the problem of who
decides what is to be done. Here we encounter something that is a
common problem in all innovations. On the one hand the inventor
makes a new technological device, which he thinks is an answer to
a real life problem. On the other hand the people who are to use
it think that the new device is an answer to all or a great deal
of their problem. They will both be disappointed: if they are
lucky the new technology will solve some problems somehow,
without being perfect. So cooperation between universities and
users should be integrated within project concerning new technology. For the field of handicapped people this is even more
important since the market-powers are not strong enough to play
the role of correction, like they do in for instance the personal
computer market. With regard to the electronic newspaper it is
equally important to have users stating what they would like to
have, as to have engineers and other experts explaining about the
limits of the present technology.
The third problem is perhaps the easiest one to answer and at the
same time the most difficult one to really solve. Of course
someone should pay the costs of development. There are a number
of possibilities here:

1. The university itself;
2. The consumers;
3. The industry;
4. The government or other funding agencies.

If we look at the financial situation of the first two parties,
we can state very clearly that none of those two has sufficient
funds to pay for expansive r & d work themselves. The third
party, the industry, will only be interested if the costs of r &
d can be gained back once the final product is on the market.
Since the market of handicapped people is both small and not very
affluent, the possibilities of the industry paying for r & d in
this field are not very large. So there only is one possible
party left: government or non-governmental agencies must be the
main parties involved in funding these kind of activities. The
reason for it is simple: new technologies can improve the quality
of life of handicapped people and nobody else will take care of
it.

## Second level: implementation

Once a new kind of technology is developed in a laboratory of
some kind, it needs to be tested in practice. Testing things in
the real life means that you try to establish a situation that
resembles reality as much as possible. In our country, it is a
century-old tradition, that independent libraries for the blind
are responsible for producing and distributing books, magazines
and newspaper in braille or on cassette. A new technology like an

electronic newspaper should be integrated within this structure, that is to say: The use of the technology as a means of giving blind and partially sighted people access to a newspaper should emphasise the involvement of publishers or libraries to really achieve the goals. In our country we have independent libraries for the blind, in other countries the publishers perhaps take care of it themselves, or libraries for the blind are directly linked with a pressure group of some sort. Whatever the structure may be, the most important thing is that someone is responsible for publishing and distributing newspapers in a format that they are readable for visually handicapped people. So the second level should be run not by the university group, although they must by involved with the project, but by some other organization responsible for the publishing of adapted newspapers.

Of course, like on the first level, it is important to involve users and r & d people in the project, so as to be sure that criticism towards the technology, can be integrated within the system. So, the parties involved in the testing of the technology in practice are:

- the r & d institute (university)
- users
- the organization responsible for using the technology in practice.

The third problem, that of who is going to pay, has a similar outlook as the same problem on the first level. If for instance a library for the blind has been made responsible for conducting a test with electronic newspapers, the funding can come from several sources:

1. The library itself;
2. The users;
3. The newspapers involved;
4. Government or non-governmental agencies.

The libraries for the blind are in most cases non-profit organisations with insufficient funds for conducting large scale experiments with new technology. They will have to receive some funding from elsewhere. As with the r & d activities, users will not be affluent enough to pay for it themselves and newspaper-publisher will not invest large amounts of money in these kind of activities. So again, financial support from governmental or non-governmental agencies is essential for experiments in the field of technological innovations for blind and partially sighted people.

### Third level: large scale adoption

Once the technology has proven itself in reality, it needs to be produced, distributed and used on a regular basis. Producing and using special technology for handicapped people involves several parties:

1. Organizations or companies who produce hard- and software;
2. Organizations responsible for exploiting services connected to the technology itself.

In the case of an electronic newspaper you need someone to produce the hard- and software required for receiving and reading a newspaper via a personal computer. Also you need someone who is responsible for producing and distributing the newspapers in the electronic format. Both parties should cooperate closely and there should be a constant review of user-demands by for instant market-surveys. In our country the Centre for Talking Magazines is responsible for producing and distributing the electronic newspaper and a commercial company produces the necessary hard- and software. The project has a European dimension, since the development and production of the software and hardware, needed for electronic reading of the newspaper is being done in Sweden. Since the main focus of activity on this level is to introduce a new service to the market, the main parties involved are the producer and consumer. It is the consumer who has to use the technology. Organizations of visually impaired people should therefore form themselves some opinion on such issues as:

- prizes;
- facilities needed;
- support needs.

They should express their ideas in such a way that the producer can integrate them in the constant improvement of the product. On the other side, the producer has to take into consideration other factors that will influence the product or service. These factors are:

- amount of money available for development and services like user-support;
- technological limitations;
- cooperation with publishers, etc.
- organizational limitations.

Once a service is established, maintaining it demands constant contact between producers and consumers. On both sides there should be a commitment to listen to each other and accept the wishes and limits of the other party.
Since the market for services for blind and partially sighted people is a limited one both in size and wealth, it will be necessary to have some support by the government. This support could be aimed at supplying consumers with computers and other hard- and software they need for reading a newspaper. After this the consumers should pay subscription fees like everyone else does.

The case of the electronic newspaper project in the Netherlands clearly shows that new developments can be introduced to people with disabilities. On all levels there should be a clear sense of the goals of the activities undertaken as well as a possibility to have government-commitment for subsidizing the costs of the extra work needed. The overall goal must be to give people with disabilities the possibility to partake in society on a more equal basis.

Drs. Harry Michels
Head of Marketing Department
Centre for Talking Magazines
P.O. Box 24
NL-5360 AA GRAVE
The Netherlands
Tel: + 31 88 60 71 234
Fax: + 31 88 60 76 535

# Different aspects of the provision of information regarding Rehabilitation Technology.

by Harry Knops O.T., and Theo Bougie M.Sc.M.E.,
Rehabilitation Information Centre 'Hoensbroeck'
the Netherlands.

**Abstract.**

This paper gives an introduction on different aspects of the provision of information in the RT market.

After an introduction about the complexity of the RT market, four levels of information provision are presented. These four levels are the basis for the work of the Rehabilitation Information Centre- 'Hoensbroeck´(RIC).

After these introductions the Information Service is presented with data collection, information provision and courses as main activities.

The paper indicates that information provision concerning the RT market is very complex. That it needs a good organisation based on national requirements is demonstrated with the Dutch experience.

## 1.    Introduction on the RT Market

* In comparison to other technology markets Rehabilitation Technology is executed and organised on a small scale. Problems to be solved occur everywhere but on a low frequency. All the actors involved can learn from the experience elsewhere. The establishment of one economic European market is a meaningful factor, however some extra attention should be paid to stimulate the exchange of experiences considering the special RT market and its organisation.

* An other remarkable point is that the core disciplines in rehabilitation have a little technological background and are not always aware of the existing possibilities and of what new is on the market. Also new technologies are not very well known by the actors and this is due to a lack in the technology transfer process from and to the actors in the Rehabilitation technology market.

* The provision of technology to individuals is influenced by arrangements regarding health and social security systems. The executing organisations of the provision system, do not only decide that technology is necessary, but also which type of device is provided.

For all the actors in the RT market it is of major importance that there is an intensive exchange of information between all the actors involved.

## 2.    Information about Rehabilitation Technology.

People use information to decrease their uncertainness in decision making. That is also the case for information on RT.

Starting point for the discussion of the information provision is a classification with four levels of information to be provide, closely related to the type of decisions that have to be taken by the users of the information.

In the following scheme the 4 levels are explained:

| level | name | description |
|-------|------|-------------|
| level 1 | Data | This level reflects the unstructured mass of available information |
| level 2 | Information | This level reflects information in a structured way. The structure depends on the request for information. |
| level 3 | Instruction | This level reflects the information that influences the behaviour of the requirer. |
| level 4 | Advice | This level is solving the problem of the user. |

These 4 levels are of great importance for the information providers, because the recognition of the level of information required by the actors in the RT market is the basis for the structure of the information service.

## 3.    Information Service for the RT market, The Dutch experience.

All four levels of information mentioned above should be provided by an information service concerning the RT market.

To fulfil this difficult task we can distinguish three main activities in the Rehabilitation Information Centre:
1. Data collection
2. Information provision
3. Courses/curriculum development

**Data collection.**

Data collection is an important activity and is the basis for the information provision. Data collection on Rehabilitation Technology is done on a systematic way and contains the following aspects, e.g.:
- existing product in the Netherlands
- market data: importers, wholesalers, retailers
- technical data
- functional data
- ongoing R&D
- provision system

Data collection is done on a systematic way and as far as possible controlled by quality assurance. This means that the data are collected within a structure and are checked through a standardized methodology.

The following part of this presentation will give an example of this.
The data collection on technical aids available in the Netherlands is based on a questionnaire which is send to the relevant organisations. We ask them for documentation and information on their products and their position in the RT market.
When the information arrives at our centre we start with processing the data.
The processing can be divided into 2 levels:

    a:    The general level:
            We add the following structure to the data:

- iso-code
- generic name
- brand name
- type/model

            This is done by occupational therapists in close cooperation with a database manager an administrative staff. This information can be related to the request: Which technical aids are available and where can I get them?

    b:    The specific level which is added to the general level:

- technical
- functional
- market

Quality control is very important in data collection.
In our centre we can see 2 control mechanisms:

1. Process control: This is done by the computer and the database manager. He is responsible for the collection process.

2. Content control: This is done by using standardized lists for generic names and brand names. Also tables are used for technical and functional data.

This control procedure gives the assurance that the information is up to date as far as possible and put on a neutral way in the structure.

The collected information is used for information provision.

**Information provision.**

The information service is mainly used by rehabilitation professionals, companies active in the RT market, and handicapped persons or relatives.
We can recognize 2 main topics in the information provision:

**- the provision of information products:**

The aim of the provision of product is to enable the users to answer a large number of questions with the same content and level.
We provide the following information products:
*       Catalogue on technical aids available in the Netherlands. This is a reference guide to the products and their availability.
*       Information system called" Techhulp". This information system can be used up to level four of the information: The individual advice.
*       The Information System "Handynet", part of the EC programme Helios

Information systems have a very important function to support the professional in the execution of his job, e.g. the assessment of the needs of the user

**- the provision of Information services:**

The aim of the Information Service is to act for the actors in the RT market as a guide to find the information or information source and to fulfil the information needs. It works like a network to connect demand and supply regarding information on matters on technology and rehabilitation.
To fulfil this task we provide in our set up the following services:

*       *Information desk* : a desk with easy access for the target group to drop their questions
*       *Facility centre:* This enables other intermediates to use our facilities like:
                - exhibition room
                - product documentation
                - expertise
                - library
        The users have to pay for the use of the facilities.
*       *Market advisory service:* Commercial organisations who want to have information about the RT market in the Netherlands can use this service.

**Courses/Curriculum development:**

As already mentioned in the introduction a lot of disciplines are involved in the RT market.
Not all the professionals have education on technical aids in their curriculum. In daily practice the need for further education of the RT market appears. The courses on technical aids organised by our centre have all the actors in the RT market as a target group. The course are bases on theoretical principles completed with the experience of the teachers.

## 4.     International information exchange:

As mentioned in the introduction the RT market is a small market. The frequency of problems is very small. Exchange of knowledge and solutions for the individual problem of the handicapped persons is important and efficient.
For this exchange of knowledge and experience an international network is necessary. For this aim existing networks can be helpfully. In this context I think of the Handynet network, The ICTA network, The ISPO network a.o.
The only problem we have to solve is how we communicate permanently and continuously. This can be done on conferences and workshops, but also by an international information service acting as a reference guide for all the actors in the RT market.

## 5.     Special influence of social security systems on the innovation

Presented will be one example from the Netherlands, demonstrating the strong influence of the social security system on innovation and information service.

It was decided fifteen years ago to regulate the provision of technical aids (from which the wheelchair was an important and first issue) by a set of measures and conditions defined at the national level. All elements of the process were studied and put under a strong regime of quality control. This regards the product, the distribution, the provision, the control after provision and the selection process. This new structure could act as a strong tool for steering research and innovation, because the national provider can ask for a large volume of new products with transparent conditions for manufacturers and importers. Information can be prepared at the national level, and can be restricted to the issues and data fields with a relevancy for the local level to support the final selection out of the preselected items.

However it happened that the complete social security system has to change because of increasing budgets and reasons of budget control. We expect now to get a system with the local Communities as main responsible level in the decision about RT for individual. This could lead to a small scale steering and operating level. Of course innovation of technology should change its policy. It is not any more the national level with large volumes, however the split up local level where the product selection happens. This means that information on products can not be restricted to a restricted number of preselected items, also should the kind of information differ, e.g. should include more commercial information.

RIC,
Zandbergsweg 111,
Postbox 88,
6432 CC HOENSBROEK
The Netherlands

# START OF CREATING AN OVERVIEW OF THE RT MARKET

by Soede M., Ph.D.
Röben P.A.M.E., M.Sc.
Institute for Rehabilitation Research,
Knops H.T.P., O.T.
Rehabilitation Information Centre "Hoensbroeck"
The Netherlands

**Abstract:** Studies in the area of the market of Rehabilitation Technology (RT) reveal that it is a market with special problems. At this moment there is no comprehensive overview of this market which explains the difficulties, describes the possibilities and relates the different parameters in a structured way. The availability of models which describe the relationships and the influences of various factors is an obvious need; and this is actually the rationale for the CORE project.
The CORE project is one of the projects within the TIDE Pilot Action programme, and is addressing COnsensus creation and awareness for R&D activities in REhabilitation Technology for the elderly and the disabled. This paper describes some of the existing problems as there are: the market is not well defined, the position of the SME's is difficult with respect to funding R&D activities, problems of distribution and legislation, communication problems, threat of the US and Asian RT industry, and the role of the provision systems in the supply and demand side of the market.
Terminology will be addressed as a major requirement for creating consensus on the necessary actions to be taken.
A description of modelling activities will be given. The modelling is based on the collection of data readily available from several national and international sources and from a questionnaire developed and uses by the CORE project.
The data collection involves the following elements and actors in the market:
Research, Development, Productions, Trade, Procurement/Financing, Service Delivery, Usage and Professional Involvement.
Finally, the paper will give some preliminary conclusions and recommendations for possible actions to improve the creation of a Single Market on RT in Europe.

## Statement of the problem:

The Rehabilitation Technology market, defined as the activities around special products for the disabled and people with special needs, is known as a complex and broad market.
It is a market with thousands of products, some of the products appearing in large varieties/models designed to meet the needs of a user. In addition to that, a considerable part of the market is the adaptation of the products to an individual's needs. In some parts of the RT market this adaptation activity seems to give a larger turnover than the sales of the product itself: for example the provision of prostheses where the fitting is largely produced in a craftsman way, and the adaptation of cars where the assessment of the needs of the future driver and the design and implementation of a personal adaptation will often be a larger expenditure than the costs of the components. An example is also that with an adaptation of a workplace for a handicapped person, the costs for assessment, procedural activities for getting the finance, and the implementation is often three or more times as much than the costs for the technical products itself. This article, however will mainly deal with the products itself.
As already implicitly mentioned, the RT market has to deal with a number of intermediaries.
The costs of the technical aids are high and therefore the majority of the aids is provided by some kind of a social security system, sick fund or private fund. This means that a there is always a route to go before an aid is actually at the place of the user: assessment, selection, application for funding, evaluation of the application, decision, ordering and delivery, adaptation, instruction and (sometimes) evaluation.
A timelag of a year is not exceptional.

Considering the whole route, it can also be said that the average duration of getting an aid (12 weeks in The Netherlands) is rather short.

Connected to this problem, is the fact that no direct feedback is given about the usability and quality of the aid from the user to the seller/producer/- designer. Or also that, right of possibly wrong, an additional feedback is coming from the (professional) intermediaries.

Due to a gradual overlap with the normal consumer market, a clear distinction of the RT market is not self-evident; however this problem is largely solved when one adopts the ISO-classification as a starting point. Finally, it is seen as a problem that the market is dominated by small and medium size enterprises. These enterprises are mostly nationally oriented; nevertheless, for some products it seems that the majority of goods is imported in many of the European countries.

**Some historical remarks:**

In The Netherlands it was felt in 1979/80 that the market of technical aids should get more attention. A quick review of the quality of the aids was done by Jonkers (1) and an insight was given in the future possibilities of having better qualitative aids on the market and a better organized market of technical aids. It was felt that this issue contained aspects which where important for several departments: the department of Health and Welfare, department of Science policy, the department of Economics and the department of Social Affairs. It was political decided to put a substantial efforts in analyzing the RT market at that time and produce recommendations for improving the RT market. The analysis was based on the development of definitions of the elements of the RT market as will be described further on. The recommendations following the analysis were to establish an Innovation programme, and information system and improve the R&D capacity. The outcome of the recommendations were the establishment of a fund to stimulate R&D, a fund for research into quality and usefulness (funded by the Dept. of Economic affairs/Dept. of Science Policy), and the establishment of the Institute for Rehabilitation Research (funded by the Dept. of Health and Welfare/Science policy, the University of Maastricht, the Lucas foundation, a rehabilitation centre and TNO, a large R&D organization). Both actions are now seen as successful actions although some further recommendations are made to consolidate and enhance the outcome or the effectiveness of the funding programmes (2).

**A Model:**

As mentioned above the start of the modelling exercise is the definition of the elements of the RT market (3).

The CORE TP 126 project has identified seven elements to be the 'basic stones' of the RT market. A market element has been defined by CORE as a market component influencing demand and/or supply. Market elements have a considerable impact on the nature and type of demand and supply for a particular RT product.

The seven identified RT market elements are:

- Research; including fundamental and applied research
- Development; conversion of knowledge into a prototype product
- Production; manufacturing of goods or the creation of services
- Trade; wholesalers, dealers, importers, retailers
- Procurement/Financing; private and public funds pay most of the procurement of the RT products
- Service Delivery; professional advice and treatment
- Usage; including the end-user and his/her supporting environment

These elements are defined as follows:

## Research

The intention is to include the research which aims directly at the improvement or/and evolution of products in the RT market and of the market itself. Sometimes rather generally applicable research should be included: for example, improvement of the functionality of the electric wheelchair can be done by doing research on batteries. Research is mostly located in academic institutions.

Fundamental research is directed to the realisation and/or adaptation of certain principles of solutions, and is not aiming at the application of a specific product.

Scientific research endeavour to discover new or collate old facts by study of a subject, course of critical investigation to gain (more) (theoretical) knowledge and understanding about the subject without having the goal to achieve an application or a product. Furthermore, scientific research is providing a basic design of a product/service which can be elaborated in the developmental phase.

## Development

Available knowledge has to be converted into RT products. The uncertainty is not the fact that the product will work but whether or not the product can be an economically feasible product. Development is often carried out within a company, but also in technical universities and by independent developers.

Development is closely related to research by evolution, elaboration and application of the research results and basic design. Development is going beyond research with conversion, production, growth and expansion of the application.

Research and development can include partly the same activities. To appoint a certain activity to research or to development is depending on whether the aim of the activity is or is not focused on a concrete product.

## Production

The production of the product or the creation of the service is done in specialised companies or is done as a special product line in a larger company.

## Trade

Various subelements exist within the trade element as there are for example importers, wholesalers and retailers. An individual company may well be both a producer and a trader of its own products as well as of other, supplementary products.

## Procurement/financing

Private and public funds are paying the majority of the products supplied by the RT Market. The rules applied constitute a strong force in the market. The rules may influence the choice of product for the individual. The need for high-quality aid may be sacrificed for budgetary considerations.

### Service delivery

Most of the aids and services are only supplied and paid for or lent to a user if there is an advice, recommendation or prescription involved, made by a (para)-medical professional.

Often forgotten in the RT Market, and thus not constituting a strong force is that the end-user can only live with the help and assistance of a nurse or of the family and relatives; the social environment of the end-user will influence choices and often should because these people have to work with the aids themselves.

### Usage

Of course, usage is the most important element in the market, but not appropriately equipped with the ability, possibility or authority to constitute a proper force in the market.

A global model which is depicting the interactions in the RT market is given below:

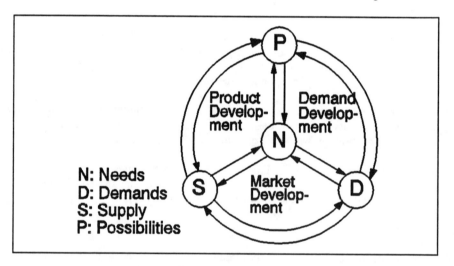

In the centre of this diagram, the needs of the elderly and handicapped user of technical aids is given. Three different processes are presented in the figure.

The Demand development is the process that describes the interaction between the user needs, the (technological) possibilities, and the (realistic) demands. Based on the user needs and knowing the possibilities which technology provides, one can define an real demand which in principle can be solved if the appropriate products are developed and marketed.

The second part of the diagram is development of a supply of products/prototypes of products. This is the process where Technology Transfer takes place.

The outcome of this process is a continuous supply of goods which enter the RT market. Again, an interaction between three variables, the needs, technological possibilities and supply of goods are determining the outcome of this process.

The third part of the diagram is the development of the market which is an interaction between the needs, supply and demand.

The market is seen as the place where the supply and demand are "regulated". Market barriers and opportunities determine the diffusion of new products on this market, and due to that, the successfulness of innovations. The general conclusion related to this diagram is that the RT market can only be developed and improved on a continuous base, if all the processes in this wheel are "moving" in the right direction.

## Awareness and Consensus:

For the creation of the RT market in Europe two of the essential activities to execute are the creation of consensus and the stimulation of awareness concerning Rehabilitation Technology. Without letting the relevant actors in this RT market know what is going on in the European area and beyond there will be very little chances to establish the necessary relationships and cooperation between the various actors in the RT field. Without cooperation and exchange of knowledge and information there will never be an European Single RT market.

Tools for these activities are used plenty, such as conferences and congresses like this TIDE Congress, publications in scientific journals and magazines, and courses on specific subjects related with RT. These are only a few examples of possible tools.

Information provision towards the RT actors is of big importance in order to let the creation of consensus and stimulation of awareness be possible.

## Role of information systems.

Information can be defined as the knowledge increasing the uncertainness in decision making.

In the RT market we can identify a lot of unstructured information flows between the actors. We also identify the need for the exchange of experience of the actors in this small market.

Information systems can play an important role in structuring this information to the users. It is an impossible task to organize all the information flows in one system for all the aspects of information in the RT market.

There exist all lot of information systems covering items of this market.

Also specialists are available in the market but not optimal accessible.

To solve these problems of referring the requirers to the right information provider, coordination and tuning of the available information will be necessary. This can be done by organising the information flows in a network with a information management function as an intermediate between request and supply side.

It has the preference that this communication network contents as much as possible the existing networks like HANDYNET,ICTA,ISPO,a.o..

## Acknowledgement:

It has to be acknowledged that the CORE project is executed by the following partners:

| | |
|---|---|
| Institute of Rehabilitation Research - IRV | NL |
| ICS-FORTH | GR |
| Swedish Handicap Institute | S |
| Infologics/Swedish telecom | S |
| National Agency for Welfare and Health - NAWH | SF |

Subcontractors are: CN-IROE (I), RNIB (GB), TNO TPD/STB (NL), RIC (NL), Swarte,MIC (NL).

**References:**

1. Jonkers L., Soede, M. ea., Technological Innovation to physically handicapped persons. PZOG. Leiden 1980.
2. Swarte, V.P.P., Technological developments in the RT market, NOTA. The Hague 1992.
3. These elements were described in a slightly different form in reference (4). The present definition comes from the CORE project which is an EC cost shared project; see acknowledgement.
4. Soede M., Jonkers, H.L., Innovation in aids for the Handicapped. Automedica, 1982, Vol. 4, pp. 169-175.

# Home Systems and
# Handicapped/Elderly people
# A Necessary Coherent Approach

Roger Torrenti
General Manager of Sigma Consultants
Buropolis - 1240, route des Dolines
F 06560 Valbonne France
Tel : (33) 93 95 85 30
Fax : (33) 93 95 84 77

We all know that technical solutions/products are not sufficient to answer the need of elderly/handicapped people (more global solutions including financial, social, service aspects have to be found). But if products are not sufficient, they are necessary.

If we now compare today markets of products for elderly/handicapped on one side, and of Home Systems (for non handicapped people) on the other side, we could say that :

. market players are quite different: one commonly find large companies and important research laboratories in the Home Systems field, (very) small companies and medical experts in the field of products for elderly / handicapped people.

. the demand for Home Systems remains quite low as the relevant product offer is important when the demand for products for elderly / handicapped is high as the product offer is weak.

When we analyse the evolution of these 2 markets we can however foresee that links between them are logical and that a coherent approach will necessarily develop. The main reason is that as far as the demand is concerned, the frontier that people use to draw between valid people and "dependent" people disappear when analyzing the problem more into detail. We could say: everyone only wants a "better life" (security, comfort, communication, etc) and everyone is "more or less dependent".

So, as far as the offer is concerned, solutions (in terms of products and services) should probably be developed for everyone. Of course, final man-machine interfaces will have to be developed (with medical / ergonomics experts) for the product to be really suited for this or that specific handicap, but this only appears as the final and logical adaptation of Home Systems to consumers.

We hope that these arguments, we will detail during our presentation, will sound obvious to most of readers and participants. We only aim at convincing marketing managers of large companies and directors of major research laboratories involved in Home Systems that they have to think to elderly / handicapped people not as an isolated / "difficult" group of persons but as an attractive market segment for which they have to invest rapid and important efforts.

# The Market for R. T. in Europe: a Demographic Study of Need

Stuart CARRUTHERS, Anne HUMPHREYS and JIM SANDHU
*Special Needs Research Unit, University of Northumbria,*
*Newcastle upon Tyne, NE7 7TW, United Kingdom*

**Abstract.** This paper describes potential consumer demand for Rehabilitation Technology goods and services in the years 1995, 2000, 2010 and 2020 for both the European Community and it's member states. The implications of projected changes in age structure over this period for European RT manufacturers is discussed. It is shown that the Community has the largest potential market for RT products and services in the developed world.

## 1. Introduction

Reliable and comparable statistics on the level of disability in the European Community are almost impossible to obtain, as only Spain and the United Kingdom use the International Classification of Impairments, Disabilities and Handicaps (ICIDH) recommended by the World Health Organisation (WHO) to record their data [1]. The R.T. industry needs to have access to reliable market information (size of market, spending power of potential purchasers, and information on the likelihood of these to purchase its goods and services) if a single market in these products is to be established.

The principal purchaser of R.T. products in most European countries is the state through its *social spending* budget. One of the main arguements used at the *political level* to advocate the development of a European R.T. industry sector is to free for other purposes some of the social spending that disabled people, particularly those who are elderly, are expected to need in the future. This arguement is especially compelling for many member states (ie. France, U.K. and The Netherlands) where pension fund and life assurance assets exceed GNP [2], and an increasing proportion of these funds contributors (state and private) are becoming recipients.

Demand for the industry's goods and services is expected to increase as potential consumers become more comfortable with technology, and as Europe's population grows older (mainly due to declining mortality and fertility rates).

The industrial and social policies of government in a *civil society* are determined to serve the *best interests* of its constituents. The resources used to implement these policies (present and future) are limited, and decisions on their distribution and application need to be planned at both the national and European level.

Consumers are unable to influence the European market for R.T., as national governments are effectively able to determine the policies for their home markets. It will be impossible to make meaningful comparisons at a European level with the statistics supplied by member states until they develop a *standard* method of data collection and analysis (hopefully one which corresponds with the ICIDH standards).

In this preliminary report the population profiles of eleven member states are analysed to estimate by age the potential number of people who might purchase R.T. products in 1995, 2000, 2010 and 2020 for a representative range of impairments and levels of severity. These estimates use the results of U.K. surveys which determined the rate, level and type of disability found in this member states population using ICIDH standards.

Information from a range of European statistical sources have also been examined to determine population projections in member states. It is hoped that this approach overcomes many of the problems associated with lack of standardisation in data collection, and that these estimates will enable both consumers and policy makers to play a fuller and more effective role in creating one of Europe's market orientated industries of the future.

## 2. Materials and Methods

Population projections of member states for 1995, 2000, 2010 and 2020 were obtained from EUROSTAT [3]. The number of disabled people in each member state (by age and impairment) for these years was estimated using statistics determined in 1988 by the British Office of Population Census and Surveys [4, 5]. These figures detail both the frequency, type and level of impairment (on a ten point scale) in Britain. People with a disability graded at level one or two are unlikely to be potential consumers of R.T. products and services - only those people with a disability graded at three or above who are likely users of R.T. are considered in this study. It was not possible to obtain projected population figures for Greece as none are available. It is likely that the potential market for R.T. products in Greece is similar to the projected markets for Belgium.

It is recognised that it would have been preferable to use estimates detailing the prevalence of disability for each member state for this study. However, only Spain and the UK use the standards determined by the WHO to determine the level, type and frequency of disability within their populations.

## 3. Demography of the R.T. Market

R.T. is an industry sector which currently has it's main consumer market in developed (industrialised) countries. These all have declining mortality and fertility rates and now have similar life expectancies [2]. It is thought that the level of disability in industrialised countries is similar [6]. Table 1 shows the population of the EFTA Countries, European Community, Japan, United States and Canada, and it can be seen that the E.C. has the largest home market for R.T. products in the world.

Table 1: Showing the Population (millions) of the Major Industrialised Countries and Trading Blocks

| Region | Population |
|---|---|
| European Community | 350 |
| EFTA Countries | 32 |
| Japan | 124 |
| USA and Canada | 277 |

The projected number of people who are potential consumers of R.T. products for eleven of the member states are shown in Table 2 for 1995, 2000, 2010 and 2020. Estimates of the

**Table 2.** Showing the estimated number of people with disabilities who are potential users of Rehabilitation Technology in 11 member states of the European Community (thousands) for the years 1995, 2000, 2010 and 2020. Sources [1], [2], [3], [4], [5].

| | B | DK | D | E | F | Ir | I | L | NL | P | UK | Total |
|---|---|---|---|---|---|---|---|---|---|---|---|---|
| **0-14 yrs** | | | | | | | | | | | | |
| 1995 | 27.7 | 14.3 | 166.6 | 108.1 | 180.0 | 13.7 | 140.0 | 1.0 | 43.3 | 30.5 | 186.0 | 911.2 |
| 2000 | 44.4 | 25.7 | 279.6 | 171.6 | 296.9 | 21.1 | 230.5 | 1.7 | 79.7 | 48.9 | 324.5 | 1524.6 |
| 2010 | 39.7 | 24.2 | 225.5 | 164.2 | 280.5 | 18.5 | 210.0 | 1.5 | 75.8 | 47.7 | 307.0 | 1394.6 |
| 2020 | 37.6 | 21.0 | 205.1 | 133.5 | 264.9 | 16.3 | 170.5 | 1.5 | 67.6 | 42.8 | 299.8 | 1260.6 |
| **15-19 yrs** | | | | | | | | | | | | |
| 1995 | 13.3 | 7.2 | 68.7 | 69.0 | 81.4 | 7.1 | 81.7 | 0.5 | 20.3 | 17.4 | 75.6 | 442.2 |
| 2000 | 9.6 | 4.4 | 52.5 | 40.6 | 61.9 | 4.8 | 48.8 | 0.4 | 14.7 | 11.1 | 58.6 | 307.2 |
| 2010 | 8.9 | 5.4 | 58.9 | 33.5 | 58.7 | 3.9 | 46.0 | 0.4 | 16.4 | 9.3 | 66.4 | 307.8 |
| 2020 | 7.8 | 4.9 | 43.4 | 33.1 | 55.0 | 3.5 | 41.9 | 0.3 | 15.5 | 9.6 | 60.1 | 274.9 |
| **20-29 yrs** | | | | | | | | | | | | |
| 1995 | 30.5 | 17.0 | 191.1 | 144.4 | 183.9 | 10.8 | 202.3 | 1.2 | 53.9 | 37.8 | 186.0 | 1058.9 |
| 2000 | 27.6 | 15.3 | 150.5 | 140.5 | 172.2 | 10.9 | 178.8 | 1.1 | 46.8 | 36.3 | 161.9 | 941.8 |
| 2010 | 25.6 | 12.4 | 155.9 | 101.5 | 165.3 | 9.8 | 128.5 | 1.1 | 43.3 | 28.4 | 166.1 | 837.9 |
| 2020 | 23.2 | 14.5 | 153.1 | 92.5 | 158.3 | 8.7 | 125.4 | 1.1 | 47.2 | 25.8 | 180.9 | 830.6 |
| **30-39 yrs** | | | | | | | | | | | | |
| 1995 | 47.3 | 22.9 | 318.8 | 178.8 | 253.2 | 15.2 | 261.4 | 1.9 | 76.0 | 48.6 | 261.5 | 1485.5 |
| 2000 | 45.7 | 23.8 | 326.9 | 192.5 | 251.0 | 14.6 | 281.6 | 1.9 | 79.1 | 51.1 | 273.8 | 1541.9 |
| 2010 | 37.4 | 20.5 | 208.2 | 189.9 | 232.0 | 14.2 | 242.8 | 1.5 | 65.7 | 49.2 | 217.3 | 1278.7 |
| 2020 | 34.7 | 16.5 | 211.7 | 137.2 | 222.7 | 13.2 | 174.5 | 1.6 | 60.9 | 38.6 | 223.1 | 1134.7 |
| **40-49 yrs** | | | | | | | | | | | | |
| 1995 | 63.1 | 34.8 | 384.6 | 218.6 | 373.2 | 20.8 | 345.0 | 2.5 | 103.9 | 58.9 | 351.1 | 1956.5 |
| 2000 | 66.7 | 32.7 | 422.0 | 234.9 | 375.6 | 21.7 | 351.0 | 2.7 | 105.7 | 64.9 | 346.2 | 2024.3 |
| 2010 | 67.6 | 34.7 | 483.3 | 284.1 | 370.2 | 21.4 | 418.5 | 2.8 | 117.9 | 76.3 | 404.4 | 2281.2 |
| 2020 | 55.4 | 29.9 | 304.6 | 280.1 | 342.4 | 21.0 | 360.9 | 2.3 | 98.0 | 73.5 | 321.4 | 1889.6 |

**Table 2.** Showing the estimated number of people with disabilities who are potential users of Rehabilitation Technology in 11 member states of the European Community (thousands) for the years 1995, 2000, 2010 and 2020 Sources [1], [2], [3], [4], [5]. *cont....*

| | B | DK | D | E | F | Ir | I | L | NL | P | UK | Total |
|---|---|---|---|---|---|---|---|---|---|---|---|---|
| **50-59 yrs** | | | | | | | | | | | | |
| 1995 | 89.0 | 51.0 | 728.3 | 338.3 | 467.7 | 27.8 | 580.8 | 3.7 | 135.7 | 91.8 | 525.1 | 3039.3 |
| 2000 | 98.0 | 60.1 | 664.6 | 361.8 | 554.3 | 32.8 | 598.7 | 4.0 | 165.7 | 96.6 | 597.6 | 3234.2 |
| 2010 | 118.4 | 56.8 | 746.9 | 243.2 | 662.5 | 38.0 | 630.2 | 4.8 | 187.8 | 116.6 | 614.5 | 3419.7 |
| 2020 | 120.0 | 60.5 | 851.9 | 503.7 | 553.9 | 37.6 | 752.5 | 4.9 | 209.6 | 136.9 | 720.1 | 4051.8 |
| **60-69 yrs** | | | | | | | | | | | | |
| 1995 | 152.5 | 65.9 | 975.9 | 580.4 | 800.5 | 36.5 | 912.9 | 5.7 | 187.8 | 147.7 | 771.6 | 4637.7 |
| 2000 | 147.7 | 67.1 | 1122.6 | 558.7 | 772.2 | 37.8 | 933.1 | 5.7 | 194.7 | 147.4 | 767.5 | 4754.4 |
| 2010 | 153.0 | 90.5 | 1031.3 | 566.1 | 872.0 | 50.2 | 959.1 | 6.1 | 260.1 | 153.1 | 925.5 | 5067.0 |
| -2020 | 185.3 | 85.3 | 1159.5 | 651.7 | 1043.8 | 58.3 | 1014.1 | 7.4 | 294.3 | 184.6 | 956.0 | 5640.5 |
| **70-79 yrs** | | | | | | | | | | | | |
| 1995 | 182.6 | 98.9 | 1189.3 | 695.7 | 950.3 | 50.7 | 1085.2 | 6.1 | 250.3 | 189.7 | 1113.7 | 5812.8 |
| 2000 | 217.7 | 97.1 | 1402.7 | 788.7 | 1205.0 | 49.8 | 1333.5 | 7.4 | 268.9 | 209.6 | 1134.5 | 6714.8 |
| 2010 | 212.0 | 93.5 | 1659.4 | 805.3 | 1180.8 | 51.3 | 1417.7 | 8.0 | 284.8 | 216.9 | 1009.6 | 6939.0 |
| 2020 | 224.3 | 126.1 | 1508.7 | 823.6 | 1363.0 | 69.5 | 1475.7 | 8.7 | 383.5 | 226.6 | 1340.3 | 7550.1 |
| **80+ yrs** | | | | | | | | | | | | |
| 1995 | 221.7 | 118.5 | 1502.8 | 703.8 | 1273.1 | 46.3 | 1195.9 | 6.9 | 275.9 | 186.1 | 1337.2 | 6868.4 |
| 2000 | 205.8 | 122.0 | 1391.2 | 745.8 | 1075.8 | 48.7 | 1125.0 | 6.6 | 293.2 | 201.6 | 1369.1 | 6584.7 |
| 2010 | 278.4 | 124.2 | 1749.0 | 934.7 | 1559.4 | 51.9 | 1661.6 | 8.9 | 351.7 | 313.9 | 1516.8 | 8551.0 |
| 2020 | 297.9 | 121.5 | 2111.0 | 959.7 | 1654.3 | 57.3 | 1897.7 | 10.1 | 379.8 | 321.0 | 1536.2 | 9346.6 |
| **Total** | | | | | | | | | | | | |
| 1995 | 827.6 | 430.7 | 5524.1 | 3037.0 | 4563.2 | 228.9 | 4805.3 | 29.6 | 1149.5 | 808.5 | 4807.9 | 25212.5 |
| 2000 | 863.2 | 448.2 | 5812.5 | 3235.1 | 4764.9 | 242.1 | 5080.9 | 31.4 | 1248.5 | 867.4 | 5033.7 | 27627.7 |
| 2010 | 940.9 | 462.1 | 6318.4 | 3322.5 | 5381.3 | 259.2 | 5714.4 | 35.1 | 1403.6 | 1011.6 | 5307.5 | 30076.7 |
| 2020 | 986.2 | 480.1 | 6549.1 | 3615.1 | 5758.4 | 285.5 | 6013.2 | 37.8 | 1556.6 | 1059.5 | 5638.0 | 31979.6 |

Table 3. Showing the estimated number of people (thousands) by category of impairment and age who are potential users of R.T. in eleven member states of the European Community. Sources [1], [4], [5]

| Impairment | Year | Age in Years | | | |
|---|---|---|---|---|---|
| | | <15 | 15-60 | 60+ | Total |
| Lower Limbs | 1995 | 81 | 1516 | 2199 | 3796 |
| | 2000 | 157 | 1529 | 2293 | 3979 |
| | 2010 | 144 | 1544 | 2611 | 4299 |
| | 2020 | 130 | 1536 | 2862 | 4528 |
| Upper Limbs | 1995 | 18 | 184 | 1178 | 1380 |
| | 2000 | 35 | 419 | 1228 | 1682 |
| | 2010 | 32 | 423 | 1398 | 1853 |
| | 2020 | 29 | 420 | 1533 | 1982 |
| Dexterity | 1995 | 31 | 631 | 1645 | 2307 |
| | 2000 | 61 | 636 | 1715 | 2412 |
| | 2010 | 56 | 642 | 1953 | 2651 |
| | 2020 | 50 | 638 | 2141 | 2829 |
| Visual | 1995 | 18 | 439 | 1732 | 2189 |
| | 2000 | 35 | 443 | 1805 | 2283 |
| | 2010 | 56 | 447 | 2056 | 2559 |
| | 2020 | 29 | 444 | 2254 | 2727 |
| Hearing | 1995 | 53 | 838 | 2528 | 3419 |
| | 2000 | 102 | 845 | 2636 | 3583 |
| | 2010 | 93 | 853 | 3001 | 3947 |
| | 2020 | 84 | 849 | 3290 | 4223 |
| Communication | 1995 | 97 | 567 | 1212 | 1876 |
| | 2000 | 189 | 572 | 1264 | 2025 |
| | 2010 | 173 | 577 | 1439 | 2189 |
| | 2020 | 156 | 574 | 1578 | 2308 |
| Behaviour | 1995 | 191 | 982 | 1316 | 2489 |
| | 2000 | 371 | 990 | 1372 | 2733 |
| | 2010 | 339 | 999 | 1562 | 2900 |
| | 2020 | 306 | 994 | 1713 | 3013 |
| Mental | 1995 | 78 | 910 | 1402 | 2390 |
| | 2000 | 151 | 918 | 1462 | 2531 |
| | 2010 | 138 | 926 | 1665 | 2729 |
| | 2020 | 125 | 921 | 1826 | 2872 |
| Other | 1995 | 218 | 1692 | 4087 | 5997 |
| | 2000 | 424 | 1707 | 4261 | 6392 |
| | 2010 | 388 | 1723 | 4851 | 6962 |
| | 2020 | 350 | 1713 | 5319 | 7382 |
| Total | 1995 | 785 | 7759 | 17299 | 25212 |
| | 2000 | 1525 | 8059 | 18036 | 27620 |
| | 2010 | 1419 | 8134 | 20536 | 30089 |
| | 2020 | 1259 | 8089 | 22516 | 31864 |

younger disabled population (<15 years) especially in northern European countries are likely to be over-estimates as the projections take no account of current and future developments in genetic counselling. The number of potential consumers of R.T. products tends to increase as the population cohorts age. It is estimated that, in 1995, 27.2 per cent of potential consumers in the eleven member states studied will be aged over 80 while only 3.6 per cent will be less than 14 years of age.

## 4. R.T. Market Sectors

The market for R.T. products (present and future) is differentiated by both the impairment (including level) and age of potential consumers. Table 3 shows the projected number of people who are likely to be users of R.T., and the nature of their impairment for three age ranges (school, employment and retirement). In 1995 it can be expected that about 26 million Europeans will be potential consumers of the industry's products, rising to about 32 million in 2020.

## 5. Conclusion

Europe is the largest potential market for R.T. products in the industrialised world. However, lack of application of a *standard* defining and describing the potential requirements of its disabled citizens at the national level is probably arresting the development of the single market. Both North America and Japan effectively have larger home markets for R.T. products than Europe at the moment, as they have a definition of disability which is applied across a larger population.

The lack of application of an agreed standard describing the level and rate of disability in Europe's member states is probably the greatest obstacle to the creation of a single market in R.T. It enables member states to determine their populations level of *need* and the amount of social spending directed towards this market.

There is an urgent need for the demography of the R.T. market to be further defined in Europe, and for agreed standards to be *applied* across member states to determine the rate, type and level of disability found in national populations. If this work is not undertaken it is unlikely that a single market in R.T. will be established.

**References**

[1]     EUROSTAT, Rapid Reports, Population and social conditions: Disabled People - Statistics. ISSN 1016-0205. Commission of the European Communities, Luxembourg, 1992.

[2]     J. Alber, The Impact of Social and Economic Policies on Older People in the European Community: An Initial Overview. EC Observatory on Older People, Commission of the European Communities, Directorate General V, Employment, Social Affairs, Industrial Relations, 1991.

[3]     EUROSTAT, Demographic Statistics. ISBN 92-826 2758 6. Commission of the European Communities, Luxembourg, 1991.

[4]     J Martin *et al.*, OPCS Surveys of Disability in Great Britain. Report 1: The Prevalence of Disability Among Adults. ISBN 0 11 691229 4. HMSO, London, 1988.

[5]     M. Bone and H. Meltzer, OPCS Surveys of Disability in Great Britain: The Prevalence of Disability Among Children. ISBN 0 11 691250 2. H.M.S.O., London, 1989.

[6]     J. Sandhu and T. Woods, Demography and Market Sector Analysis of People with Special Needs in Thirteen European Countries: A Report on Telecommunication Usability Issues. ISBN 0 906721 43 1. Newcastle upon Tyne Polytechnic. 1990.

# Market Penetration
# Economic Support a Necessity
# for the Viability of R&D-results

Jan-Ingvar Lindström
*Swedish Telecom, Centre for Telematics and Disability,*
*PO Box 510, S-16215 Vällingby, Sweden*

**Abstract.** Market penetration in the field of rehabilitation technology depends upon financial support in several steps in the process from innovation to marketing . There are several reasons for this. One is the limited financial capacity of the customers. Another the small scale production. Consequently, viability of R&D results depends upon political decisions in terms of regulation and legislation. Examples of such methods are given.

## 1. Introduction

Through history, people with disabilities have belonged to the poor part of the population. There is much evidence for this in art and literature. In our time, this fact is verified by statistics. Even in the rich part of the world, people with disabilities are in general poorer than the main part of the population. In most countries this is true for the elderly as well.

Various action plans within the EC point out, that the groups of elderly and people with disabilities are large. This means that there is a potentially large market, hampered by the lack of financial resources of its members.

## 2. The consumer groups

According to available data, the number of people who are old and/or disabled amounts to at least 60 million in the Community. We must, however, remember that from the market point of view there are some more millions in the EFTA countries, not to mention the Eastern and Central European countries where the need for proper equipment is at least as high as in the Community.

There is a strong correlation between age and disability. A rule of thumb is that about 70% of people with disabilities are to be found in the groups of retirement age, ie 60 or over. The current trend implies that by the year of 2020, one in four in the Community population will be 60 or above.

Three groups of people with disabilities are discernable. First, there is the group of young people, who in many cases were born with a disability or have acquired an impairment in an accident or sudden disease. This group has often got adapted to advanced technology and has often become  motivated and skilled during an early stage of their lives. They are often highly motivated to use new technology, and less concerned about costs and other barriers.

The second group is constituted by the "young elderly", ie people between 60 and 75. Already now, there are surprisingly many of those who have acquired tastes and habits for consuming the new technological tools and services. It's also to be noticed, that even in this group a large number belongs to those who have contributed to the creation of the modern attitude of integration and equal rights to people independent of abilities or disabilities. In other words, they are prepared to fight for their right of access to technology and services on their premises.

The third group, ie the old elderly (75+) may have the same or even more need for devices and services facilities. However, they form a much less powerful group for two reasons. One is that disabled people's rights were formed when they had left the active part of their lives and have never assimilated the current policy. Another reason is that they form the poorest part of the group and also have the most limited experience and taste for advanced technology. Also, with growing age perceptual and cognitive capacities decrease significantly which makes it difficult to adapt to new procedures and change habits.

There are several studies which verify the abovementioned statements. In general, with growing age disabled people have a more negative attitude to new technology and also have less capacity to acquire it.

## 3. Market penetration

Given the abovementioned limitations in purchase power, the development, manufacturing and marketing of devices and other facilities are impeded. Experience shows, that the uncertain market prevents manufacturers from taking several important steps in a developmental process, and that they hesitate to take these streps without finacial support.

To start with, financial resources must be made available for research and development. The main reason is, that often enough firms involved belong to the category of small and medium size enterprises, where very little risk capital is available. Then, even after the development of a prototype, costs may be insurmountable for taking the step from prototype to first serial production. Companies often request help in financing tools and equipment for the benefit of large scale production. This in turn can significantly decrease the prices of the goods as a result of large scale production. But even so, support may be needed in order to achieve the financial benefits of large series. In Sweden, a special guarantee has been made available for this purpose. The provider makes an agreement with the manufacturer that a certain amount of devices will be sold within a restricted time intervall, say 18 months. If this does not occur, the provider will buy the remaining products in store.

Claiming economic support for the abovementioned steps does not per se mean that the money should be given to the manufacturer. Often enough, loans on decent conditions are enough. In case the enterprise becomes successful, a pay back of risk capital will take place in a pace slow enough not to increase the retailer price significantly. If not, no refunding is requested.

This process is important in order to promote an innovative market in the field of technical devices. However, in order to create an interesting market, a consumer group who can afford the devices must be identified. Experience shows that it is not possible to produce goods cheap enough to activate regular market forces. There are two resons for this: one has already been mentioned, ie the low purchasing capacity of the consumer groups. The other is related with the nature of the devices in question. They are often - at least as far as IT devices are concerned - rather sophisticated technically, and thus comparatively expensive. As an example, text telephones for the hard of hearing are often several times more expensive than an ordinary telephone, not to mention videophones to be used for deaf persons' sign language communication. - A braille display used as a substitue for a VDU for blind persons cost at least ten times as much as a visual alternative.

## 4. Which are the forces?

Under normal conditions, the main market force is the demand of the consumer - may it be "natural" or provoked by advertising ao. Given the discrepancy between cost and purchase capacity of the customer in this case, some additional forces must be allocated. One is regulation or legislation eg in a form developed in the US with the Americans with Disability Act (ADA). This act states that it is discriminating, and thus against american law, to prevent anybody from getting access to society, and that those who provide facilities to the general public should also be responsible that corresponding facilities are given to people with disabilities. The full effect of the ADA has not been seen yet, and some people doubt that it will solve but part of the problem.

Another possibility is to provide disabled persons with the necessary financial resources to be able to purchase the goods needed. This however, has two drawbacks: one is that there is then no guarantee that the money is used for the purpose. Second is, that no control of the quality of the goods is provided, and that  the consumer leaps the risk of spending money upon devices of doubtful quality.

A third possibility is that the government makes technical procurements and thus provides approved devices free of charge or to reduced prices to the consumers. This method has been used successfully in Sweden for about two decades.

In Sweden, more than SEK 2 billion (about ECU 250 million) is spent per year by the government   in providing RT devices to people with disbilities. This has created an interesting market and - together with risk capital for the abovementioned steps in the process - made it possible even for SME:s to act.   -  In the final report from the 1989 Commission on Policies for the Disabled, this method is accepted and implemented in the new area of Telematics and Disability. The Commission states, that special money is needed for the creation of a market in this field. The idea put forward is to charge all operators in the telecommunication market in Sweden with a fee to build up a special fund, from which money could be allocated for R&D, manufacturing and marketing of products and service facilities. This is considered as very important, not only for the quality of life for people with disabilities, but for the viability of R&D results.

## 5. The future

Legislation is another tool for the provision of RT. So far this method has been used to a very limited extent in Sweden and most other European countries. The way of stimulating the market by providing devices and services facilities free of charge has proven to be prosperous. The need for and experience from legislation, however, should not be neglected, and it might be that a combination of financial stimulation and legislative measures will turn out to be the most efficient guarantee for the viability of R&D results.

### References

1. J. Sandhu and Thomas Wood. Demography and Market Sector Analysis of People with Special Needs in Thirteen European Countries: A report on Telecommunication Usability Issues. Special Needs Research Unit, Newcastle Polytechnic, Newcastle upon Thyne, 1990.

2. L. Scadden, Stimulating the Manufacturing and Distribution of Rehabilitation Products: Economic and Policy Incentives and Disincentives. Electronic Industries Foundation. Washington, DC, 2000. 1987.

3. Age and Design, Age & Cognitive Performance Research Centre, University of Manchester, 1990

4. K. Cullen and R. Moran. Technology and the Elderly. The Role of Technology in Prolonging the Independence of the Elderly in the Community Care Context. Work Research Centre and Ekos. Dublin. 1990

5. A. Tinker. The Telecommuications needs of Disabled and Elderly People. An exploratory study. Age Concern Institute of Gerontology. Kings College London. 1989

6. G. Fagerberg and B. Lundberg, System for providing Assisitive Devices and other Rehabilitation Engineering Solutions to Individual Users in Sweden. *ECE/IFMBE Workshop on Rehabilitation Engineering*. Fagernes. Norway 1991.

7. A Society for All, Final Report of the 1989 Commission on Policies for the Disabled (Summary). Swedish Government Official Reports . 1992:52

# INFORMATION NEEDS OF ELDERLY AND DISABLED PERSONS IN CONNECTION WITH NEW TECHNOLOGY IN TRAFFIC AND TRANSPORT

Ralf RISSER                    &    Agneta STAHL
FACTUM,                             DTPE, Lund Institute
Danhausergasse 6/8                  of Technology, Box 118
A-1040 Vienna                       S-221 00 Lund
Austria                             Sweden

Abstract: It is likely to assume that in future traffic organisation and traffic planning everything will be done to encourage elderly and handicapped to take part in social life. I.e.,
traffic and transport structures will have to be such that they
can be used by these groups. However, to those members of
society that have difficulties to take part in traffic for
individual reasons (disease, mobility handicaps, etc.) several
types of support can be given. One important area in this
respect is tele-communication. With the help of new technology
in this area the requirements of elderly and disabled persons
can be met in a very specific way with respect to various
scenarios of life. Several VTX-systems exist in Europe already
that offer a large number of services. However, there is some
evidence that knowledge about these services is not good at
all, especially among the groups we want to address in this
present context. Moreover, the use of the system is very often
a difficult task that needs good explanation and guiding. In
this respect, several short-comings can be identified. Our aim
is to look upon these problems as a main concern for experts
that develop and implement different tele-communication services. Especially as far as information to potential users of
services on all levels is concerned, much work has to be done.
Among other things, these experts should be better trained and
instructed in order to be able to meet the information needs of
customers.

## 1. Introduction

It can be assumed that in future traffic organisation and
traffic planning everything will be done to encourage elderly
and handicapped to take part in social life. I.e., traffic and
transport structures will have to better meet the needs of
these groups. However, to those members of society that today
cannot, or have difficulties to take part in traffic because of
individual reasons (disease, mobility handicaps, age, etc.)
several types of support can be given.
   One specific area where support can be given in the
respect mentioned is tele-communication. With the help of new
technology in this area the needs of elderly and disabled

persons can be met in a very specific way and thereby support
interaction between elderly and disabled and the various scenarios of life.

An important aspect in this respect is that the
proportion of elderly and especially of "very old" people (as
people over 74 years are called in Gerontology) will increase
sharply already until the year 2000. Table 1 and 2 shows the
expected increase of people 65 and above and 80 and above,
respectively, in Sweden.

Table 1   Proportion of old-age pensioners aged 65 and above

| Year | Per cent of total population | People |
|------|------------------------------|--------|
| 1980 | 16.4 | 1.360.000 |
| 1988 | 17.8 | 1.504.000 |
| 2000 | 17.2 | 1.507.000 |
| 2020 | 20.7 | 1.860.000 |

Table 2   Proportion of old-age pensioners aged 80 and above

| Year | Per cent of total population | People |
|------|------------------------------|--------|
| 1980 | 3.2 | 263.000 |
| 1988 | 4.1 | 345.000 |
| 2000 | 5.1 | 447.000 |
| 2020 | 5.0 | 446.000 |

During this century people in Sweden is growing older and today
(1992) about 18 % of the population are 65 years or older. The
number of persons in the age group 65 and over (65+) will not
change between now and the year 2000, yet between 2000 and 2020
it is expected to increase by almost 25 %. On the other hand,
the numbers of the very oldest in the population are continuing
to rise, as they have been doing for some time. The age group
80+ has increased in number by 31 % since 1980, with prognoses
showing that between now and the year 2000 the age group 85-89
years is expected to increase by just over 40 % and those 90+
by just over 75 %.

Age is the factor which demonstrates the strongest
link with consumption of social services and health and medical
services. In all probability, therefore, the increase in the
numbers of the very oldest will be accompanied by a growing
burden on the various elements of the services for the elderly.

## 2. Available services today

At present, a considerable number of services, aiming especially at supporting elderly and disabled, is available, e.g., on
VTX:

home shopping
home banking
ordering of special transport services
classified advertisements
etc.

However, the purchase and the use of such new technology cause problems, especially for the elderly group. In the
following it will be described what we have been doing, so far,
in order to tackle these problems.


## 3. Information and handling problems

There is some evidence that knowledge about VTX services
available today is not good at all, especially among the group
we want to address in this present context. Moreover, the use
of technology-based aids, including tele-communication, is very
often a difficult task that needs good explanation and guiding.
In this respect, several short-comings can be identified. Many
experts are kept busy with the working up of informational and
instructional material for the (potential) final users of such
aids in order to help them solve their "new" tasks without any
problems. This in the future will become a primary precondition
for the undisturbed settlement of everyday's duties even more.
        In the forseeable future we can expect the develop-
ment of new products with high technical/technological standard
in diminishing intervals. Those persons who produce supporting
informational and instructional material for the final users
will certainly need appropriate psychological know-how in order
to be able to cope with this job. In this respect, the problems
of elderly and disabled will have to be focussed especially.


## 4. The use of new technology in the area of traffic/transport

As the traffic/transportation sector is not left untouched by
the quickly preceding technological innovation (e.g. international programs like PROMETHEUS, DRIVE, etc.), people in this
area will have to deal with more and more complex systems:
Today, this means for instance the whole area of stationary
information systems like the signposting in subway stations.
The transferring of money value to magnetic cards used in
regional traffic, or the use of interactive navigation systems
in cars, etc., are examples of much more complex handlings.
        Experts are often confronted with unusual tasks in
connection with new developments: At the moment there is no
routine for designing and implementing information in connection with new technology in the traffic/transportation field.
It is necessary to refer to basic perceptional and psychological knowledge available in order to be able to develop materials in a professional manner. Up to now there is a lack of
expert knowledge that has been prepared in an appropriate way
in these areas.

In other words: Strategies for information and instruction have to be developed that can be understood in a
distinct and reliable manner. Know-how from the field of
marketing has to be introduced. Work in this respect has to
become professional.

To those persons who prepare such information and
instruction material on and for various levels, regularities
should be pointed out, in order that they can generalize the
transmitted knowledge, which means that they can transfer the
knowledge on to other fields, to other target groups etc, as
well.

## 5. A pilot project in the frame of the COMETT[1] program

In autumn 1992 a pilot course was prepared and held in the
frame of the COMETT programme. This course, which we regard as
a pilot project for the planned activities in connection with
the use of tele-communication services as described below, was
dealing with information problems in traffic/transport.

Some generally applicable training packages on the
basis of a rough survey on new interactive guiding and navigation systems were developed. Attempts for fundamental statements were made on the issue how, on what level, and on what
aspects persons must be supplied with information in order to
transform the information or instructions of the areas in
question into real - and adequate - actions.

All partners in the pilot project - institutions from
Austria, Italy, Sweden, and the UK - also participate in some
way in the programs PROMETHEUS, DRIVE, and in other international projects. This fact and various contacts to managers of
public transportation systems allowed us to both select some
exemplary new technical systems and to prepare them for the
training course of the present project. The didactic materials
were prepared on basis of rather simple but frequently used new
technological "gadgets". We looked for some "typical" systems
which already had reached a certain range of distribution (for
instance computer-based information systems for railway time-
schedules, route guiding systems, ticket-selling machines,
etc).

Representatives from companies and institutions, for
whom the above mentioned problems are of immediate interest,
i.e., who place new interactive systems on the market, participated in our course: 2 persons from Sweden, 5 from England and
1 from Austria. The course consisted of two days of seminar
with four hours each.

---

[1] COMETT is an EC-programm that enhances international
cooperation on the development of training courses for
development and implementation of new technology, and for
the support of users.

The course was accepted well by the attendants. One impressive statement from a transport company representative was: "Actually we do not know too much about the needs of the users and largely live from guesses". This only means that in the area dealt with adequate user information is not known as an important aspect when implementing new technologies. This is strange, because on the other hand everybody knows about the necessity of good advertising, and experts in this sector usually know about the importance of considering user needs well.

In addition, public relations and marketing experts also do know that the potential purchaser's suspicion that he/she might not be able to handle a sophisticated product well might cause a higher threshold for the purchase of a product than is necessary. Potential customers have to be informed about the existence of any product in a clear way, so that they can make up their mind whether they need this product or not. They have to be told how they can get the product (equipment, tickets, instructions, etc.). And it has to be clear that the use of the product will be easily possible to them.

These statements were generally acknowledged. The participants agreed that courses of the type as performed here reflect a special need on the industry's side quite well. The contents of the course, presented right below, can thus be looked upon as being relevant, at least as far as the experts opinions and attitudes are concerned.

The following aspects were presented and discussed extensively in the pilot course (summarised in Clark et al. 1992):

1    Some marketing aspects connected with good informa-
     tion (in non-profit areas as public transport, it is
     often forgotten that products can only be bought if
     they are known; in order to be cost-effective, howe-
     ver, methods in order to address the relevant peer
     groups have to be applied)

2    Some basic rules for motivation in marketing and
     their connection to good information of users (e.g.,
     it is often omitted to explain what products are good
     for, and to point out their advantages)

3    The motivational background of information (info has,
     e.g., the function to underline identification and
     image aspects, etc.)

4    Characteristics of efficient information (e.g., short
     but still containing the relevant aspects - which
     however requires that one knows about the relevant
     aspects, i.e. the aspects the potential users are
     interested in; that means that, among others, som
     know-how about user needs and interests is required)

5    Examples for efficient preinformation, guiding in-
     formation, and on-line information (some practical
     examples from the partner countries that reflect the
     aspects named so far were given)

6    9 Rules for good quality information (see CLARK et
     al.)

7        Detected problems and shortcomings in today's prac-
         tice of user information (especially in non-profit
         areas there is too little knowledge among potential
         users about available options, high thresholds for
         purchase and use are the rule rather than the excep-
         tion, etc.)
8        Assessment of information systems (methods like in-
         terviews, on-line registration of handling processes,
         checklists, etc., are discussed here)

The didactical methods applied in the frame of the
course consisted of a mixture of verbal presentation of know
how, demonstrations with the help of video and soft-ware,
practical exercises with existing soft-ware, role plays,
discussion, and team work in order to produce own ideas for
identification and the solution of problems.

## 6. Information in connection with the use of tele-communication services

The know-how resulting from the pilot project discussed in
detail above can be generalised to problems inherent to user
information in connection with new tele-communication services.
    In the frame of a more extensive project - financed
in the frame of the COMETT-programme, as well - experts from
six institutions in four European countries (the same countries
as the partners in the pilot project: Austria, Italy, Sweden
and UK) have recently started a new project dealing with
development and implementation of training courses. The aim is,
to instruct experts who develop and implement tele-communication services to decide which information should be given to
customers, at which places, at which time, and in which mode.
    The courses will be so-called long courses: Partici-
pants will have to attend approximately 30 hours. Half of the
time the course will deal with the special problems of elderly
and disabled.
    Course materials and course structure will be develo-
ped following analyses of the user information presented
together with new tele-communication services today: How can
pre-information, guiding information and on-line information be
judged in this area.
    It is in principle planned to stick to the training
structures and the didactic methods developed in the frame of
the pilot course. In addition it is decided that the courses
will be offered in many different countries and cities in the
future: Thus, European cooperation will be intensified by
inviting persons from other countries than the ones participating in the development of the courses, as well.

## References

Clark J., Raso E., Risser R. & Ståhl A. 1992, How to inform travellers
according to modern standards. Training program for Persons who plan and
install the information and instruction systems for different traffic
modes, A COMETT-C$_2$ project, Vienna

# The Role of Evaluation in the Development of Rehabilitation Technology Products

Jim SANDHU, Ian MCKEE, Stuart CARRUTHERS
*Special Needs Research Unit, University of Northumbria,*
*Newcastle upon Tyne, NE7 7TW, United Kingdom*

**Abstract.** This paper emphasises that not all disabled people need rehabilitation technology but they all need good design. Product evaluation is critical to evolving good design, and to obtaining user feedback for further product enhancement. For manufacturers it is the most effective means of enlarging their markets. A user-based strategy is described centring on two familiar products.

## 1. Introduction

In Japan design power has been widely accepted as being market power for decades. In the typical Bushido code good design is seen as the creation of a product that is totally right - made in the right way to meet user needs, of the right material, at the right price, to the right specification, to deliver the right performance.

Crucial concepts like ease of use, value for money, safety, easy maintenance and effective operation are all part of the design imperative, alongside the functional and aesthetic requirements: carefully designed products must also look the part.

However, product success depends not just on marketability or design gimmicks. Like Swatch, we need innovative design principles to crack world markets. Like Sony and Yamaha, we need a succession of design variations to maintain a product lead. In the context of special needs an integral part of variability is the 'generic' approach to rehabilitation product design. Fall behind in these principles and you fall behind in both quality and perceived quality. Perhaps, what we really need is a form of the Bushido code for rehabilitation technology products.

## 2. Evaluation

Central to establishing quality both during and after the design process for a product is the iterative or usability evaluation phase. Amongst other product-related activities this is precisely what SNRU has been undertaking for clients over the past 12 years. To date we have evaluated just over 400 items ranging from wheelchairs, cookers, washing machines, plugs, microwave cookers, kitchens, handles, workstations, software, switches to playgrounds, and public transport systems.

It is significant that a substantial amount of our time has focussed on 'usability' rather than iterative evaluation. This has largely been dictated by our clients and funders Research Institution for Consumer Affairs, Consumers Association, British Gas, Tyne & Wear Passenger Transport Authority, etc. It is also a reflection of the fact that a large proportion of users with special needs make do with 'ordinary' products to the best of their ability. This is due to lack of choice in product selection as well as lack of foresight amongst designers. Whether focussed on specialised or mainstream products evaluation case studies can provide useful guidelines for product design as well as clarify user requirements. This is illustrated later with reference to cookers and microwave cookers.

## 2.1. User Panels

An integral and unique feature of SNRU's evaluative work is our voluntary panel of disabled testers which has been operational since 1981 - starting with the evaluation of the Tyne & Wear Metro System. Over the years the panel has grown to a core of 250 panel members with access to more volunteers if need be. Although considerable attention is paid to keep the range of handicaps proportional to the national average as established by SNRU for the Commission's RACE programme [1] it is not always possible. The size of the panel makes sampling of various handicaps empirically viable. Despite the social and economic differences which have tended to keep disabled and ageing populations apart, some similarities in functional characteristics are evident in our panel grouping: physically handicapped including wheelchair users, visually impaired, hearing impaired, those with poor coordination, or general weakness. Just over half the panel is over 60 years old.

The number and range of impairment categories selected for a specific exercise largely depend on the following:

* conditions imposed by the contracting organization, such as a request to concentrate on the visually impaired market;

* the nature of the product, e.g. specialized easy-to-wire plugs compared with gas or electric cookers (which require more extensive and exhaustive data collection);

* the overall budget which dictates what can be achieved in a given timescale; the honoraria we can afford to pay our volunteers; the geographical and impairments spread of volunteers; and so on.

## 2.2. Usability Issues

An important feature of SNRU's approach to evaluation is to learn from panellists about their experiences with products. What design features make a product work for them? What features render a product inaccessible? The reason for this emphasis is that, traditionally, disabled and especially elderly consumers have not been the subjects of market research. Very few studies exist describing their attitudes towards the equipment they use. In this sense SNRU studies are not directly geared to establishing design guidelines but rather to evolving *meta-rules* for clarifying the functional specifications of products in the process of being used.

The prime concern in evaluating a product is to find out the extent to which the product is convenient to use by people with special needs. We have little interest in technical evaluations because these have usually been carried out exhaustively by SNRU's contractors. Our approach to usability can best be described by Figure 1 where it is shown that success in use is dictated by three main ingredients.

The value of this approach to the evaluation process can best be illustrated by Figure 2 which outlines microwave cooker elements which need to be examined. These elements form the basis of detailed convenience checklists which are used to measure the usability of each product for a range of people. Another important stage in evolving the final checklist is to examine all tasks necessary to use the product and the overall evaluation criteria as shown in Table 1.

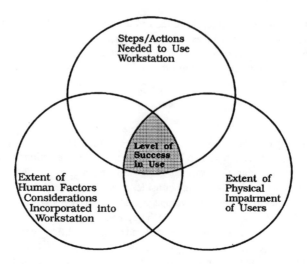

**Figure 1** Factors affecting successful use of products by disabled people

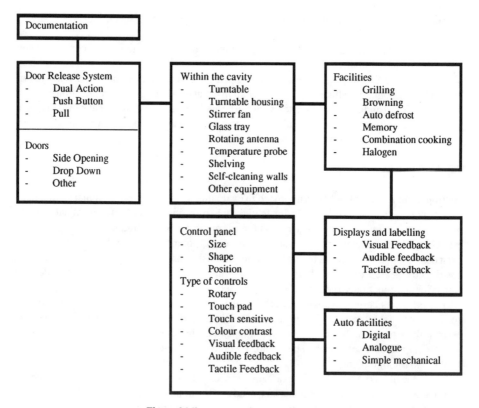

**Figure 2** Microwave cooker taxonomy chart

**Table 1 Evaluation of Microwave Cookers**

*Establishing User Tasks*
Task sequence involves three main areas of operation
  Loading; Programming; Unloading
Task sequence can involve the following actions
  Grasping; Lifting; Pulling; Pushing; Turning
The standard sequence of operation is
  Opening door; Placing an object in the cavity; Closing door; Setting programme; Starting programme; Finishing programme; Switching off; Opening door; Removing object/utensil; Closing door; Cleaning any spillages
*Factors considered in arriving at overall evaluation*
  Ease of use overall and within each separate task; Comfort of user whilst using appliance; Ease of understanding instructions; Effort required to carry out each individual task; Absence of any sharp edges or dangerous components e.g. safety; Ease of cleaning; Audibility of signals, timers etc; Colours, contrasts, lettering, light etc.

Depending on the type of product and range of models which need to be tested, an evaluation session can last from 90 minutes per volunteer for three makes of easy-to-wire plugs to 5 hours for 16 makes of cookers.

## 2.3. Results

In view of the complexity of factors involved in the success or failure of a product as characterised in Figure 1 the extensive results of our evaluations are expressed in qualitative rather than quantitative terms. Although the results as described here only refer to two products, are synoptic in description, and only describe the negative features, they highlight an important fact - that quite small improvements can make products much more accessible to elderly and disabled users. Moreover, these very small considerations also improve the product for 'ordinary' users. The negative features provide a useful 'what-to-avoid' checklist for designers and manufacturers.

**Table 2 Summary of some of the poor features of 14 microwave cookers**

Guide
  Programme guide unreadable to visually impaired; Programme guide too complicated and confusing
Labelling
  Very small lettering on panel; No instructions on how to set time; Need to bend and squint at labelling; Labelling became covered during use; Labelling around digital display area difficult to see
Controls
  Easy to go past the programme one needs to set; Confusing pre-timer for light and fan; prior to programme setting; Control panel difficult to understand; Temperature setting confusing; Poor colour definition on control panel; Poor contrast between lettering and background; Controls awkward to set; Controls much too close for arthritic hands; Controls difficult to set with shaking hands; Controls need a lot of physical and mental effort; No quick way of stopping the sequence without opening door; Controls require a lot of pressure
Display
  Faint digital readout; Very small digital display area
Door
  Labelling on door release misleading: should be on control panel; Door button not obvious; Indent on door release controls too small and shallow for large fingers; Door release button requires too much pressure; Some force required to close door; Door does not open effectively; Door catch protrudes: could catch clothes; Door swings closed; Door swings open, knocks into hands; Door panel too dark to see food cooking; Door panel too small; Sharp edges on door
Cavity
  Stripes on glass panel make it difficult to see food cooking; Need to bend to look inside cavity; Sharp edges on internal cavity racks; Oven cavity too small to manoeuvre food easily; Cavity height could be higher to

bring it more to body level; Cavity needs to be wider to be able to remove turntable easily; Loading and unloading resulted in excessive bending; Cavity tray difficult to remove; Cavity turntable too heavy to handle; Cavity lining difficult to clean
Feedback
Poor audible feedback while setting programme; Completion audible signal too short and too quiet; Completion signal inaudible from the next room; After completion fan continues causing confusion to some users

**Table 3 Summary of poor features of 27 different makes of cookers**

Hob
Glass lid difficult to get into the safe open position; Pan supports restrict sliding of the pan from one to another; Difficult to reach rear burners; Hob controls/area gets too hot; Pan supports too large for easy removal/cleaning/replacing; Burner rings/caps and trim difficult to remove/clean/replace; Hob top far too heavy to lift and support; Sharp edges on hob area; Dirt traps on hob area
Grill
Door difficult to open or close; Two hands needed to open door; Some force needed to open or close door; Poor or awkward grip on door handle; Grill-pan far too heavy; Grill-pan unbalanced or uncomfortable to hold; No stop or ineffective stop on grill-pan supports; Grill-pan components difficult to remove/clean or replace; Grill/second oven door does not open horizontally; Grill-pan has only one handle; Insecure grill-pan handle; Difficult to engage/disengage grill-pan handle; Sharp edges within grill compartment
Oven
Far too low for easy access; Totally inaccessible for normal use; Poor or awkward grip on door handle; Two hands needed to open door; Far too much force needed to open door; Awkward rod shelving supports for sliding or removing; Rod shelves fall off rails too easily (safety); Sharp edges on some components in oven compartment; Difficult to clean oven compartment
Controls
Poor access to control panel; Difficult to operate controls to give accurate heat settings; Poor visual feedback of heat setting indicators; Fine control needed to set heat; No automatic ignition on some functions; Simmer control difficult to disengage; Main controls difficult to grip; Some force needed to operate main control functions; No/limited audible indication; No/limited tactile indication (detents)
Auto-Timer
Control knobs/buttons; too small to enable easy setting; Gaining access to the controls difficult; Display in awkward position to see from all angles; Limited audible feedback; Two-handed/two-fingered operation for setting functions

## 3. Conclusions

The next few years will witness a growing awareness of the needs of disabled and elderly people. There is also strong evidence [2] that this group is potentially the fastest growing consumer market in the developed world. Designers, manufacturers and rehabilitation engineers should make it their priority to undertake evaluative research with end users at all stages of the design process and, in particular, prior to launching the product. Not all disabled people need rehabilitation technology but they all need good design.

### References

[1] Sandhu,J.S. and Wood,T. Demography and market sector analysis of people with special needs in thirteen European countries: a report on telecommunication usability issues. A RACE-TUDOR report. ISBN O 906721 43 1 Newcastle Polytechnic, 1990, pp 1-116.

[2] Carruthers,S., Humphries,A., Sandhu,J.S. The market for rehabilitation technology in Europe: a demographic study of need. TIDE Congress Paper. Newcastle: Northumbria University, 1993, pp 1-5.

# Product Duplication

Stuart CARRUTHERS, Anne HUMPHREYS and Jim SANDHU
*Special Needs Research Unit, University of Northumbria,
Newcastle upon Tyne, NE7 7TW, United Kingdom*

**Abstract.** This paper critically examines the prototype products being developed by the European Commission's TIDE initiative. It is suggested that lack of knowledge about the availability of R.T. products originating from member states, America and Japan is arresting the commercial development of products in Europe which have strong commercial potential. It is also suggested that TIDE's remit gives it a responsibility to ensure that all technological research and development work funded by the Commission, and which *might* be made directly available to disabled and elderly people, takes their needs fully into account.

## 1. Introduction

If a commercial market for a product exists, it is accepted within a market economy that entrepreneurs will develop it as required by consumers. The cost of technological development is now high. National governments and trading blocs throughout the world have developed methods of *subsidising* the development of new products and services by their industries to maintain the competitiveness of their technological industries.

The main aim of the European Community's research and technological development policy is to maintain and strengthen the international competitiveness of its industry in high technology sectors, in the face of competition on global markets, above all from the USA and Japan [1].

This policy is realised in three main ways: *i) establishing cross-border cooperation, coordination and mobility between industry and science; ii) supporting basic research which is becoming increasingly important, and for which medium-sized companies frequently do not have the necessary personnel or capital; iii) integrating research and technology into the concept of completing the single internal market in Europe.* This applies especially to standardisation, which often requires high levels of research and development.

TIDE is the Community's initiative in the area of Rehabilitation Technology. The principle objective of the TIDE programme was described in the initial call for proposals as '*the development and matching of technology to the abilities of elderly and disabled people in order to satisfy their needs*' [2]. TIDE's purpose is to develop European standards, and stimulate the transfer of existing and emerging technologies to products targeted specifically at this market.

We have estimated that there are about 26 million people living in Europe who are potential consumers of these specialist R.T. products [3]. In Britain the majority of *high technology* goods currently available to consumers of this market would appear to originate from the United States of America [4].

TIDE as a *market oriented* programme of the European Commission needs to take account of both the requirements of potential R.T. users and the international competitiveness of this industry sector. In this preliminary report, the international competitiveness of the prototype
considered, and suggestions are made which could enable European industry to achieve an increased share of both the home and international market.


## 2. Sources of Product Information


The *information system* developed to describe Rehabilitation Technology products and their markets in Europe is *HANDYNET* (funded and maintained by the European Commission through DG V). It maintains information on each product's functional and technical specifications, its manufacturer, distributors and cost, and on regulations governing its availability in member states [5]. *HANDYNET* restricts its attention to European products and has only made the information available since the beginning of 1992 despite having been in the process of development since the 1970s [6].

The TIDE pilot project CORE (TP126) is developing a *new* information system to enable policy makers to gain an understanding of the R.T. market, and enable specific sectors to be analysed [7]. In the pilot phase of TIDE no implementation of the information system was to be effected.

Many member states maintain databases on the R.T. products available in their country. Most of the organisations responsible for these activities are also members of their national *HANDYNET* consortium, and are supplied with product information by manufacturers and retailers of R.T. products who have an active presence in their national market.


## 3. Priorities for R.T. Product Development


Funds for R.T. product development are available mainly from statutory and charitable sources. In the U.K. these funds are allocated on a competitive basis without any definition or description (as far as we are aware) of funding priority areas. The majority of R.T. products developed in this country that reach the market would appear to do so because an entrepreneur has identified a market opportunity. These do not normally obtain funding for product development on a non-commercial basis.

In the United States of America the government's General Services Administration advises on its telematic resource requirements. It identified areas of unfulfilled need for people with special needs in 1988 [8]. These included development of a *graphic user interface* access method for visually impaired users, and a method of overcoming the problems associated with the *terminate-stay-ready-software* used by switch users.

The member states of the European Community effectively developed an action plan for R.T. development (market opportunities) with the launch of the product based TIDE pilot phase in 1991. Following consultation with national experts and industry actors a further 43 pre-normative and pre-competitive tasks were identified and adopted by the Commission in 1992 [9].

The Commission is now probably the largest single source of funding for research into R.T. and the development of products for people with special needs in Europe. Funding for the R.T. industries is now consequently based mainly at the European level.

In the pilot phase TIDE may be either stimulating the development of competitive R.T. products and services, or maintaining through subsidy an industry sector which is unlikely to become competitive in the future.

## 4. Product Duplication

Using the currently available information sources it is difficult to gain an overview of the availability and distribution patterns of different R.T. products around Europe. The fact that HANDYNET considers only products manufactured in the Community [10] means that the level of penetration of its R.T. market particularly by American manufacturers has gone largely unnoticed [4]. In the UK an American R.T. product may be supplied where a European alternative exists simply because information flow is often more efficient across the Atlantic than across the Channel.

The failure of member states to adopt a uniform standard describing the level and rate of disability in their population [3] gives added impetus to this phenomenon, as it enables member states effectively to regulate their markets for R.T. through their social spending programmes outside the framework of the single market. It also enables distortion of the size of the market for R.T. particularly by lobby groups representing the interests of people with particular impairments, in their search for scarce resources for the benefit of their constituents at both the national and European level.

## 5. TIDE Pilot Projects

TIDE pilot projects were required to address the issues involved in developing telematic R.T. products specifically for disabled and elderly people through multinational consortia. In all but one of the TIDE pilot projects these activities are directed towards the production of prototype devices and systems. Projects were required to involve potential consumers of these goods and services in their work. In the second phase they will be required to deliver statements of end user requirements, and detail the anticipated benefits of the technological solutions to the end users.

Europe has the largest home market for R.T. products and resources in the world. However, our estimates suggest that the market size is sometimes overestimated by as much as 100 per cent. Many commentators on the size of the potential European market for R.T. indicate that it is between 60 - 80 million [7]. Using incidence figures from the OPCS survey of disability in the UK [11] we estimate that, while 68.5 million Europeans may be elderly or disabled by OPCS criteria only about 26 million of them are likely to have a disability severe enough to require a specialist technical aid [3]. The remainder would be more effectively helped by measures to promote good general product design practices.

The majority of TIDE pilot projects have failed to take full account of the increasing prevalence of disability with age [3]. This will have an inevitable effect upon the commercial viability of many of the products and services being developed as part of the pilot action, and potentially in the next phase.

There is a measure of overlap between TIDE pilot projects in the subjects they address and in the products they aim to develop. For example, the problems of the Graphic User Interface and terminate stay ready software identified by the American GSA in 1988 are each targeted by two TIDE projects.

Within the programme, overlap in itself need not be detrimental to progress. Investigation of a problem in two or more different contexts can lead to a fuller understanding of its nature and possible solutions. However the TIDE pilot action has not provided adequate opportunities for sharing and co-operation between projects and the chance to benefit from subject overlap has not been exploited, either commercially or academically.

Instead, because of the emphasis on the development of viable and marketable products, TIDE projects potentially find themselves in competition. At a more general level it has been observed that '*while EEC expenditure in total is almost double that of Japan much of its R&D efforts are duplicated*' [12]. The next phase of TIDE could benefit greatly from a programme management structure encouraging a high degree of contact and co-operation between projects.

## 7. Conclusion

The European Community, in developing a formal research and technological development programme, implemented a policy to subsidise prenormative and precompetitive research by its high technology industry sectors which would *maintain and strengthen their competiveness in global markets.*

The Commission's TIDE initiative is responsible for implementing this policy in the area of Rehabilitation Technology (R.T.). As has been shown, TIDE's pilot phase has been hindered by inadequacy of market information relating both to consumers and to products, and by a lack of programme cohesion. All these can readily be remedied in future.

Greater emphasis needs to be placed on the *global market* potential of future TIDE prototype products. If this does not occur the Commission will effectively be maintaining a market sector through subsidy, and will not be fulfilling the requirements of its research and technological development policy. It is suggested that the commercial potential of all future TIDE project proposals be assessed independently, in the light of all available product information sources, and that these assessments be considered in the project selection process.

The definition of R.T. currently used by the Commission through the TIDE programme is *technologies provided directly to elderly and/or disabled people, to enable them to live more independent lives and become integrated in the social and economic activity of their communities, preferably outside of institutional care* [7]. This potentially covers a much wider area than that addressed in the TIDE pilot projects as it takes in all products - including those from the mainstream - which might allow disabled and elderly people to live more independent lives.

TIDE consequently has two formal roles within the Commission's R&D programme through its *special responsibility* to develop a single market in R.T.: *i)* to develop prototype products and services through shared cost projects, *ii)* to ensure that technology research initiatives undertaken or funded by the Commission, and which *might* result in products or services being made directly available to disabled and elderly people, take account of their special needs.

Effectively **all** of the member states have implemented a social dimension into the research activities that they fund at the European level. It remains to be seen how this policy responsibility devolved to the TIDE programme by member states and the Commission will be effected (it is likely that most are unaware of the implications of their definition of R.T.).

TIDE has the potential to restructure the European R.T. industry. If implemented its responsibility to enforce market orientation across all Commission funded R&D programmes should make many items specifically developed for people with a disability unnecessary. Science and technology will be forced to adopt a human scale, and the potential market for telematic products in the single market will be enlarged.

## References

[1]     L. Krickau-Richter and O. von Scwerin. EC Research Funding: A Guide for Applicants. Directorate General XII, C.E.C., Brussels. 1990.

[2]     Commission of the European Communities. Background Information for the Call for Proposals for the TIDE Pilot Action. Brussels, March 1991.

[3]     S. Carruthers *et al*. The Market for R.T. in Europe: a Demographic Study of Need. In: Studies in Health Care and Informatics. IOS Press, Amsterdam, 1993.

[4]     S. Carruthers *et al*. Rehabilitation Technology in the United States and its Impact upon the Creation of a Viable European Industry Sector. In: Studies in Health Care and Informatics. IOS Press, Amsterdam, 1993.

[5]     P. Daunt. Meeting Disability: A European Response. Cassell Educational Limited, London. 1991.

[6]     J. Pierre. STOA Exhibition on Technologies for the Disabled. ADAPTH, Luxembourg. 1992.

[7]     Commission of the European Communities. TIDE initiative for disabled and elderly people: Pilot Action Synopses. ISBN 92 826 4570 3, Directorate General Telecommunications, Information and Innovation, Luxembourg, 1992.

[8]     SNRU. Rehabilitation Technology. Legislation, Regulations, Policy and Provision: A Preliminary Study of Current Status in the United States. The Market for Assistive Services (3). University of Northumbria, Newcastle upon Tyne. 1992.

[9]     TIDE. TIDE: Initiative Overview (from Pilot Phase to 2nd Phase), C.E.C., Directorate-General XIII, Brussels.

[10]    A. Wagner, STOA Exhibition on Technologies for the Disabled. ADAPTH, Luxembourg. 1992.

[11]    J. Shermer, Director of SRS Systems *pers com*, 1992.

[12]    James B.G. Trojan Horse: the ultimate Japanese challenge to Western industry. London: Mercury Books, 1989.

# Analysis of
# the Rehabilitation Technology sector
# in the Netherlands

V.P.P. SWARTE

Swarte, Consultants in Medical Technology
Bakenessergracht 52, 2011 JX Haarlem, The Netherlands

**Abstract**. The Dutch RT market show actors that have several strong interrelations, clustered in four mutual networks. Five of the actors influence the RT market by introduction of interventions. These interventions are based on three policies and they attack in three different battlefields. Indicators of the Dutch RT market motivate the introduction of interventions. Changing circumstances adapt the policies. Because of a stronger basis in the RT market, interventions can be more effective than ten years ago.

## 1. Introduction

### 1.1 Survey

An extensive research on the Dutch market of rehabilitation has been executed. Aim of the research is to investigate how effective interventions can influence the rehabilitation, RT, market. Methods to analyse the market have been developed [1] [2]. A wide spectrum of data from 1980 and 1990 have been collected [3] [4].

To understand the effectiveness of interventions, one has to understand the RT market structure and some parameters that characterize the RT market. These parameters motivate actors in the RT market to introduce interventions. In the Netherlands three policies formed the basis of interventions the past ten years. Recently conditions change, so does the RT market. These changes introduce threats and opportunities as well.

### 1.2 Interventions

An intervention will be defined as a specified interposition to stimulate, discourage or change the direction of the product- and moneyflow in the RT market. Not only government introduces interventions, also other actors in the RT market do. The interventions show a basic distrust in a free and competitive economic RT market.

## 2. The Dutch RT market

Figure 1 shows ten different actors in the Dutch RT market. They all have their own position and relations within the RT market. During the past ten years these relations strongly intensified. Most actors only are related to one or two other actors. It appears that these relations are clustered in four networks of strong mutual interrelations [4].

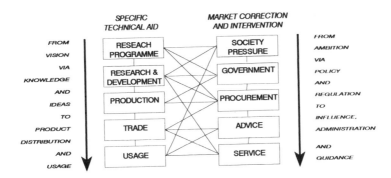

figure 1: Productcycle and market interventions

One network represents research and researchplanning. Research centres, government, social groups, research programme institutes and some industry take part in the network. A second network represents the pricing of technical aids. Social security, health insurance, industry, trade and advisors take part in this network. A third network represents selling, buying, and usage. Trade, advisor, service delivery and individuals with a handicap meet each other regulary. Government policy forms the last network, in which government, procurement and social groups are represented. Procurement, represented by health insurance and social security, has a central role in the Netherlands. They take part in three of relation networks. Only planning of research and productdevelopment is not within their scope. The actors are devided in two groups. Figure 1 shows that five actors form the hard-ware process from idea via product development to sell, buy and use. It is the basis for a free market. The other actors try to influence the RT market on their own way and with their own interest. While procurement tries to slow down prices and control the budget to meet the needs, other actors influence research or purchase decisions.

Some twelve percent of the Dutch population has a severe impairment. Nearly 50% of these people have severe impairments within more than one category. Eighty percent of the users of technical aids have more than one aid and from different categories [5].

In 1990 the Dutch spent 427 million ECU on technical aids. Ninety percent was payed for by social security, health insurance and hospitals. Price-quality rate is unsatisfactory, the average quality and usefullness of technical aids is low compared to general consumer goods. Last decade the Dutch RT market had an annual growth of ten percent, but within categories there are peaks and regressions. Recent government tries to slow down budgets [8]. Price will become a more important issue. The Dutch import of industrial constructed aids is more than three times as large as the export. Never the less, past decade export has grown to 50 million ECU. Most of the producers are small sized enterprices [6]. They are strong at very specific areas. Most of them are quite new companies, that only recent form mature organisations.

In the Netherlands, each year an average of fourteen million ECU is spent on research in rehabilitation technology and the development of technical aids. Research mostly is done at universities and research institutes. The connection between Dutch research and productinnovation is weak.


## 3. Why Interventions

Interventions of any kind often are ment to improve the potential for strategic product innovation and economic activity in the long term. In the RT market interventions also have a social component: to improve the quality and usefullness of the products. In the Netherlands four motives triggered initiatives to introduce interventions during the past decade. Unsatisfactory quality and usefullness of the technical aids lead to comparative testing by userorganisations. A negative quality/price ratio lead to the introduction of quality marks by social security and bargaining about prices. Because the fast growing market and relative weak position of industry, the Dutch minister of Economic affairs stimulated economic activity by focussing the intervention at subsidising productinnovations and structural networks between industry and research centres. A few years later the ministers of Health Care and Social Security introduced closed budgets to slow down the market-growth because of the immense costs of the health care and social security in the Netherlands. A lack of timing of the introduction of the interventions weakened the effect of each other. In case of a sequence of interventions a better result could be expected.


## 4. Basics in Intervention policy

Actors in the RT market have different motives and policies to introduce interventions. Three policies formed the basis of interventions during the past decade in the Netherlands.

The first policy started from the need of people with handicaps. It was a market pull strategy. The intervention was designed as comparative testing and public information about technical aids. The intervention appealed to the purchasing process and influenced trade, advisors, service and individuals with a handicap directly. After four years of publications, it appeared that the product information leaflets were wide spread and a strong way to influence the purchase desisions. In some cases the effect even was too strong. This kind of intervention needs a long time and balanced strategy.

The second policy started from the technology. It was a technology push strategy. The intervention appealed to research and product development and tried to introduce needs of people with a handicap in an early stage of design. At the same time the intervention stimulated economic activity. Research centres, social groups and producers were target groups with the intervention. Only to a selected group of industry the innovation stimulation programme fit into their business strategy. From those who took part of the programme, most of them still benefit the results.

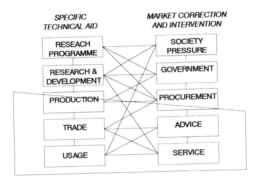

figure 2: The intervention battlefield in comparative testing

The third policy restructured the RT market. The aim was to get an overall control by introducing a new social security law in the Netherlands in 1976. Social security, health insurance, industry, trade and advisors were the target group. The introduction of a quality mark raised the bargaining power of procurement and changed the attitude of the manufacturers, even outside the Netherlands. At the same time the RT market gets less flexible and the costs of a quality structure seems to be substantial.

A side effect of the combination of interventions based on structural control and technology push was a strong growth of the export activity.

## 5. Perspectives

Dutch society changes and also government adapts its policy. Recent Dutch government announced the total reorganisation of the procurement of technical aids that must be realised in 1994 [8]. The key issues are cost-reduction, control and decentralisation. The budget to buy technical aids will be reduced. The new regulation must form an integral and coherence advisory route. Government wants to give full responsibility to the decision making units. The expectations are that only at the short term activity in the Dutch RT market will stabilize. Demographic developments, like the strong growth of the number of elderly people in the Netherlands, will introduce a strong pressure at the new system. Merging of companies can be expected, and also a strong accent on export. At the same time, Dutch companies grow mature. Interventions to stimulate research and product development will be more effective, when they link up with mature industry that know how to handle research and development.

The Dutch RT market is relative small. Small scale production will give problems in the future, when the RT market gets mature and prices will become an important marketing strategy. Production at an European level will give competitive advantage. Harmonisation and standardisation accellerates this process.

## 6. Discussion

In the Netherlands, interventions have been executed in parallel. Because of contra-productive interests, the effect was not as optimal as possible. Never the less, the RT market has become much more dynamic and mature. Introduction of new interventions might have a better basis to effective stimulation. Stronger network relations, more activity, more knowledge, more information and information channels, mature industry, they all are conditions to effective interventions. The Dutch survey shows that one of the problems that industry phases, is the lack of information about RT markets in other European countries. Practical knowledge of the dynamics in the European RT market is needed to execute surveys adressed to industry and the other actors in the RT market. At this moment the CORE [9] project is modelling the European RT market.

## 7. References

[1]    Porter, M.E., Competitive Advantage of Nations, MacMillan Press. London 1990
[2]    Nelson R., Winter G., An evolutionairy Theory of Economic Change. The Belknap Press of Harvard University Press. Massechusetts and London 1982.
[3]    Swarte, V.P.P. Strategic Interventions in RT. Internal document. Haarlem 1992.
[4]    Swarte, V.P.P., Technological Developments in RT. NOTA. The Hague 1992.
[5]    CBS, Statistics in the Netherlands. CBS. The Hague 1991.
[6]    Alders, B.C.M., Reaction at the Preliminary document regarding the Modelling of the RT market. STB-TNO. Apeldoorn 1992.
[7]    Swarte, V.P.P., Judgement of Quality and Usefullness of Technical Aids for People with Handicaps in relation to Product-choise. IG. Utrecht 1991.
[8]    Swarte, V.P.P., The procurement of Technical Aids. SDG, Utrecht 1992.
[9]    CORE is a TIDE subsidised project on consensus and awareness for R&D activities in technology for disabled and elderly people. Participants of the consortium are: IRV, RIC, STB-TNO, Swarte, Consultants in Medical Technology, The Netherlands; ICS-FORTH, N. Vernardakis, Greece; Handicap Institute, Infologics, Sweden; NAHW, Finland; RNIB, M. Fairhurst, United Kingdom; CNR, Italy.

# Rehabilitation Technology in the United States and its Impact upon the Creation of a Viable European Industry Sector

Stuart CARRUTHERS, Anne HUMPHREYS and Jim SANDHU

*Special Needs Research Unit, University of Northumbria,*
*Newcastle upon Tyne, NE7 7TW, United Kingdom*

**Abstract.** This paper describes the state of the Rehabilitation Technology industry in Britain. It is shown that North American R.T. manufacturers already have a considerable commercial presence in Britain, and that the USA probably has the most developed R.T. industry sector in Europe. The implications of the Americans with Disabilities Act (1990) for the development of a single European market in R.T. are discussed with particular reference to North American industry.

## 1. Introduction

The European Commission formally acknowledged in the early 1980s that lack of information about the availability of Rehabilitation Technology products was arresting the creation of a single market in this area. It implemented the development of the *HANDYNET* system to provide the market information needed by manufacturers and potential purchasers to stimulate the creation of a single market in rehabilitation products and services [1]. One of the Commission's main reasons for developing the *TIDE Pilot Programme* in the early 1990s was because it recognised that Europe's R.T. industry was threatened by American and Japanese competitors [2].

Since the early 1980s databases on R.T. products have been established and maintained in most countries in the European Community. These databases detail the availability of products in member states. In Britain the Special Needs Research Unit has maintained the *BARD* series of databases since this time, and is a member of the British *HANDYNET* Consortium.

*TIDE* has a strong market orientation and is aiding the development of prototype products and services which have good commercial potential [2]. The European Commission sponsors research and development: 'to maintain and strengthen the international competitiveness of European industry in high technology sectors, in the face of competition on global markets, above all from the USA and Japan' [3].

A significant market for R.T products and services exists in Europe. We estimate that there are currently about 26 million potential consumers living in Europe, and that this market will grow to about 33 million people by the year 2020 [4]. In this preliminary report, the state of the rehabilitation technology industry sector in the United Kingdom is assessed using the records contained on the *BARDTEC* database to determine the likely impact of the single market on this industry sector. The contribution of British industry to the *TIDE Pilot Programme* is also assessed to provide an indication of the state of the European R.T. industries and their ability to compete particularly with North American manufacturers.

## 2. Materials and Methods

### 2.1 Database Search

The Special Needs Research Unit maintains databases of R.T. telematic hardware and software available to consumers in the UK. It is recognised that these databases will never provide a complete record of all the products available in this country. However, their contents are a representative sample of the U.K. market for R.T., and probably contain between 80 and 90 per cent of all commercially available products.

Records of R.T. products from BARDTEC (a database of telematic hardware commercially available in the United Kingdom) were analysed and each product's cost, manufacturer and country of origin recorded. BARDTEC contains records of over 1,100 products actively marketed by R.T. manufacturers and retailers to British consumers.

### 2.2 Analysis of TIDE pilot programme participants

The organisations participating in the TIDE Pilot Programme were determined from the Synopses [2]. The country of origin of participants and their type (*industrial, research, university or other*) were recorded.

## 3. Manufacturers of Rehabilitation Technology in the UK & USA

BARDTEC records were analysed to determine the number of R.T. manufacturers active in the United Kingdom, their region of origin, and the number of telematic hardware products marketed by manufacturers from each economic region. The results of this analysis are shown in Table 1.

**Table 1.**    Showing the Number of Telematic Hardware Manufacturers Commercially Active in the United Kingdom, their region of origin and the number of products originating from each economic region.

| Region | Manufacturers | Products |
|--------|---------------|----------|
| UK | 123 | 563 |
| USA | 110 | 509 |
| EEA | 8 | 19 |
| **Total** | 241 | 1091 |

EEA: European Economic Area excluding the U.K.

## 4. Product Cost and Origin

BARDTEC records were analysed to determine the cost of products and the economic region from which they originated. The result of this analysis is shown in Figures 1 and 2. Thirty two per cent of the records on the database contained no pricing information.

Priced products were sorted into six price categories. About seventy five per cent of these products cost less than ECU 500. The country of origin of priced products for each price category was determined (Fig. 1). Lower priced products (<ECU 100) tend to originate from the U.K. while more expensive products (>ECU 500) are mainly manufactured in the United States.

The total value of all priced products described on BARDTEC amounted to ECU 524,987. Products manufactured in Britain accounted for 28 per cent of this figure. The remaining 72 per cent of total product value contained on the database orginated from the United States.

Figure 1. Showing the Country of Origin and Number of Products Maintained on Bardtec and Commercially available in the UK for Specified Price Ranges

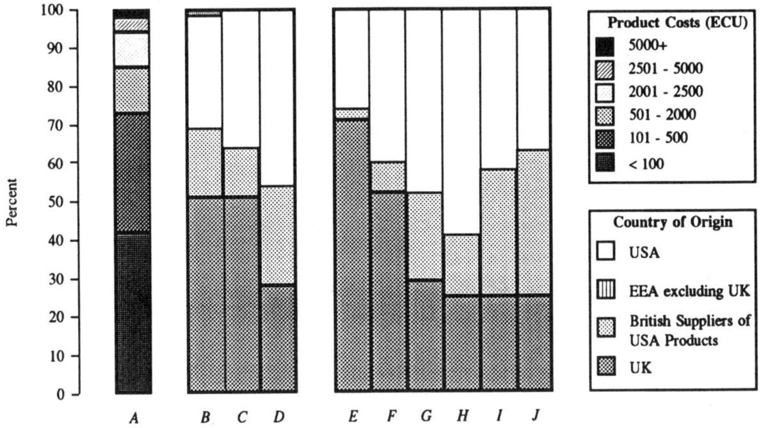

a: Showing the price distribution of R.T. products, b: Showing the country of origin of products, c: Shows the country of origin of priced products, d: Shows the value of priced products and country of origin, e: Showing the country of origin of products costing < 100 ECU, f: 101 - 500 ECU, g: 501 - 2000 ECU, h: 2001 - 2500 ECU, i: 2501 - 5000 ECU, j: 5000+ ECU

## 5. European Industrial Base

The TIDE Pilot Programme due to its inherently competitive character as part of the European Commission's R&D programme, required consortia of organisations drawn from European member states and EFTA countries to submit proposals for funding of projects which would develop R.T. prototype products and services with good industrial potential [2]. Analysis of the nationalities of the organisations involved in consortia which were successful in securing TIDE funding should give an indication of the state of the R.T. market within these countries due to the competitive nature of the programme.

Components of the R.T. market include consumers, developers (researchers), manufacturers and retailers. European policy for R&D programmes places the greatest emphasis on those components of the market which will maintain, increase or develop the manufacturing base of Europe. Analysis of the nationalities of the industrial partners in

TIDE should, due to the programme's competitive nature, indicate in which member states Europe's R.T. industries are strongest. The results of these analyses are shown in Fig. 2.

**Figure 2.**    Showing the Involvement of Member States and EFTA Countries (percentage) in the European Commisssion's TIDE Programme

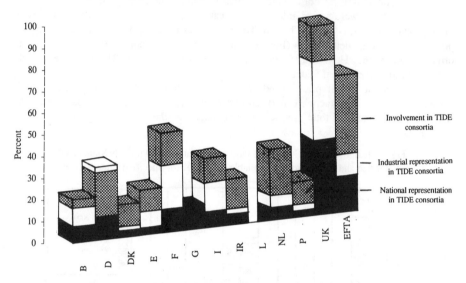

The United Kingdom has the greatest number of representative organisations taking part in the *TIDE Pilot Action* (29 per cent of participating organisations). It has the greatest industrial involvement (31 per cent of the industrial participants) and these organisations are involved in 67 per cent of *TIDE* consortia. It is also participating in more TIDE consortia than any other country or Bloc (81 per cent, of TIDE consortia).

These results suggest that the United Kingdom has the best developed RT industry sector within the European Community, and that its manufacturers should be best placed to take advantage of the single European market.

## 6. The Americans with Disabilities Act

The Americans with Disabilities Act (1990) (ADA) recognised that disabled people in the USA were subject to discrimination. By specifying that all work and leisure opportunities must be fully accessible to these people it has ensured they now have effective civil rights.

One of the stated aims of the ADA is to *regulate commerce*. In the USA business and service providers are now forced to take account of disabled consumers at a policy level. In 1990 British consumers spent about ECU 225 billion on consumer goods and services [5]. Assuming equivalent spending levels throughout Europe, consumers with special needs who are potential purchasers of R.T. products directly spent about ECU 100 billion on products or services where choice exists. Although special needs consumers are the exclusive users of products such as wheelchairs, screen readers and hearing aids, they are also active consumers of everyday products.

The USA through the ADA has implicitly recognised the importance of people with special needs to its national economy. European member states have yet to enact similar civil rights legislation.

## 7. Conclusion

One of the main reasons for the creation of the TIDE Pilot Programme was to counter the threat posed by the American and Japanese to the future competitiveness of the European R.T. industries.

Japanese companies in the high tec industries are already reporting in their promotional literature and company reports details of the steps they have taken to incorporate the needs of people with special needs in their products.

At the TIDE Pilot project CORE's meeting in London on 20th November 1992 a representative of National Cash Registers (a subsidiary of the American multi-national AT&T) reported that their company had incorporated the requirements of many disabled people in their automatic teller machines (ATMs) but had no intention of implementing this technology. The Japanese technology multinational Fujitsu in an advertising feature in Business Week makes a point of stating that it: *was the first company in the world to design and install these machines with voice guidance and braille features to accommodate visually impaired customers.* These are already installed in both the U.S.A. and Japan [6].

The United States has now regulated through the ADA that its business community must take account of the needs of disabled people. It would be logical to assume that the Japanese multi-national Fujitsu will soon develop a larger share of the American market in ATMs.

In the U.K. the majority of *high tech* products developed for the R.T. market and available to consumers would appear to originate from the U.S.A. Currently, there is neglible import penetration from the Far East. The U.K. would also appear from its representation in TIDE to have the greatest industrial involvement in R.T. in Europe. Over 40 per cent of European Community industrial involvement in the pilot programme originates from this country. There can be little doubt that the European R.T. industry needs to be strengthened if it is to maintain (or develop) its competitiveness on global markets in this area of high technology.

Europe is the largest single market in the developed world. The second largest is the USA. If Europe's competitiveness on the global market in high technology is to be maintained its industry needs to have access to the American market, and this now requires through the ADA that the needs of disabled people are incorporated within products. The Community needs to meet this challenge to its research and development programme as soon as possible.

## References

[1]    P. Daunt, Meeting Disability: A European Response. ISBN: 0 304 32386 1, Cassell Educational Limited, London, 1991.
[2]    Commission of the European Communities, TIDE initiative for disabled and elderly people: Pilot Action Synopses. ISBN 92 826 4570 3, Directorate-General Telecommunications, Information Industries and Innovation, Luxembourg, 1992.
[3]    Commission of the European Communities, E.C. Research Funding: A Guide for Applicants. D-G XII, Luxembourg, 1990.
[4]    S. Carruthers *et al.* In: The Market for Rehabilitation Technology in Europe and the United States: a Demographic Study of Need. Studies in Health Care and Informatics. IOS Press, Amsterdam, 1993.
[5]    R. Adams *et al.* Changing Corporate Values. ISBN 0 749 94074 2, Kogan Page Ltd., London, 1991.
[6]    Anon. Fujitsu: Technology is only the Beginning. Business Week. 6 April, 1992.

194

# Some Social Dimensions of Computer Support to Handicapped Persons in the Workplace
Report from a Nationwide Study in Sweden

Stig LARSSON, Ph. D.
*NOPUS, Box 12133, S-402 42 Göteborg, Sweden*

**Abstract.** This article is based on a sample of 713 out of about 11.000 persons in Sweden who have general financial disability support as the only benefit from the general insurance system, which means that by definition they are seriously handicapped and engaged in full time study or work. A vast majority (72.2%) of the population had their employment in the ordinary labor force. The others were employed thanks to various state subsides to employers. The category of visually impaired had the lowest degree of employment in the ordinary labor force (64.6%) and the group with "other" handicaps the highest (79.4%). Computerization in society in general has obviously also affected the group of seriously handicapped persons in their daily work situations: 42.1% of the population in the study stated that more than 10% of their work was computer-based and 25.7% stated more than 40%. The rate of computerization in the work situation was relatively equal in the various groups of handicaps. Only 8.2% of the respondents had received special computer equipment for handicapped persons. Over and above these, 19.2% of the total population declared that they wanted technical applications for work with computers. A number of other data on social dimensions of computer use of handicapped persons in the workplace is presented.

This article is based on a report written as part of a broad research project [1] made possible by grants from the Swedish Work Environment Fund. It describes the circumstances in which a nationwide survey [2] of severely disabled people was conducted and some findings which should be of interest in an international perspective. We thought such a survey was urgently needed, since there has as yet been no systematic analysis -- neither in Swedish nor in international research -- of the needs that severely disabled people may have for computers in their work. The use of a questionnaire can of course be discussed, as this method has a number of limitations [4, 5]. To obtain a population representing persons with severe disabilities who are in full-time employment, there is probably no better approach in Sweden than to take the category of people receiving disability allowance as their only pension benefit according to the National Insurance Act. To receive disability allowance one must have a permanent functional impairment. Only people over 16 and under 65 qualify.

At the end of 1988, a total of 47,047 people were receiving disability allowance in Sweden. Of these, however, only 10,538, or 22.4%, received it as their primary benefit, the others had either a half or two-thirds disability pension or temporary disability (sickness) benefit and were thus only partially in gainful employment.

The questionnaire was distributed in the spring of 1989. The form of the questionnaire was based on experience gained from a number of trial interviews. Without taking any extra measures apart from a number of reminders, we received replies from 78.1% of the subjects. When we analyzed the dropouts we found certain differences between the people who had and those who had not responded.

This presentation of the findings is based on data obtained through the questionnaire. A total of 557 responded, 58% of them men, 42% women. Most studies of the conditions of the handicapped show that they live alone to a much greater extent than the population as a whole. This can be explained to a significant extent by the age composition of the groups with disabilities of varying severity. The number of persons with mild or serious disability increases with age. In the 16--44 age group, for instance, only 1% is physically disabled (those with impaired mobility), whereas the corresponding figure for the Swedish population aged 75--84 is as high as 45% [7].

The proportion of people living alone is 27.5% in our material. For comparison we may mention that the figure for people aged 16--64 living alone is 14.8% of the population as a whole. Of the people in our study, 26.6% have only compulsory education. Compared with the 1985 study of the Swedish labor force, our data indicate that the education level is generally higher for people in our material than is the general case in Sweden. The corresponding figure for the labor force aged 20--64 was 39%. The proportion of persons in our survey with an academic qualification or a university education was 15.9%, whereas the labor force study had a figure of 11%. The intermediate categories of education do not allow full comparison. Nevertheless, on the basis of the low proportion with only compulsory education and the relatively high proportion with a university education, we can safely say that the level of education is higher among people in gainful employment with disability allowance as their only benefit than it is among the labor force as a whole.

There are, however, great differences from one handicap group to another. Twenty-five percent of the visually handicapped have a university degree, whereas the figure for those with impaired hearing is only 6%. In the group of physically disabled, the figure is 21.4%, and in the group with other handicaps it is 17.9%. This spread among the different groups can perhaps be interpreted as showing that impaired sight or mobility make it necessary for a person seeking entry to the labor market to have a higher education as a compensation for the disability. There is a large number of handicap groups in our population, and they are not always easy to distinguish. One handicap often entails another. Nor is it always easy to draw the line between chronic states of illness and the impaired functioning that can result from them.

Over a third of the persons in our material have been severely disabled since infancy (under the age of 1). Moreover, it is remarkable that less than a third (30.7%) suffered their severe disability after the age of 20. Naturally, the higher the age group, the lower is this proportion. However, this figure may be considered noteworthy. It indicates that, among the people who have such serious handicaps that they are entitled to disability allowance, relatively few who acquired their disability as an adult can support themselves completely through their own work.

If we examine the different handicap groups separately, 33.9% of the visually handicapped acquired the disability in infancy, 62.2% of those with impaired hearing, 23.5% of the physically disabled, and 19.3% of those with other handicaps. The distribution of the various handicaps in our study is: vision 10,1%, hearing 33,5%, mobility 35,5% and other handicaps 20,9%.

Since the subjects of our survey have only disability allowance, there are by definition none who have retired early with disability pension. This does not mean, however, that they all support themselves by working, much less that they all have a permanent job. In our material there were 79.3% who had a permanent job, more of these being men than women. There were 5.8% in temporary employment, more women than men. There is also a small group of self-employed (3.4%). People are constantly exposed to a process of socialization into work. Yet working conditions also influence the way workers perceive and evaluate themselves. For people with severe handicaps, deskilling tasks at work can mean that those who have already received a blow to their self-esteem as a result of the social stigmas that a handicap often involves, have their negative self-images reinforced. For this reason the questionnaire included a question in which we sought to elicit how the subjects perceived the competence level of their working tasks. More than one in five said that their tasks were below the level of the occupational skills that they felt they had. The proportion is so large that we could hardly expect to have obtained these figures if we assumed a roughly even distribution of the tendency to over- or underestimate one's own ability. It is naturally a highly complex matter to ascertain what a satisfactory work environment means in mental terms [7,8,9,10].

To obtain a rough measure of the way our informants perceive their work in a broad psychosocial perspective, the questionnaire posed the simple question: "Are you satisfied with your tasks?" The result shows relatively widespread discontent. The fact that only 60.1% said they were fully satisfied must be seen as a serious indicator that the work environment in a broad sense is relatively poor for full-time employees with severe handicaps. According to a recent nationwide survey [11], 32% of all those employed in Sweden used computers in their work. Computers are being used increasingly in the manufacturing industry, as well as in the service sector. Of people employed in banking and insurance in Sweden, 90% are computer users, while the business with the smallest proportion, agriculture, has only 10%. It is very difficult, however, to say how big a role computers play for individuals in the exercise of their profession. We therefore chose to ask the informants in our survey how much of their regular work they would describe as work with computers.

A clear majority (58.9%) use computers for less than 10% of their working time. It appears that the extent of computer use at work is fairly low among people with severe functional impairments if they are compared with the population of Sweden as a whole [11]. Even though computer use at work is lower among the severely disabled than among the population as a whole, our survey shows that computerization has had a greater effect on the working life of this group. Increased computerization has meant that many disabled persons come into contact with computers at work in a variety of ways.

There are large differences, however, between different handicap groups. The visually handicapped have computer-based technical aids in their work to a much greater extent than other disabled persons. As many as 42.9% of this group use computer-based aids in their work. For the deaf and hearing-impaired the figure is 7.9%, for the physically disabled 1.7%, and for people with other handicaps 2%. These figures are somewhat deceptive, however, since the visually handicapped are a relatively small group among the disabled. There is a significant group (19.2%) who have not had the opportunity to use computer-based aids in their work but who would like to.

Since there are a great number of actors in the rehabilitation arena (doctors, social workers, psychologists, technicians, educators, insurance administrators, and many more), the decision-making channels can be diverse, making it very difficult to achieve well-functioning, coherent communication with the individual to find the most appropriate technical solution. This is not the place to go into the problems inherent in the interplay between the various actors in the rehabilitation arena. It will suffice here to say that we had a question in the survey, "Are you satisfied with the way (administration, delay, procedure, etc.) in which you received your computer-based technical aids?" Only about half of the informants answered positively. It is obvious that the problems in handling the decision-making and delivery process concern more than finding an adequate technical solution. A similar conclusion has been drawn by another Swedish study [12].

We thought it reasonable to include in the survey a question about the informants' attitude to training in the use of computer-based aids: "Are you satisfied with the training in the use of computer-based technical aids?". The persons who were not completely satisfied with the training they received were in a majority. Generally speaking, the data from our survey indicate there is much to do in the sphere of training to make it easier for the disabled to use computer aids in their work. It must be emphasized, however, that training is often a complex matter; if it is to be successful it often requires continuous follow-up and feedback from work experience. Our survey included also a question: "Are you satisfied with the follow-up as regards technical support with computer-based aids?" Those who were completely satisfied with the service they had received after the installation of the equipment were in a distinct minority.

The extent to which the social network at the workplace functions as social support for the individual disabled person working with computer aids is probably one of the most decisive factors if a successful solution is to be achieved with the aid of new technology. Some studies suggest that people with handicaps have looser ties to their workmates than people in general [13]. Partly for this reason, but also against the background of our experience of trial interviews, it was natural for us to include in the survey a question about the possibilities of obtaining help with problems with computer equipment at the workplace. Roughly one person in four persons with computer-based technical aids always had access to someone in the immediate vicinity who could help with the equipment. The same number of people had such support most of the time. Nevertheless, there was still a majority who had access to such support only occasionally or almost never.

The question is, however, how often one needs access to technical assistance with computer aids. It was therefore natural for us to include a question that would provide an answer to this. A majority of the informants felt that they rarely needed help with the application of computer technology in their work, but one-third said that they needed it at least once a week. If we compare those who have good access to people capable of giving support with the extent of the need for computer-based technical aids, we see that roughly half of those who need help at least once a week only need technical aids rarely, and in some cases never. As regards the distribution according to handicap group of answers to the question of how often they needed technical assistance with computers, the following needed help at least once a week: visually handicapped 27.3%, deaf and hearing-impaired 41.9%, physically disabled 20%, those with other handicaps 50%. As we have said above, it was of special interest for us to try to shed light on the extent to which the groups of studied persons feel that their working tasks have been changed as a result of receiving computer-based aids. The background to this is the discussion about deskilling but also on coping [14,15]. In the questionnaire we had a question where we had the informants choose among set alternatives describing how their tasks had changed.

More than half considered that their tasks had improved as a result of being given computer-based aids. There was a clear difference between the sexes here. It appears that women more than men have unchanged tasks even after the introduction of computer aids. This is probably due in large part to the fact that many women do secretarial work and that their tasks did not change significantly when word processors replaced typewriters. With the use of computers for word processing, however, there are many more opportunities for handling text in a variety of ways; the fact that many people working with word processing have not been given better tasks may indicate the unwillingness or inability of the management to utilize the many possibilities of computer word processing.

Seven percent of the informants said that their tasks were worse as a result of the introduction of computer-based aids. This is a low figure, but still high enough to indicate that there is a risk that the use of new technology can mean deskilling in working life for the severely disabled. It seems obvious, however, that computers more often enhance competence and stimulus in working life, as our figures clearly show.

The overall picture is very clear. Thus far it seems that persons with severe disabilities working full-time have mostly seen an improvement in their working tasks as a result of being able to use computer-based technical aids. The fears that the new technology would entail deskilling have hitherto proved unwarranted, but this does not mean that we can ignore them, especially since it is reasonable to assume that the disabled people who have hitherto received computer aids are those who are highly active and among the most conscious in their handicap groups of the importance of having access to the aids that can compensate for their own disabilities.

**References**

[1] **Larsson, S:** *Disabled Persons Computers and Work: Perspectives on Psycho-Social Analyses* in *Computers for Handicapped Persons* (eds: Reiteter, H et al), R Oldenbourg, Wien, München, 1989
[2] **Larsson, S:** *Handikappade, arbete och ny teknik* (Disabled Persons, Work and New Technology), Hadar, Malmö, 1991
[3] **Kaplan, A:** *The Conduct of Inquiry. Methodology for Behavioral Science,* Harper & Row, New York, 1963
[4] **Sudman, S & Bradburn, N M:** *Asking Questions,* Jossey-Bass, San Fransisco, 1981
[6] **SOU 1990:19:** *Handikapp och välfärd* (Handicap and Welfare), Allmänna förlaget, Stockholm
[7] **Lennerlöf, L:** *Arbetsmiljön ur psykologisk och sociologisk synvinkel* (Work Environment from psychological and sociological perspectives), Allmänna förlaget, Stockholm, 1986
[8] **Hamburg, D A, Coelho, G V & Adams, J V:** *Coping and Adaptation: Steps towards a Synthesis of Biological and Social Perspectives* in *Coping and Adaptation* (eds: Coelho, G V et al), Basic books, New York;
[9] **Syme LS:** *Control and health: a personal perspective* in *Stress, personal control and health* (Steptoe A, Appels A, eds), John Wiley & Sons, Chichester, 1989
[10] **Karasek, R A & Theorell, T:** *Healthy Work. Stress Productivity, and the Reconstruction of Working Life,* Basic books, New York, 1990
[11] **Gärdin, O:** *Datorvanor 1990* (Computer Habits 1990), DF förlags AB, Stockholm, 1990
[12] **Hagström, T:** *Psykosocial förundersökning - arton provarbetsplatser* (Psychosocial preexamination. 18 test-workplaces), Tuffa-rapport 1989:1, AMS, Stockholm 1989
[13] *Synskadades levnadsförhållanden* (The living conditions of visually impaired persons), SRF, Stockholm, 1990
[14] **Lazarus, R:** *Psychological Stress and the Coping Process,* McGrow-Hill, New York, 1966
[15] **Burish, T G & Bradley, L A (eds):** *Coping with Cronic Disease,* Academic Press, New York, 1983

# Computer Technology for Impaired or Disabled Persons in an Occupational Environment. Experiences from a Five Year Project in Sweden.

Thomas Malmsborg BSc (occup. th.), TeleNova, Stockholm
*Box 1023, S 122 22 Enskede, Sweden, Phone: +46 8 399090, Fax: +46 8 395880*

Jan Breding MSc (eng), Swedish Labour Market Board, Stockholm
*S 171 99 Solna, Sweden, Phone: +46 8 7306000, Fax: +46 7306055*

Ulf Keijer PhD, Royal Institute of Technology, Stockholm
*S 100 44 Stockholm, Sweden, Phone: +46 8 7674720, Fax: +46 8 7678140*

**Abstract.** This paper presents experiences from the TUFFA project. TUFFA is in Swedish an acronym for Technical Procurement for Disabled Persons in Work Life. The regular deliveries according to the project started 1988 and till today approximately 1200 workplaces have been installed, of which all include advanced technology and computers. The paper describes a model for cooperation between different competences and a method for writing specifications of requirements, based on functional needs and environmental conditions. Two elucidating practical cases are presented.

## 1. Introduction

The TUFFA project started 1987 with a commission from the Swedish government to the Swedish Labour Market Board, (AMS). The background was a wish to widen the vocational field for disabled persons. In contradiction to the hopes of more and better jobs there was at this time a growing fear amongst persons with different kinds of disabilities, that new technology in general and information systems in particular would become a barrier for them, if nothing radical was done.

The project was run as a technical procurement. However, it was clear from the very beginning that a successful project would have to encompass more than technical development and manufacturing. Training of staff, development of the organization forms and development of knowledge of the physical work place and its psychosocial environment, were among the subjects that were identified. A holistic approach was adopted from the start and this became more pronounced over time.

After an extensive analysis of the demands, the specifications of requirements were written. The specification was based on competence and experiences at the Employability Institutes with special resources for disabled persons (Ami-S) in four handicap areas, i.e vision, hearing, physical impairment and intellectual handicap. The result became a list which contained both technical aids, standard computer components, standard software and components, or functions, that were not available at the market at that time. From this point of view it was clear that the functions and possibilities for the disabled person at the worksite, were more important than the actual technical aids. Therefore it was natural that the project very early was oriented towards procurement of a principal supplier.

## 2. Realization

The realization was carried out in two parallel phases, viz. the prototype testing and the regular deliveries. A formal contract was written between AMS and the principal supplier, TeleNova, a company at that time a subsidiary to Swedish Telecom. According to the contract, the principal supplier was to deliver 1000 complete adapted worksite within a period of 4 year. On the other hand the AMS took the responsibility for strengthening their organization as to make it possible to analyse and procure the presented number of worksites. This meant education, training and developing a new perspective in the means of purchasing advanced technology.

In the middle of 1992 the 1000th worksite was delivered and installed. These worksites are spread over a wide vocational field and concerns a huge number of different occupations, e.g., a blind physical therapist, a musician with cerebral pares, a deaf lorry driver, a statistician with aphasia, a blind lath operator, and many others. Today, 300 - 400 persons get their worksites adapted each year, which means 1 - 2 advanced installations of turn-key adaptions, each work day of the year.

### 3. Holistic Model and Organization

One of the essential issues of the TUFFA concept was to use the computer technology in order to let the disabled use his abilities productively. By not focusing on the difficulties, but on the contrary strengthen the individuals' capacity at the worksite, both the employer and the employee could benefit from the adaption. This approach demanded for a holistic view on the adapting process and a need to focus on all functions at the worksite, instead of looking at the technical aids isolated from the rest of the environment.

A model for this task was formed by the supplier and the Ami-S, and involved competence from three spheres, i.e. handicap, psychosocial and ergonomic competence (Ami-S), production and labour management competence (the employer), and finally, technical and project managing competence (the supplier), see fig 1.

### 4. Methods

A general method of adapting individual worksites with advanced technology has been established during these years and consists of three parts:
- the analysis phase; it results in an individually based, functional specification of requirements and tendering.
- the solution phase; it results in a solution, including an offer and a schedule.
- the realization phase with purchase, configuration, testing, adapting, training and installation.

### Holistic Model and Organization

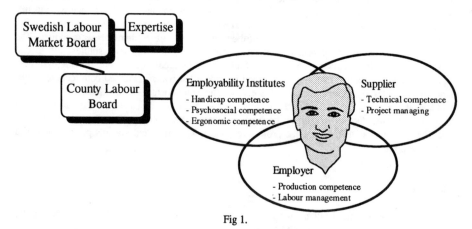

Fig 1.

If the analysis phase is carried out in a structured way, and really involves different competences, it has proved possible to put functionally based demands before technical, product orientated, ones. A procurement founded in a functionally based specification of requirements, can be focused on the main goals, instead of certain products. The TUFFA concept leaves to the principal supplier to choose the solution and the products. It's not in the interest of the purchaser what products are chosen as long as the main goals in the specification are attained to a reasonable cost. The main point is that the Employability Institute buys a "function" and the supplier is obliged to offer what is called a functional guarantee. Thus, he is required to alter the arrangements until the worksite functions according to the specification, on his own cost.

In this kind of procurement it is necessary that the supplier is free to choose whatever computer, software or technical aid he founds most suitable, regarding to production, environment, ergonomics and personal preferences of the individual concerned.

## 5. Encountered Problems

During these five years we have encountered some problems worth discussing. Most of them described and defined already at the start of the project.
- The systems' ability to define the problems at the work place, take the right measures required and describe functions rather than technical equipment.
- Getting the employers interested in employing disabled persons.
- The balance between the necessary cooperation and the distinguishing roles of purchaser and supplier.
- Making advances into non-traditional job areas, e.g. moving out from offices and trying other approaches such as workshops, services, etc.

We have continuously tried to find methods of further training for our personnel in the area of making the best possible use of the new technology. The reluctance of employers to employ or even try out disabled persons on different jobs is a major problem. There is an urgent need for new approaches in this area.

There has been an emphasized distinction between the purchaser and the supplier from the very beginning of this project. Without any doubt, this has been one of the explanations behind the success. Due to this division, there have been two motive powers in pulling the project forwards, i.e. the purchasers wish to help more persons and the suppliers wish to deliver more worksites. On the same token, there has been a great need for cooperation during all phases of any individual adaptions. Without cooperating competences it would have been impossible to attain a high technical level at the worksites, and still not loose the holistic view involving the rest of the environmental, ergonomic and psychosocial needs.

## 6. Conclusion and Future Prospects

The TUFFA project has so far been a success. About 1200 disabled persons have been able to get a job or keep their former employments due to adaption of their worksites with advanced technology. Furthermore, a joint venture between governmental and private bodies has been established and proved to be successful for the disabled person. A holistic model in analysing worksites and forming specifications of requirements according to functional goals, has been developed, and become a useful method for non-technicians to effectively purchase advanced technical solutions, get a secure guarantee and a possibility to measure the results against well defined goals, and still use their own vocabulary.

The different types of adapted worksites is spread over a wide field. The access to information and accessibility to information technology have, with no doubt, opened a wider vocational field for persons with disabilities. In addition, we believe that these, well adapted worksites, will increase the possibilities to accomplish new tasks and a chance for many disabled persons to offer their services in the production at their actual educational level.

The majority of the worksites, so far, are delivered to visually and mobility impaired persons. Still some important advances have been made for other handicap groups. Solutions and new ideas in using computer technology to support intellectual disabled, are perhaps one the most interesting prospects for the future. Although only a handful worksites for this group have been developed, there is obviously a great benefit achieved in allowing these people to take part in the production, instead of being subjects to allowances. It will be an inspiring challenge to continue these efforts.

Instead of being an obstacle, the information technology has proved to be a new opportunity to disabled persons. In both case studies below, it would have been extremely costly to adapt the worksites if modern information technology hadn't already been at hand. Accessibility to information systems have proved to be a ticket to new possibilities for a large number of disabled persons.

## 7. Case Studies

### 7.1. A Blind Library Assistant

The user, (L), is a woman, employed at a school library. During the last years her eyesight has gradually been reduced, to the point that she can only distinguish between light and dark, i.e she is functionally blind.

Her former tasks at the library consisted of lending and receiving books, give informations on the books and put them back onto the book shelves.

When the analysis phase started, the county library had recently invested in a central database which contained information on the books, authors and abstracts on the books. A barcode had been provided on all books and the customers registration cards. The facts above formed the functionally based demands on the adaption:

---
*Functional demands*
L, who is blind, shall be able to continue her work with lending, receiving and placing books in the shelves. She should be able to register the lendings into the database at the county library.

---

### 7.2. Solution

A small radio transmitter was developed, which was able to send data from all points of the library to a personal computer in the office. The computer was equipped with a modem and an emulation program for communication with the computer at the county library. The personal computer was also equipped with at synthetic voice, a loudspeaker and a radio transmitter. Finally the shelves were marked with barcodes at certain critical points and a book trolley was manufactured with a barcode reader and the radio transmitter attached to it, see fig 2.

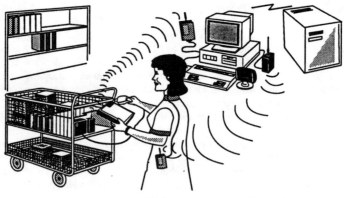

Fig 2.

L is now able to register the lendings and put the books back in the shelves. She reads the title of the book white the barcode reader. The transmitter sends the data to her computer and uses it to search for information in the database, via the modem.

The information is sent back the same way, from the database to the computer, is read by the synthetic voice and transmitted to a tiny radio receiver attached at L's ear. In about 2 seconds time she gets the information according to the book she is holding in her hand.

With the barcode reader and the software in her personal computer she is also able to register the lenders and the books they lend or bring back, in the central database.

### 7.3. An Intellectual Disabled Petrol Station Attendant

The second case study, describes a intellectual disabled man, (S), who was unemployed and received a pension when the adaption work started. He was not able to read or write and he could not count. The petrol station would benefit from his work if he could be able to put prices on the goods for the store and place them in the shelves. The main part of the goods was marked only with an article number when delivered from the supplier, and because S' disability to read, he often placed the goods at the wrong shelves in the store.

> *Functional demands*
> S, who is intellectual disabled, should be able to put prices on the goods at the petrolstation and correctly place them on the shelves in the store.

### 7.4. Solution

A portable barcode reader was connected to a very small micro computer and adapted with one green and one red lightbulb. A software was developed, which compared two barcodes and lightened the green lightbulb if the readings were similar. A personal computer was placed at the stock, containing a database from the supplier of the goods. In addition to this computer, a software was developed which, if it got a correct input of article number, immediately wrote a label with a barcode and the price, stored in the database. Finally the shelves in the store was marked with barcodes corresponding to the goods.

With his portable micro computer with the attached barcode reader, S is now able to place goods in the store at their correct places. With the database he is capable of putting the right price on each article.

When S is working at the computer he "copies" the article number, figure by figure, from the article to the keyboard. If he copies the number incorrectly, no label is produced and he has to try again. Due to this he attains a high level of security in his work, gains self confidence and gets a chance to develop his skills.

S, himself, when putting the barcode at the goods, is therefore in a way producing his own technical aid.

**References:**
[1] Breding J, Keijer U., 1992, Computer-based Technology for Disabled Persons in Work Life: A Holistic Approach. In New Technologies and the Employment of Disabled Persons, (eds. Hunt & Berkowitz). International Labour Office, Geneva 1992.
[2] Ami-S, Employability Institutes with special resources for disabled people, Swedish National Labour Market Board, 1987.

# MODEMA - A Knowledge Based Browsing System to Facilitate the Employment of People with Disabilities

Jill HEWITT, John SAPSFORD-FRANCIS
University of Hertfordshire, Hatfield, Herts, ENGLAND
Greta BOLSTAD, Olav EFTEDAL
SINTEF Unimed, N-7034 Trondheim, NORWAY
Philip HALFORD
Compris Consulting Limited, 56 Boycroft Avenue, London, ENGLAND
Dirk VERVENNE, Michael VERHEYEN
BIKIT, Plateaustraat 22, 9000 Ghent, BELGIUM

**Abstract**. This paper describes the stages of the MODEMA project which have been carried out to establish the user requirements for a computer system and to implement a prototype version. Sections describe the Market and User Analysis, the Knowledge Extraction methodology, modelling and implementation and the evaluation procedures. Finally, potential exploitation possibilities and future developments are discussed

## 1. Introduction

The MODEMA group is building a computer based system to assist with the integration of people with disabilities into paid employment. It is intended to provide help to three categories of user - employers, employment advisors and people with disabilities who are seeking work. The knowledge to be encapsulated in the system includes legislation and advice relevant to people with disabilities seeking employment, as well as details of specialist equipment to augment the abilities of 'differently able' people in various employment tasks. The system utilises multimedia technology to provide video and photographic information to enhance its information base. While supporting general database browsing facilties, the system also offers a task and user-profiling structure which provides a guided route through the data bases to enable the user to home in rapidly on the required information and to browse through relevant areas via a hypertext facility.

In the early stages of the project, a market and user analysis was carried out to establish the potential market for the system and the existence of relevant information in the participating countries. In order to ensure that diverse user requirements were met by the system an iterative prototyping approach was followed, allowing maximum exposure of the emerging system to potential users and enabling evaluations to be carried out throughout the project. The knowledge embodied in the system was captured through a program of structured interviews and questionnaires, designed to capture both general knowledge about working environments and the more detailed and diagnostic knowledge held by disability experts.

## 2. Market and User Analysis

In the process of collecting and compiling information which could serve as background information for subsequent knowledge extraction for the computer based system as well as describing the potential market for such a model, it became evident that the relevant data were either lacking or only available in a form not adequate for the MODEMA system. Data describing the number and distribution of people with various types of disabilities, their level of education, current employment rate, legislation concerning disabled people as well as information on various available services, were collected in England, Belgium, Spain, Portugal and Norway, by the respective partners in the consortium. The initial aim of the work was to compare these data, treat them statistically and present them in a manner suitable for comparing living and working conditions for disabled people with those of the corresponding able-bodied populations in the five countries. However, it was apparent that available data suffered from various weaknesses.

In most of the five countries important information, such as level of education and annual income, was lacking. Other types of data may exist, but were not suited to be compared with corresponding data from other countries because the underlying basis and/or the statistics were not comparable. Even when based on the same survey, different publications may report different numbers describing the same topic. For instance for Spain, three different publications report that 7.6, 10 and 14.98% of the total population are disabled [1,2,3]. One report [4] argues that the number of people with reduced functions defined by fairly objective criteria is considerably larger than the number of people who acknowledge that they are disabled when asked about it. The information collected has been fed into a database, but due to the inconsistencies in the available data, the results are presented separately for each of the five countries.

The aim of the user analysis was to identify and describe the various categories within the frame of the project. Two main groups of user were identified: 1) users of the workplaces, i.e. the disabled person applying for work, and 2) users of the computer model. Potential users of the computer model may be: Advisors for and employers of disabled people, equipment producers or the disabled themselves. The informaiton collected through the user analysis is focussed on physical characteristics and performance and perception abilities for the different user categories. A brief discussion on how these characteristics and abilities may influence the funcitonal abilities of the person is also included, to help decide which tasks the particular disabled person may or may not be expected to perform adequately.


## 3. Knowledge Extraction

Three types of knowledge model were required for the system - models of working environments and their adaptation for people with disabilities, models of 'expert' knowledge relating to all aspects of the integration of disabled people, and models of the potential user groups. In each case, it was important to use a knowledge extraction technique suitable for the task in hand and to develop a method which would:
* be portable across international boundaries
* allow knowledge extraction by practitioners with varying degrees of expertise
* be usable in a wide variety of settings
* be capable of testing existing hypotheses about the knowledge base
* capture knowledge in a form that is readily convertible for input to the computer system

To build generic models of working environments, it was important to cover a wide range of scenarios in all the participating countries, and a task checklist approach - TOX [5] was considered appropriate since this gave a broad but shallow coverage of many work places. The elicitation of an expert's knowledge however could not be undertaken without an in-depth interview, so it was recognised that a smaller number of cases would be studied, but in much more depth. The models of users were developed through the prototyping and evaluation cycle, which are discussed in sections 4 and 5.

### 3.1 Task Oriented Cross Referencing (TOX)

This method utilises an iterative approach to building a generic model and is designed to be operated over several iterations, using a checklist that has been refined where necessary to better reflect the generic model. In addition to the checklist, a short questionnaire is provided to elicit such details as job title, disability, length of employment, type of organisation etc.

A preliminary task analysis is carried out for a specified environment to develop a set of hypothesised generic objects and actions. These are represented on a "cross referenced checklist" which is used in subsequent knowledge capture interviews. The left hand side of the checklist contains lists of typical actions, grouped according to the 'role' to which they belong, so for example 'supervise staff' comes under the managerial role, whereas 'take minutes' and 'arrange meetings' is under 'administrative'. The role headings are there for guidance, but in practice most office jobs involve tasks from a number of roles, although they tend to cluster around one or two. In the shop floor environment, some jobs involve only a single task (e.g. 'counting'), although others such a 'maintenance engineer' encompass many different activities. Along the top of the form are a list of typical tools used to carry out the tasks, e.g. telephone, pen & paper, typewriter, memo etc. - but in the case of disabled employees these may need to be augmented by compensatory equipment - recorded on the right-hand side.

Once the forms have been completed they are sent back to the 'expert' knowledge elicitors who use the information to refine and build the generic models of the workplace, and where necessary to amend the forms for the next knowledge extraction round. After the first knowledge extraction round it was decided to prioritise tasks on a scale of 1 to 5 rather than just marking them as core or peripheral. In addition, the vertical columns were discarded in favour of free-format text describing tools used for the job. The analysis of these forms is currently taking place.

The revised models of the working environments are fed into the prototype computer system which is used to validate the model against the knowledge of the end users.

### 3.2 Knowledge Extraction from 'Experts'

Two methods of recording an expert's knowledge were used for this project. The first, based on ADESCIRA [6] is designed to be used in conjunction with a fast prototyping approach. It uses a rule-based approach to create dependency trees and rule tables from raw interview transcripts. The steps of the method are as follows:
- **chunk** the information and if necessary pretreat any graphical data
- build a **topic tree**, which is useful for offering an overview of content and making a list of reference points useable in later phases
- build an **object-attribute-value** table - this is the main database of the model and records all entities with their prime functions their attributes and attribute values
- build an **object hierarchy** from which inheritance relationships can be derived
- build a **dependency tree** which shows interdependence between objects
- build a **rule table** to express the protocol's knowledge in the form of rules
- build a **lexicon** which defines all terms used in the model

This method is suitable for use on experts with extensive knowledge of a particular area - e.g. legislation relating to the disabled, however there was not enough time available in the project to use this method widely, so a second method based on a structured interview format was used to get a wider but shallower coverage of experts' knowledge in the major aspects of the system domain, these are the following:

Legislation: All aspects concerning legislation related to the integration of disabled people. e.g. What is the employment quota of disabled people?

Financial support: All aspects concerning grants related to the integration of disabled people. e.g. What grants are available to help an employer to adapt the workplace and buy compensatory equipment?

Service Institutions: All aspects concerning services and support related to the integration of disabled people. e.g. Which are the experts in the field who could advise?

Training and education: All aspects concerning training and education related to the integration of disabled people. e.g. What training courses can be followed?

### 4.    Modelling and Implementation

At the heart of the system are currently three databases - compensatory equipment, legislation and advice. These can be browsed in 'normal' database mode, but the strength of the system lies in the fact that it allows a multiperspective view of the information, based on the task models of the working environment and disability profiles. In this mode, a user will:

- select a disability profile (e.g. severe visual handicap)
- select a working environment (e.g. office)
- select a task from the list of tasks presented (e.g. arrange meetings)
- be presented with a list of activities related to this task for which further information is offered for the selected disability (e.g. reading, writing, telephone use)
- select an activity (e.g. reading)
- be presented with a page of free text (the equivalent of an expert's knowledge) with hypertext words which can be selected to take them to relevant parts of the information base.

The prototype systems are written in Knowledge Pro to run under Microsoft Windows on any standard PC. Photographs of equipment are included in the equipment database, and video clips show compensatory equipment in use in working environments. Case studies relating to disabled employees can be accessed to provide further insight into various aspects of the knowledge base.

## 5. Evaluation

Evaluation took place in each of the five participating countries. It was essential that the evaluation procedure would be applied uniformly. Accordingly, validation organisers for each country attended a validation workshop. Here the method of evaluation was explained and the organisers participated in example evaluation sessions.

An early decision in the project was that validation and evaluation should be carried out by samples taken from the population of the narrow domain experts that provided the expert knowledge in the first place. The confirmatory bias of hypothesis testers is well established e.g. [7,8]. One way of avoiding this bias is to have the evaluation carried out by people who did not generate the hypotheses. We have seen that these knowledge sources are numerous and widespread and that to carry out an effective validation, narrow domain experts in all participating countries would have to be approached. Furthermore an adequate selection from the three main types of narrow domain experts should be approached: people with disabilities, employment advisors and employers. Access to experts has provided a major bottleneck in this project since there are relatively few experts and each one typically has expertise in one aspect of the field. Accordingly it was decided that knowledge extraction would proceed in tandem with system evaluation and validation.

An important part of scenario based evaluation is the selection of appropriate and representative scenarios. To use a scenario that has been the source of current knowledge does not adequately test the validity of a knowledge model, so for this reason test scenarios were collected from local contacts independantly of the main knowledge extraction process. Scenarios provide rich contexts that enable problem solvers to access knowledge that may otherwise be hard to reach (e.g. [9]).

Within each evaluation session, three short scenarios were used to train the validators to use the prototype. They were then asked to carry out three specified test scenarios and comment on the usefulness and accuracy of the information provided. The evaluation session finished with the completion of a structured interview designed to ensure the evaluator's views were captured as accurately as possible. Transcripts of the evaluator's responses were collated along with the evaluator's name, experience, area of expertise, any useful background information, country and locale of testing, name of the evaluation organisor, date and version of the prototype.

The integration of this mass of data from five countries presented something of a challenge. Conflict resolution can be a serious problem when extracting knowledge from multiple experts, on the whole however, conflict resolution has not been a problem in the MODEMA project. The key to effective conflict resolution was the maintenance of audit trails to enable us to track knowledge representation deceisions back to the knowledge extraction or validation processes that gave rise to those decisions and the main factors that influenced those processes. To maintain and use these audit trails, the following were important:

- recording the characteristics of the evaluator: name, experience, area of expertise, nationality and locale on which that expertise is based
- recording the characteristics of the evaluation session: name of the organiser, date of the evaluation and version of the prototype
- documenting all conclusions drawn from evaluation reports and referencing them to the reports on which they were based
- documenting all decisions about changes to the knowledge structure and cross referencing them to the conclusions above
- all documents were annotated with counterindications from evaluation and knowledge extraction sources.

## 6.0   Exploitation and future developments

By the end of the project, the team will present a working demonstrator system with the following features:
- customised interfaces for the three user groups, to take into account expert and novice modes
- specialist interfaces for blind and motor handicapped users
- examples of all types of information, with approporiate photographs and video clips

If the funding becomes available, the work of MODEMA will be extended to provide a system that will support pan-European information flow. This will incorporate Structured Annotation to allow users to update information, support for management of the data by domain experts, the further development of non-standard interfaces for use by people with disabilities, and a generic system that will assist in the translation process for data input to the system, facilitating translation by language experts with no system domain or computer expertise.

In order to implement such a system, there is a need to establish an infrastructure for a pan-European information system, based on centres of expertise, with clusters of sites attached to each centre.

## 7.0   References

[1]   Ministerio de Asuntos Sociales: Las personas con minusvaia en Espana, Madrid, 1989.
[2]   The United Nations: The United Nations Disability Statistics Microcomputer Data Base (DISTAT), Version 1, 1988.
[3]   Alfonsin E.T, Ferruelo M.G: Survey of impairments, disabilities and handicaps in Spain, in: International Journal of Rehabilitation Research, Vol. 12, No. 2, HVA. Edition Schindele, 1989.
[4]   Fredriksen J, Martin M, Puig de la Bellasca R, Von Tetzcner S : The use of telecommunication: The needs of people with disabilities. Fundesco and Telefonica, COST 219, Madrid 1989.
[5]   Hewitt, J. and Sapsford-Francis, J. 1992 A Knowledge Extraction approach for capturing dispersed knowledge and its application to the modelling of working enviornments for people with disabilities. International Cybernetics Conference, Namur.
[6]   Vandamme, F. Vervenne, D. 1991, The Adescira versus KADS/SKE KT Methodology. BIKIT Library Bulletin Vol 5. nr. 6 pp 98-103
[7]   Sanford, J. 1987 The Mind of Man, The Harvester Press.
[8]   Baron, J. 1988 Thinking and Deciding, Cambridge.
[9]   Sapsford-Francis, J. Britton, C. and Brown, J. 1992 Problem Solving (..in Computer Science) ISTIP '92, Proceedings of the 5th UK Conference.

# Session 3:

## Methodology of R&D Programmes

# A Method to Analyse the Strain of Memory of Elderly Persons Working with Information Technologies

Andreas GOURMELON

*Projekt VAG-CT, Univ. Erlangen, Glückstrasse 6, D-8520 Erlangen, Germany*

**Abstract.** The demands on human memory are a major barrier for elderly persons in the interaction with information technologies. Moreover, these demands are increasing, while memory capabilities are decreasing. With the help of ANI - Analysis of Identifiers - the strain of memory which occurs if two or more programs are used can be measured. ANI promises to be a reliable, economic and valid method.

## 1. Information technologies and the human memory

Information technologies (IT) have become the gate to modern social life. For example, if you want to catch a train you will have to buy your ticket at a machine; the money which is needed for this purchase will be handed over by a cash dispenser.

The use of IT is widespread and increasing. But a lot of people - especially elderly people - have difficulties to interact with IT and this may result in a reduction of social activities. Rudinger observed in his field study people (more than 60-years-old) using ticket-machines [1]. Twenty-four percent of the elderly failed to buy a ticket, 66% reported problems in using the machines, 80% bought a ticket which was too expensive for its purpose. Interestingly enough, younger persons had problems with the ticket machines, too (10% failed, 51% reported problems). Notice that the elderly persons who failed to use the machines were members of an already positively biased sample. It may be argued that many elderly persons stay at home and do not even try to use a ticket machine.

In a qualitative field study, von Benda, Staufer and Jamnig investigated the problems elderly employees (45-65) have working with computers [2]. Not surprisingly many employees mentioned bad illumination conditions, small screen sizes, noise and unsuitable furniture. The elderly employees also complained about reduced control over the working-process, time pressure, autocratic introductory processes and negative stereotypes concerning ageing which resulted in modest training opportunities. However, the main finding of the study was that a lot of employees experienced a massive strain of memory: statements like "... it is difficult to change from system A to system D or vice versa, ... each program has its own command names", and "In my age I forget facts easily, but as I have mentioned earlier there have been a lot of facts to remember" indicate this strain. For elderly persons this strain of memory is harder to compensate than for younger ones  because they usually have only weak prior computer knowledge: "Older persons ask questions which younger persons wouldn't have asked", "You really become angry ... these young guys are more familiar and quicker with the technology ... they know the coherences" [3][2]. In addition, elderly persons have difficulties in learning new materials. The encoding of new information is not so pronounced as it used to be, more time and expenditure are needed to transfer the learning material into the long-term store. Also, the capacity of the short-term store diminishes, basic cognitive processes slow down. In many cases the retrieval of formerly learned material fails.

## 2. The increasing demands on the memory

As described above, the strain of memory seems to be the major barrier in the interaction with IT. Moreover, persons who already experience a decline in their cognitive capabilities are confronted with increasing cognitive demands. Take for instance the increasing complexity and functionality of a text-processing program as it is shown in table 1.

Table 1: Increasing complexity and functionality of a text-processing program [4]

| features | WordPerfect 4.2 | WordPerfect 5.0 | WordPerfect 5.1 |
|---|---|---|---|
| year | 1987 | 1989 | 1991 |
| pages of reference guide | 417 | 631 | 972 |
| amount of functions | 250 | 350 | ca. 400 |

Table 2: Different ways of interaction in several programs [4]

| function | program | keys/command names |
|---|---|---|
| help | Harvard Graphics 3.0 | press F1-key or klick the help button |
| | WordPerfect 4.2 | press F3-key |
| exit | Brain 3.0 | press ESC- or '0'-key |
| | WordPerfect 4.2 | press F7-key |
| | Windows 3.0 | klick the field 'file' in the menu bar |
| | Harvard Graphics 3.0 | klick 'exit'-button or press 'E' |
| copy file | MS-DOS | copy |
| | UNIX | cp |
| list files of a directory | MS-DOS | dir |
| | UNIX | ls |

In four years the complexity of the program has doubled. The demands on the memory functions are even higher if the elderly person has to use several programs because usually the ways to interact with IT are different (table 2).

## 3. Possible solutions

After describing the problem of increasing memory demands on the one hand and decreasing memory capabilities on the other I will turn to possible solutions. One strategy is to improve the memory of elderly persons and to qualify them for interaction with IT. It has been demonstrated that this strategy can be successful, but the costs for training are enormous [5]. Furthermore the studies showed that trained elderly persons can be lifted up to the level of younger untrained persons, but having the competence of a younger person does not mean to be able to master successfully every important demand (remember Rudinger's ticket machine study). The second strategy is to reduce the memory demands. To reach this goal, one must first know what the specific demands on the memory are. We have to analyse and measure the strain of memory. Promoted by the German ministry of youth, family and seniors our research group, which consists of cognitive psychologists and computer scientists, are developing a method to tackle this task. In the next paragraph a method will be presented that analyses the strain of memory which occurs when two or more programs are used.

## 4. Analysis of Identifiers

The strain of memory experienced by a person working with several programs may be defined by:

$$SM = \sum_{i=0}^{n} sm_i + I_{sm}$$

In this definition SM indicates the total strain of memory, $sm_i$ the strain of memory caused by the program i and $I_{sm}$ the strain of memory which derives from the usage of n programs. If the user-interfaces of the n programs are perfectly identical, $I_{sm}$ would be zero. In practice, software-packages which integrate several programs within one kind of user interface (for example MS-WORKS) may aproximate to this value.

With the help of the Analysis of Identifiers (ANI) the value of $I_{sm}$ can be estimated. ANI is based on a model of knowledge-transfer [6]. A transfer of knowledge how to interact with one program to another program will be successful, if

- the interaction of both programs is based either on recognition or recall,
- command names and/or icons are similar,
- the places where a memory output is necessary are corresponding and
- the actions of the users and their chronological order are the same.

Therefore, the first step of ANI is to check whether the identifiers of a chosen set of functions meet the requirements of a successful transfer. An identifier of a function may be a command name, an icon or anything else which makes the function work. Because it is not possible to compare all functions of two programs, we have chosen the functions "load file from permanent memory into working memory", "help", "print file", "save file" and "finish program". These five functions seem to be available (and necessary) in most programs. The result of the first step is a list of elements which documents what the user must do to start the function (table 3).

Table 3: The lists of elements representing the necessary mnemonic operations to start the function "load file from permanent memory into working memory" in WordPerfect 4.2 and Harvard Graphics V 3.0

Function: loading a file from permanent memory into working memory

| *Reproduction or Recognition* | *Where do I have to remember?* | *Which name or icon do I have to remember?* | *What do I have to do?* |
|---|---|---|---|
| WordPerfect 4.2 (german version) | | | |
| recognition | function-keys | Dateiverzeichnis | press F7-key |
| reproduction | III (quadrant of monitor) | A: | keyboard input + return |
| recognition | variable | name of file | cursor |
| recognition | III | laden | keyboard input |

(continuation of table 3)

| Reproduction or Recognition | Where do I have to remember? | Which name or icon do I have to remember? | What do I have to do? |
|---|---|---|---|
| Harvard Graphics V3.0 (german version) | | | |
| recognition | I | Datei | keyboard input or return or mouse klick |
| recognition | I | Graphik laden | keyboard input or return or mouse klick |
| recognition | I | A: | keyboard input + return |
| recognition | I | name of file | keyboard input |

The second and final step is the comparison of the element-lists of two or more programs and the computation of $I_{sm}$.

The advantages of ANI are that the time to learn and apply ANI is short, it is easy to use and it offers both objective qualitative and quantitative results. The disadvantages of ANI are that the application of ANI is restricted to user interfaces which are internally consistent and that ANI is still in preparation. But we are hoping that the studies to prove the reliability and validity of ANI will be finished by the end of 1993. Then we will also present a method to estimate $sm_i$.

**References**

[1] Rudinger, G. (1992). Abschlußbericht zum Projekt "Alter und Technik" (ALTEC): kognitive Verarbeitung moderner Technologie. Bonn: Universität Bonn, Institut für Psychologie.

[2] Benda, H. von; Staufer, M. & Jamnig, S. (1989). Ältere Arbeitnehmer und moderne Bürokommunikation. Erlangen: Universität Erlangen, Institut für Psychologie I.

[3] Staufer, M. (1992). Technological change and the older employee: implications for introduction and training. Behaviour & Information Technology, Vol. 11, 1, pp. 46-52.

[4] Benda, H. von (1992). Anforderungen an Gedächtnisleistungen bei der computergestützten Arbeit von älteren Arbeitnehmern. Vortrag auf dem Kongreß "Erwerbsarbeit der Zukunft", 3.-4. November in Berlin.

[5] Hartley, A. A.; Hartley, J. T. & Johnson, S. A. (1983). The older adult as computer user. In: P. K. Robinson, J. Livingstone & E. Birren (Eds.), Aging and technological advances (pp. 347-348). London: Plenum.

[6] Anderson, J. R. (1990). Cognitive psychology and its implications. New York: Freeman.

# In What Ways Can the Psychology of Perception Contribute to the Development of Rehabilitation Technology?

Gunnar Jansson

*Department of Psychology, Uppsala University*
*Box 1854, S-751 48 Uppsala, Sweden*

**Abstract**. Even if rehabilitation technology is mainly a technical enterprise, the usefulness of an aid is highly depending on its adaptation to the characteristics of the human users, not the least their sensory equipment. The psychology of perception may contribute to increasing this adaptation in three ways: by providing stored knowledge, by producing new knowledge, and by suggesting methods for evaluation. It is argued that stored and new knowledge may be especially useful early in a project by saving time and effort in finding the most promising options, while the evaluation methodology can contribute at a later stage. At short sight, economic constraints and time limits are the most severe obstacles for a full utilisation of the knowledge of perception; at long sight, it may be wise to invest in acquiring this knowledge.

## 1. Introduction.

The development of rehabilitation technology is, as all technology development, mainly a technological enterprise. This may be seen as self-evident, but it is not the whole truth when there is a human operator, as it always is in the case of rehabilitation technology. The human operator and the technical device form a system with two contact surfaces: (1) the information input from the device to its user and (2) the output from the user by which he/she controls the equipment. This is standard knowledge in human factors and human engineering contexts [1]. However, it seems not seldom to be forgotten when technical inventions are discussed and devices evaluated. The aim of this paper is to give an overview of the contributions that one of the basic sciences, the psychology of perception, can make in order to make a technical device better adapted to the user.

The emphasis in this paper is on the input side, that is on the information provided by the device to its user. How successful the input is depends to a high degree on how well it fits to the properties of the human sense involved. A complication in the case of rehabilitation devices is that the information may have to fit a not perfectly functioning sense or a sense not normally handling the kind of information in question.

That the perceptual side is emphasised does not mean that the output side is meant not to be important. On the contrary, it should be considered very important, not the least because of the close interaction between perception and action; cf. the theory of perception developed by Gibson [2].

Perception is the oldest subject area within experimental psychology. Knowledge in this area has been collected since the middle of the nineteenth century. This means that many data can be found by reviewing the literature. However, there are many lacunas in our knowledge about the senses which means that knowledge in many cases has to be found by new investigations. This is often the case in applied contexts where the knowledge wanted about specific kinds of information can not be discovered in, for instance, studies of basic problems. The experience of making experiments on the perception of human subjects may also be useful in the evaluation of final versions of rehabilitation equipment. The three kinds of utilisation of knowledge from the science of perception (stored knowledge, new knowledge, and methodological knowledge) will be further discussed below.

## 2. Stored Knowledge

The standard method of finding stored knowledge in perception is to search in a suitable data base, *Psychological Abstracts* being the first choice. For both a first orientation and later more detailed studies, handbooks such as the one of Boff, Kaufman, & Thomas [3] may be helpful. A handbook specifically aiming to be used in human engineering contexts has also been edited [4]. If you are lucky there may be a book discussing the specific kind of rehabili-tation equipment you are interested in. Examples from my own field of study are books on electronic travel aids [5] and on themes related to tactile pictures [6].

What can be found in handbooks of this kind is basic data about the functioning of the senses, such as their sensitivity to different kinds of stimulation, including absolute thresholds, difference thresholds, and optimum stimulus values, but also data on a more complex level, for instance perceptual organisation and spatial orientation. I think that a search of the literature on relevant topics early in the building of a prototype may save much time and money. Technological devices with poor adaptation to the properties of the senses may be sorted out before too much work has been devoted to them and too much money spent. However, I have got the feeling that a systematic search of knowledge of this kind is seldom made, but the technological development is started without it.

## 3. New Knowledge

It often happens that the information wanted is not found even if a careful search is made. This may be the case both when the knowledge wanted is general and when it is specific for a special device context. One option is to guess an answer and hope that the device will be useful with the choice of parameters made. This is risky, of course. A safer alternative is to make an experiment on your own. Preferably this is made, in the case of a general problem, as an ordinary perception experiment, or, when the problem is more device-oriented, as a simulation study where the relevant parameters are investigated without building a real device. Astonishingly enough, this alternative is not very often used in rehabilitation technology, in spite of its apparent advantages. The existence of all those prototypes that were not successful because of insufficient usefulness should suggest the advantage of an early detection of the problems including the perceptual ones. However, the attention is too often focused on the technical problems of building a prototype.

Making an investigation to get new knowledge might prove very worthwhile in terms of both work and money. It may show that the version originally planned will not work as expected, but, maybe, that an alternative should function better.

## 4. Methodological Knowledge

When the device has got its final form, or is close to it, some kind of evaluation is usually made, preferably before the aid reaches the market. However, such evaluations can have very different forms.

One alternative is to give the aid to some handicapped persons asking them to make a judgement after having used them freely at home. This may seem to be a straight-forward way to make an evaluation. However, there are difficulties with this method. If the instructions are very general, the evaluators may consider quite different aspects of the functioning of the device, and many aspects may not be judged at all. If more specific instructions are given, an analysis of what the important aspects are must be made. This may sometimes be a quite demanding task requiring much both theoretical analysis and empirical work. Further, it must be decided how the user should give his/her judgement, for instance by a free state-ment, or by answering a series of specific questions, which can be made quite sophisticated.

However, the aim to get information about the functioning of an aid may not be reached by asking for verbal descriptions by the user. It is a very difficult task for a user to give a fair statement by just observing oneself. A safer method is to make experiments where the users' performance is measured under well-controlled conditions.

Such methods are developed within experimental psychology. It is in the present context suitable to remind about two main kinds of experiment, laboratory and field experiments [7]. The laboratory experiments are the most controlled ones, often suitable in the above-mentioned search for new knowledge. When the task is to evaluate final versions of an aid a field experiment is an interesting option.

I will give only one example by mentioning a method developed for travel aids for the blind [8, 9]. With this method the users' performance in natural contexts is videotaped and carefully analysed in a number of aspects. The difference between the performance with and without the aid can be objectively evaluated. When making a field experiment of this kind some of the control of the environment is lost, but, hopefully, the investigation gains in relevance for the understanding of the use of the aid in practice. Unfortunately, there are not many examples of methods of this kind developed in the context of rehabilitation technology.

## 5. The Ideal Situation and Difficulties in Realising It

From the point of view of the psychology of perception, as I see it, the ideal situation for the development and evaluation of products in rehabilitation technology, where perceptual information is essential, should include three phases: (1) a careful review of relevant literature, (2) new experiments, often laboratory experiments, about problems for which no solution was found in the literature, (3) experiments evaluating final products or close-to-final prototypes, often of the field experiment type.

There are probably few cases, if any, where the development of a rehabilitation device has strictly adhered to such an ideal situation. There is often a jumping between the different phases. For instance, there may be an original idea about a technological product and the work starting with the building of a prototype (phase 3). If this does not work as expected, a following step may be to search in the literature (phase 1) and/or making an experiment on a basic problem (phase 2).

The realisation of the ideal situation may also be blocked by economic constraints, as well as by time limits. These can, of course, not be neglected, but the result may be products that are less useful than it could have been if both stored and new knowledge in perception had been taken into account. I argue that the probability of developing a useful device increases with attention given to this knowledge, as well as that a more reliable evaluation can be made by measuring the performance of users in controlled conditions. In the long run, the time and money spent on including knowledge from the science of perception may be a wise investment.

## Acknowledgements

The author's ongoing research in this area is funded by the Swedish Council for Social Research and the Swedish Work Environment Fund.

## References

[1] M.S. Sanders & E.J. McCormick, Human Factors in Engineering and Design (Seventh edition). McGraw-Hill, New York, 1993.

[2] J.J. Gibson, The Ecological Theory of Visual Perception. Houghton Mifflin, Boston, 1979.

[3] K.R. Boff, L. Kaufman, & J.P. Thomas (Eds.), Handbook of Perception and Human Performance, Volumes I and II. Wiley, New York, 1986.

[4] K.R Boff & J.E. Lincoln (Eds.), Engineering Data Compendium. Human Perception and Performance, Volumes I - III. Harry G. Armstrong Aerospace Medical Research Laboratory, Wright-Patterson Air Force Base, OH, 1988.

[5] D.H. Warren & E.R. Strelow (Eds.), Electronic Spatial Sensing for the Blind. Nijhoff, Dordrecht, the Netherlands, 1985.

[6] W. Schiff & E. Foulke (Eds.), Tactual Perception: A Source book. Cambridge University Press, Cambridge, England, 1982.

[7] G. Jansson, Development and Evaluation of Mobility Aids for the Visually Handicapped. In: P.L. Emiliani (Ed.), Development of Electronic Aids for the Visually Handicapped, Nijhoff/Junk, Dortrecht, the Netherlands, 1986, pp. 297-303.

[8] Armstrong, J.D., Evaluation of Man-Machine Systems in the mobility of the visually handicapped. In: R.M. Pickett & T.J. Triggs (Eds.), Human Factors in Health Care. Lexington Books, Lexington, MA, 1975, pp. 331-34.

[9] A.G. Dodds, D.D.C. Carter, & C.J. Howarth, Improving Objective Measures of Mobility. *Journal of Visual Impairment and Blindness* 77 (1983) 438-442.

220

# The design and evaluation of rehabilitative computer technology for blind people: the need for a multi-disciplinary approach

Helen Petrie, Technical Research Department, Royal
National Institute for the Blind, 224 Gt. Portland St.,
London W1N 6AA, United Kingdom

Thomas Strothotte, Institut für Informatik, Freie Universität
Berlin, Nestorstraße 8 - 9, D - 1000 Berlin 31, Germany

Gerhard Weber, Institut für Informatik, Universität
Stuttgart, Breitwiesenstraße 20 - 22, D - 7000 Stuttgart 80,
Germany

Frank Deconinck, Vrije Universiteit Brussel, Laarbeeklaan
101, B - 1090 Brussels, Belgium

**Abstract.** If rehabilitative technology is to be of maximum use, a multi-disciplinary approach to its design and evaluation should be adopted. This paper will outline research from disciplines such as psychology, ergonomics, computer science and human-computer interaction that can contribute to the development of more effective rehabilitative technology. This approach will be illustrated with examples from the GUIB Project (Graphical User Interfaces for Blind People), a TIDE project to develop multimedia systems to adapt graphical user interfaces (GUIs) to computer to make them accessible to blind people.

If rehabilitative technology (RT) is to be of maximal use to disabled people, a multi-disciplinary approach to its design and evaluation needs to be adopted. In this paper research from a number of different disciplines such as psychology, ergonomics, computer science and human-computer interaction will be discussed to illustrate how these disciplines can contribute to the development of more

effective RT. Examples will be given of how a multi-
disciplinary approach to design and evaluation is being used
and further developed within the GUIB Project (Graphical
User Interfaces for Blind People), a TIDE project to develop
multimedia systems to adapt graphical user interfaces (GUIs)
to computers to make them accessible to blind people. GUIs
raise severe accessibility problems to blind people in terms of
both input to and output from computers [13]. The research
areas to be discussed in this paper will be:

(a) methods of evaluation of multimedia computer
    systems,
(b) the integration of design and evaluation in
    developing computer technology,
(c) modelling computer interfaces by formal and
    informal methods,
(d) users' mental models of computer systems, and
(e) blind people's understanding of graphical
    information.

To evaluate the usability of rehabilitative computer
technology, we are building on techniques developed by
research in the disciplines of ergonomics and human-computer
interaction [7]. These techniques offer a variety of methods,
such as questionnaires, surveys, observational studies and
experiments for conducting scientific evaluations of computer
software and hardware. However, such techniques have
generally been developed for the evaluation of single medium,
visual systems. Systems for blind users such as GUIB system,
which deal with the complexity of information provided in
GUIs, need to be multimedia, including speech, sound and
tactile information. We need to evaluate the usability of each
different information channel, but also how the usability of
the total system is affected by the interaction between the
different information channels. Is a multimedia system simply
the sum of its parts, or more or less than that sum? This
question has implications for multimedia technology both
within and beyond the RT field and techniques for the
evaluation of multimedia and hypermedia computer systems
are only beginning to emerge in human-computer interaction
research [12]. In the GUIB Project we are developing new
evaluation techniques suitable for such multimedia systems,
which will be transferable to the evaluation of other
multimedia and complex systems in all RT domains.

Researchers in the field of human-computer interaction
argue that design and evaluation of computer technology need
to be integrated in an iterative cycle. Analyses of the tasks
which users want to perform and the problems they encounter

in performing those tasks produce a rationale for the (re)design of computer technology; the evaluation of this technology in use produces further information for (re)design of the technology. These two processes of (re)design and evaluation should iterate to produce more and more effective computer technology. Carroll *et al.* [2] have referred to this cycle as the *task-artifact cycle*, the artifact in this case being the item of computer technology. This is an important, if controversial, concept that needs to be considered in the development of RT. One way of informally modelling the tasks which users perform which can also be applied in the area of RT is through the development of *scenarios*. Nardi [11] has characterised scenarios as "a description of a set of users, a work context and a set of tasks that users perform or want to perform". Thus scenarios are a way of grasping the interaction between users and computers that avoids the difficulties of formal modelling techniques developed in computer science, although the concept is not without problems [1,8]. Scenarios can be developed with respect to the needs of disabled users as well as those of their more able bodied colleagues. If such scenarios are included in mainstream human-computer interaction practice as well as in specifically RT work, the development of more accessible computer systems would be greatly facilitated [10].

Within the GUIB Project more formal modelling of the interaction between users and systems is also being developed. Modelling such interaction has been studied in the light of formal methods for the construction, description and evaluation of user interfaces [4]. Models based on relations over sets of input and output units, grammars or symbolic descriptions have been proposed in the past. For example, a formal rule-based model described by an Event Response Language (ERL) has been implemented for a drawing program [6]. This approach is being further developed for studying interaction between blind users and computer systems using an ERL [14] known as the GUIB-ERL. This type of language is well suited to model event-driven user interfaces. Any input or output (e.g. key press, mouse movement) fits into the event model of the ERL. One of the advantages of an ERL is that simultaneous input of two input devices (e.g. mouse and keyboard) can be expressed. This is particularly important in a multimedia system. This type of modelling assists in making design of RT less manufacturer-specific, and a more co-operative procedure between manufacturers, rehabilitation specialists and users.

A further consideration in the design-evaluation cycle that has come originally from psychology is the concept of a *mental model.* Users form mental models of how computer systems work through their interaction with the system and their prior experiences and beliefs about computers. The study of mental models has proved useful in understanding how people solve problems and undertake tasks involving complex systems such as computers [5, 9]. In the GUIB Project the concept is being used both in terms of understanding what mental models users have of a GUI, and of how their mental models develop by interacting with a system. The concept is also useful in investigating blind people's understanding of graphical information. What mental models do blind people have of spatial metaphors like the computer interface? If we are to provide alternatives useful to blind people to the graphical information presented in GUIs, we need to know what limits the understanding of graphical information by blind people, in order to be able to reorganise this information in ways which will make computer systems more easily understandable to these users. Classical computer vision or image understanding approaches often reduce the understanding problem to a perception or classification task. In understanding blind users' exploration of computer interfaces, this approach is too limited and one has to take non-computable information, such as task context, cultural and emotional factors into account [3]. These factors are also being included in the design-evaluation cycle of the GUIB Project.

All these lines of research are contributing to the multi-disciplinary approach adopted within the TIDE GUIB project. They can aid in the development of more useful, acceptable rehabilative technology in many other areas.

This research is supported by the Commission of the European Communities under the TIDE Pilot Action (Technology Initiative for Disabled and Elderly persons).

References

[1] R.L. Campbell, Will the real scenario please stand up? *SIGCHI Bulletin* **24** (1992) 6-8.
[2] J.M. Carroll, W.A. Kellogg and M.B. Rosson, The task-artifact cycle. In: J.M. Carroll (Ed.), Designing interaction: psychology at the human-computer interface. ISBN: 0-521-40056-2. Cambridge University Press, Cambridge, 1991, pp. 74-102.
[3] F. Deconinck, C. Stephanidis and G. Weber, Access to pictorial information by blind people. In: J. Cornelis and S. Peeters (Eds.),

Proceedings of the IFMBE North Sea Conference on Biomedical Engineering. 1990.

[4]    M. Farooq and W.D. Dominick, A survey of formal tools and models for devloping user interfaces *International Journal of Man-Machine Studies* **29** (1988) 479-496.

[5]    Gentner and A. Stevens, Mental Models.    Lawrence Erlbaum, Hillsdale New Jersey, 1983.

[6]    R.D. Hill, Supporting concurrency, communication and synchronization in human-computer interaction - the Sassafras UIMS, *ACM Transactions on Graphics* **5** (1986) 179 - 210

[7]    J. Karat, Software evaluation methodologies.   In: M. Helander (Ed.), Handbook of Human-Computer Interaction.   Elsevier Science Publshers, Amsterdam, 1988, pp. 891 - 903.

[8]    C.-M. Karat and J. Karat, Some dialog on scenarios, *SIGCHI Bulletin* **24** (1992) 7-17.

[9]    D.E. Kieras and S. Bovair, The role of a mental model in learning to operate a device, *Cognitive Science* **8** (1984) 255-273.

[10]   W.W. McMillan, Computing for users with special needs and models of computer-human interaction. Proceedings of CHI '92. ACM Press, New York, 1992.

[11]   B.A. Nardi, The use of scenarios in design, *SIGCHI Bulletin* **24** (1992) 13-14.

[12]   G. Perlman, Evaluating hypermedia systems, Proceedings of CHI '90. ACM Press, New York, 1990.

[13]   H. Petrie and J. Gill, Current research on access to graphical user interfaces for blind people. *European Journal of Special Needs Education*, in press.

[14]   G. Weber, Modelling interaction of blind people using graphical user interfaces. In: F.H. Vogt (Ed.), Personal computers and intelligent systems - Information Processing '92, Volume III. Elsevier Science Publishers, Amsterdam, 1992.

# Information for People Planning Technical Research for Visually Disabled Persons

J M Gill

*Royal National Institute for the Blind, 224 Great Portland Street, London W1N 6AA*

**Abstract.** The TIDE CORE project is studying the information needs of the different groups within the rehabiliation technology field. However there is already some experience at Royal National Institute for the Blind with information provision for research workers in the field of visual disability. The most common types of information asked for, by research workers, are:

| | |
|---|---|
| (a) | What research and development needs to be done? |
| (b) | What research and development is being done? |
| (c) | What research and development has been done? |
| (d) | What are the sources of funding for research and development? |

The paper emphasises that nobody in this field can afford complacency in information provision since the nature of the market and the rehabilitation technology actors relationship with it are constantly changing.

## 1. Introduction

The TIDE CORE (Consensus Creation and Awareness for R&D Activities in Technology for Disabled and Elderly People) has identified seven main groups of actors in rehabilitation technology as:

1. Research
2. Development
3. Production
4. Trade
5. Procurement / financing
6. Service delivery
7. Usage

The CORE project found that most rehabilitation technology actors made little use of on-line computer-based information services, but mainly relied on paper-based services; this is compatible with the findings of surveys among those undertaking technical research for visually disabled persons which indicated a desire for printed information on:

1. Research and development needing to be undertaken.
2. Sources of funding for this research and development.
3. Ongoing research and development.
4. Existing products for visually disabled persons.
5. Existing techniques.
6. Published papers and "grey" literature.
7. Exploitation of research and development.
8. Demographic data.
9. Standards.
10. Organisations concerned with visually disabled persons.

The Royal National Institute for the Blind (RNIB) is in the process of integrating its information services for research workers to better meet the changing information needs of this group. There has been an increase in the number of small companies who do not have the resources or expertise to access on-line information services, as well as many of the information services being inappropraite to their needs. This has led to an increase in the gap between information rich and poor.

## 2. R&D Needed

The identification of research needed by the visually disabled population has been tackled in collaboration with the Research Committee of the World Blind Union, the European Project on Technology and Blindness, and the EC COST project on Telecommunications and Disability. Various areas have been identified as priorities for future research taking into account the probability of the work being of long-term practical benefit to visually disabled persons. The current task is to convert the data into a structured form suitable for storing in a database format.

A related area is to bring these unmet needs to the attention of the research community including those who have had no previous connection with rehabilitation technology. So far, this aspect has been tackled by writing articles and giving lectures in universities and research departments of companies.

## 3.     Sources of Funding

In the present economic climate, it is essential for most research workers to find external sources of funds for their research work. As yet, little systematic work has been done on data collection in this area, but there is an increasing unmet need to inform research workers of relevant calls for proposals in sufficient time that they may prepare an application. There also is a need to advise research workers on how to prepare grant applications to the various grant giving bodies; for instance, some research workers have had difficulty with the style and format of applications required by the European Commission.

## 4.     Ongoing R&D

The database, which dates back to the early seventies, covers ongoing non-medical research and development for visually disabled persons throughout the world; the main mode of dissemination is as an annual printed publication. A newer database, funded by TIDE but located at RNIB, covers core actors in rehabilitation technology in Europe; this database is produced in print as well as on computer diskette.

## 5.     Existing products and techniques

A computer-based system has been developed which includes information about devices which are already on the market; the scope is limited to those groups of devices of greatest interest to research workers concerned with visual disability. This system will be superceded by the European Community Handynet system when it becomes fully operational.

In addition, a technique is a method of doing something which may not involve any technical device (eg with a long cane, the technique is more important than the device for efficient pedestrian travel). However information services have avoided attempting to create databases in this area since techniques are very difficult to classify and to describe concisely. But, it is in areas such as techniques that the research worker needs to be aware so that their prposed research does not re-invent the wheel.

## 6.     Published material

Traditionally, research workers relied on published papers as their main source of information, but in the fast changing area of technology the information is often out of date by the time it is published.  Also much of the useful reports in the field of visual disability appear in "grey" publications which may not be covered by the main bibliographic databases.  Therefore specialist bibliographic databases are seen by many research workers as less important than they were ten years ago.

## 7.     Exploitation

Academics working on technological research for visually disabled persons are increasingly aware of the problem of transferring their research to being of practical benefit to visually disabled persons.  Therefore they often ask for infomation about methods of exploiting research results; in general, the earlier this information is requested, the more likely that the research results in a useful product or service.  In the blindness area, the market is often very distorted by substantial subsidies from non-profit organisations; this can mean that a new product has to compete against an existing product which is being sold for less than its manufacturing cost!

## 8.     Demographic data

Demographic data about the incidence and prevalence of visual disability, age and income distribution, and prevalence of additional handicaps is often requested by persons new to the field.  More reliable, but incomplete, data is now available for the visually disabled population in the UK.

## 9.     Standards

As well as requiring information on national or international standards which apply to various types of assistive device, research workers often want precise specifications for areas for which there is no formal standard (eg the spherical radius for a braille dot).

## 10.    Organisations

Research workers often want contact with local organisations concerned with visually
disabled persons; most often this is so they can gain access to experimental subjects for
evaluation purposes.


## 11.    Conclusions

The information needs of any given group are a constantly changing target. Information
systems and services must be designed so that they provide appropriate information in a
suitable format. This means that the content and method of delivery must be constantly
reviewed to ensure that they are still optimum for the changing needs.

# Tools for Living: Design Principles for Rehabilitation Technology

Ian Craig, Paul Nisbet, Phil Odor, Marion Watson
*CALL Centre, University of Edinburgh, 4 Buccleuch Place, Scotland*

**Abstract.** This paper addresses some issues of design of rehabilitation technology. We argue that the complexity of configuration and use, of emerging R.T. systems must be managed if systems is to be practically useful. We suggest that the nature of the market demands open, modular systems. A modeless, object-oriented design developed for an intelligent powered wheelchair is presented by way of example. The approach provides an open, cost-effective technique for designing and developing complex R.T. systems.

## 1. Introduction

Developments in materials science, production techniques and, in particular, information technology provide new possibilities and challenges for rehabilitation technology (R.T.). R.T. systems can be designed and built to tackle tasks which were simply impractical or beyond the technologies of even a few years ago.

For disabled and elderly people, the benefits are systems which are more sophisticated and capable of a wider range of tasks in home, work and school than were previously possible, and which are accessible by a greater number of more severely disabled people.

However, in order to deal with such breadth of function and application, R.T. systems are becoming more complex and a central task for designers is therefore to limit or manage this complexity to produce a system which is usable by both professionals and by disabled and elderly people.

This paper presents one approach to the problem of design for use, developed as part of the design of the CALL Centre Smart Wheelchair. The Smart Wheelchair was originally developed as a motivating educational and therapeutic resource for use by and with severely and multiply disabled children [1]. The chairs are not designed simply as mobility aids (although they do perform this function), but as tools for assessing and developing physical, cognitive, social and communicative skills. Thirteen chairs have been built to date and evaluated in three locals schools, another was built for a young adult in a residential hospital, and another three systems are to be produced for adults in pre-vocational training establishments.

The Smart Wheelchairs are adapted, computer-controlled powered wheelchairs (the system can in principle be fitted to any powered wheelchair) driven with a wide range of devices such as switches, joysticks, laptop computers and voice-output communication aids. They are fitted with sensors to safeguard the pilot and environment and enhance uses and applications. The number of different possible chair configurations is large, yet the developers, practitioners and users require to configure the system to meet individual and specific needs quickly and easily. The system is therefore representative of a class of R.T. equipment which is becoming increasingly common.

## 2. Design principles, constraints and considerations

### 2.1 Design aims

Our approach to design was intended to produce systems which could be:

• *extensible* - use of augmentative mobility for education and therapy is a relatively novel concept and the development team anticipated revising and extending the initial specification as experience in use and applications was gained. Therefore, our architecture should permit development of new facilities without significant re-design of the existing system, and subsequent configuration of a chair incorporating these new features had to remain straightforward.

• *open* - the potential Smart Wheelchair 'market' is characterised by unusual breadth and heterogeneity in relation to overall size. An open system design makes use of existing components and standards and allows other developers to contribute to the range of compatible systems, giving efficient development and dissemination.

• *usable as a system component in larger integrated designs* - for example, in combination with *smart house* solutions to independent living; augmentative communication aids; or keyboard emulators.

• *tailorable* - an extensible, open system developed for use by children with widely varying needs, skills and environments will necessarily offer a very wide number of individual system configurations (56 in the original Smart Wheelchair specification defined in 1987, not including variations in control devices) and if the system is to be at all useful in a busy school environment, it must be quickly configurable by staff, carer or child.

### 2.2 Modularity

Each of these aims implies modularity of mechanical, electronic and software design. A modular system simplifies addition of new functions by the developers or third parties; eases and reduces the cost of constructing individualised systems by eliminating unnecessary items; and helps to create a *modeless* system. As Odor [2] points out, moded systems can impose unnecessary structural complexity upon the user, can hinder the development of new modules which do not fit neatly into the system modes, and require the user (whether parent, carer, professional or chair pilot) to retain a needlessly complex mental "map" of the system with which to deduce how the desired system configuration might be achieved. Modularity of design applied to the Smart Wheelchair also implies:

• *distributed processor design* - wheelchair motor control is handled by one of a number of commercially available motor controllers; the pilot's control device can be an augmentative communication aid or laptop computer offering many different styles of user interface; and the Smart hardware and software is based upon a multi-processor design.

• *adoption of object - oriented techniques* - taking advantage of message passing protocols between hardware/software modules, re-usability and extensibility.

• *continual review of emerging external standards, components and systems* - to enable these to be incorporated into the design where appropriate.

## 3. Implications of design principles

### 3.1 Object orientation and modularity

Usually, object-oriented methods are used to guide the *internal* design and development of systems. In some systems (such as WIMP environments) the internal architecture can also be reflected at the user level. The Smart Wheelchair adopts this principle in an attempt to design for the *encapsulation of functional modules* (referred to as tools)*as objects*. In other words,

Smart Wheelchair tools are both externally, functionally distinguishable and mode-free user features, *and* internal representations and associated data structures with messages. Therefore, the implication is that (especially in distributed processor systems) object oriented emphasis and interest lies more in the opportunities for designing flexible polymorphic message passing and the simple incorporation of new objects which add new functions, than in, say, benefits of inheritance or reusability of code. However, designs like ours, with mode-free arbitrarily combinable tools, must provide clear indications to users of what the system is doing. The approach is through a combination of transparency of chair behaviour, and an explicit subsystem (called the *Observer*) reporting to the user.

## 4. Relationship to other development programmes

### 4.1 Behaviour-based systems

The concept of the Smart Wheelchair as a bag of tools, each of which performs a specific, definite functional task or behaviour has close parallels with the *subsumption* architecture developed by Rodney Brooks and colleagues [3]. Brooks' architecture decomposes the system into layered co-operating task-achieving behaviours, rather than along classical functional lines. His approach offers . While the Smart Wheelchair tools exhibit some of the characteristics of Brooks' behaviours, it is important to note that Brooks' intention is to build *autonomous* robots while ours is to build a fail-safe aid for a human being.

### 4.2 The COMSPEC project

The COMSPEC [4] team is developing an open, modular, object-based, extensible, system-as-component architecture to provide an open protocol for building augmentative communication systems. A key aspect of COMSPEC is the adoption of a *language model* defining the specific content, grammar and structure of the system's capabilities and function. Aspects of this have informed the Smart Wheelchair power-up procedure, where the distributed processors inform each other of their capabilities (tools) and corresponding internal objects. The Smart Wheelchair will eventually reply to COMSPEC system requests for these functional profiles.

### 4.3 Smart House

The development of interconnection standards for smart houses requires a common message-passing system emphasising distributed, cooperative, multi-vendor processors. The hardware and message-passing protocols developed for the Esprit Home Systems bus are relevant to the Smart Wheelchair design, but more important is the possibility of integrating Smart Wheelchairs with smart houses to provide a seamless system for the user.

### 4.4 ISO Wheelchair Control standard

ISO Working Group 7 [6] are currently defining an interconnection standard for powered wheelchair components based on a fast serial bus. The hardware and message-passing protocol is currently being evaluated by the TIDE M3S project.

## 5. The Smart Wheelchair system architecture

The interface between the Smart Wheelchair processors and the host motor controller is via digital to analogue converters with configurable voltage levels to match several commercially available units (for example from Controls Dynamic or Penny & Giles). The user interface is bi-directional offering a range of inputs with the chair *Observer* responding and reporting its perceptions via a speech synthesiser or the pilot's input device. The Smart Wheelchair software, running on multiple 80C552 processors communicating via an I2C serial link, monitors user commands and sensors according to the currently selected tools. The software architecture is currently under revision to enable software objects to be mounted on any hardware processor within the smart configuration, with the available objects being established upon power-up by mutual interrogation between processors.

Figure 1 illustrates how objects or groups of objects form modules (tools) which encapsulate specific functional tasks. Selection of a tool is best illustrated by an example. In (a), the activated objects enable switches to drive the chair directly (the *Motion Tool* object provides momentary, timed or latched control over the chair). If the user selects the 'Bump and Turn' tool (b) (either with discrete switches or via the RS232 link), the Modifier object re-arranges the topology of the system (c) by activating the relevant bump objects and linking them into the current set. Development of new tools, such as *SlowDown* (d), involves building the object and associated possible links and adding it to the set of objects available.

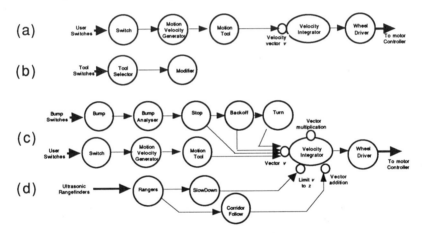

Figure 1 : Smart Wheelchair software architecture

The system was developed using *chipForth* [7], a polyForth-based development environment for microcontrollers. The system is multitasking with each object defined as a separate task and message passing handled automatically by the multitasking scheduler.

## 6.  Benefits of tool - based, modular designs

Modeless designs reduce memory demands for able people, and this is even more important for young disabled children.

• Tool - based systems make the chair easy to learn and to teach. A well-designed tool performs a recognisable task; is named accordingly in terms of what it does rather than its components; is more predictable either in isolation or when combined with other tools; and is freely combinable with other tools to create a system with overall predictable characteristics.

• The modular design enables cost-effective solutions to be provided for a wide range of individuals with differing needs, by specifying only those modules required.

• A degree of *future-proofing* is provided by the clean functional distinctions between object definitions

• The open system design avoids the need to re-invent other designs and enables incorporation rather than replication and permits multiple design team development programmes.

## 7. Problems and issues

The experience of the authors to date indicates the need for substantial investment of design resources in choosing a metaphor to underpin the message-passing system and the messages themselves. Both must simultaneously avoid waste by accommodating existing designs and components; reflect the tools needed for central aims of the chair itself; and flex to fit new concepts and systems.

This robust and unconstraining message passing and tool definition protocol must also not prejudice system integrity and safety; must allow for multiprocessor designs (including designs with multiple communication protocols as illustrated by the use of both I2C and RS232 links in the Smart Wheelchair); and must not overload the communication bandwidth available, even when multiple tools are engaged. The issues of safety are particularly important when dealing with a powered wheelchair: the message-passing protocol must be completely reliable to avoid losing potentially vital messages (eg. STOP!).

Modelessness does not guarantee tool orthogonality: there will always be tool interactions. While orthogonality of tools is a design aim, it is not always possible in practice either when configuring the chair or in use. For example, for safety reasons it is not always desirable to enable any tool to be combined with any other tool. Alternatively, consider our previous example with the single switch user tool and *bump and turn*: when a collision occurs the bump tool usurps the pilot's control momentarily while reversing and then turning away from the collision. A more complex example, might be a corridor follower combined with remote collision sensor where conflicts between two chair tools can occur. The designer's job is to identify such interactions, and ensure that

• the user is never left in doubt as to why the chair acts as it does (the role of the Observer tool is vital here), and

• the user tool is never over-ridden except for safety reasons, and then neither for long, nor reducing degrees of freedom unduly.

Orthogonality, modelessness, user priority and safety should not be prejudiced by the integration of non-chair tools such as communication aids, or external computers. This has implications for the location and power of the safety-monitoring components, which can never be *relegated* to external systems, only *supplemented* by them.

## 8. References

[1]   Nisbet, P.D., Odor, J.P., Loudon, I.R., *The CALL Centre Smart Wheelchair*. Proc. 1st Int. Workshop. on Advanced Robotics for Medical and Health Care, Ottawa, Canada, 1988. CALL Research Paper 7.

[2]   Odor, J.P.,*Computer Toolkits in Special Education* Pres. Int. Conf. on Technology and Education, Edinburgh, 1988. CALL Research Paper 10.

[3]   Brooks, R.A., *A Layered Intelligent Control System for a Mobile Robot*, IEEE Journal of Robotics and Automation, Ch. 8., 365-372, 1986.

[4]   Odor, J.P. *Connecting External Systems to COMSPEC Aids*. A report to the COMSPEC Working Group, 1992.

[6]   ISO Working Group 7  *Serial Interface for Electric Wheelchair Controllers*, (draft), contact Sven Linmann, Permobil AB, Gottsundavagan 13, S-184 92 Akersberga, Sweden.

[7]   *chipForth microcontroller development environment* available from Computer Solutions Ltd., 1a New Haw Road, Addlestone, Surrey KT15 2BZ, England.

# Networking, Consensus and Awareness

Gunnar FAGERBERG

*The Swedish Handicap Institute, Box 510, S-162 15 Vällingby, Sweden*

**Abstract.** Rehabilitation technology is a growing, yet fragmented field. Clinicians, researchers, industry are separated by national boundaries and sectorial thresholds. Closer contacts and cooperation would benefit everyone. Limited national resources could be joined to attain synergistic effects. Larger markets would result in better, less expensive products. Experiences and knowledge could be shared for mutual benefits. Persons with disabilities would know what services to expect when travelling between countries. Some of the means to achieve this are different meetings, publications and a rehabilitation technology member society.

## 1. Background

Rehabilitation technology is a rapidly growing field. In some countries, the increase in production and consumption is close to 20% per year [1]. Despite the present slow economy, indications that the growth will continue can be seen in the demographic changes, recent technical developments and political decisions. The increasing strength of the disability organizations is also an important factor in this development.

But the field is also one of fragmentation [2]. Small companies address local, regional, sometimes national markets and specialize in narrow market segments with little interaction with other producers.

National systems vary from country to country depending on tradition, policies and priorities. Although rehabilitation technology is now widely recognized to be a multi-disciplinary area involving many different actors, there is too little interaction between the actors.

For example, in a survey of different actors in the rehabilitation technology field, carried out by the CORE (Consensus creation and awareness for research and development activities in technology for disabled and elderly people) project [3], "understanding of end-users needs and requirements" and "user requirements and available information" were ranked highest among all factors identified as having influence/affect on the different elements in the rehabilitation technology market.

Earlier observations [4] that almost all international collaboration efforts take place between institutions, backed by governments or official authorities, are still valid.

Furthermore, these contacts are limited to a small number of persons and countries, whereas the reabilitation technology field now involves a broad and large spectrum of actors, growing in number.

From this background, it is clear that there is a need for increased contacts between individuals at the grass-roots level and in particular multi-disciplinary contacts. These individuals, whether they work in industry, clinics or research labs or whether they are end-users, family members or assistants, all have a definite need to share experiences and to give and receive information.

To meet this need, networking activities should be launched. These may include more meeting points, publications, computer databases and conferences, information systems and an international organization with individual membership.

## 2. Meeting points

Even in this increasingly electronic world, nothing can replace personal, eye-to-eye meetings for the sharing of information and experiences and building understanding and confidence. More opportunities should be provided for people to meet.

On a pan-European level, the ECART (European Conference for the Advancement of Rehabilitation Technology) serves such a purpose [5]. It will now be held every two years, its venue circulating in Europe. In addition, there should be more national and regional meetings, seminars and workshops where all different actors can get together. One particularly desirable but too infrequent confrontation that should be facilitated is between manufacturers and consumers (end-users).

It is therefore important, that employers, personnel officers and others are made aware of the need for interaction between individuals, continuing education and knowledge updates in a rapidly developing field. Resources for attending such meetings should be made available.

Meetings should be coordinated as much as possible, in order to avoid conflicts of time. International meetings should be announced well in advance, so other international and national arrangements can be scheduled accordingly.

## 3. Publications

There is a need for information in print on several levels. Brief news, events, publications, job opportunities are items suitable for publication in frequently appearing newsletters, intended for a broad range of readers. One recent example of a newsletter with an official character is the TIDE News [6], scheduled to appear approximately bi-monthly with news mainly from the TIDE programme of the European Community. It could well be complemented by other newsletters with different focusses. For readers less familiar with English, newsletters in their native language should be available.

On another level, the rehabilitation technology field needs a scientific journal that can provide a solid base of knowledge and methodology for researchers, manufacturers and clinicians. Today, most of the research results is published in journals that cover rehabilitation technology only marginally. Although attempts are being made to publish such journals in North America, such as RESNA's Assistive Technology, rehabilitation technology research and development in Europe has now reached such a level of quality and volume that there should be material and a market for a European journal.

## 4. Society

To initiate and maintain activities such as the ones mentioned above, a focal point and a driving force is required. It is an advantage if such an entity emanates from the individuals concerned - bottom-up rather than top-down - although international institutions established by government agencies may serve important functions in specific areas. An association based on individual membership provides a sense of belonging, helps in forming consensus, gives a recognition of the area and raises awareness about the field.

The time has come to start a European rehabilitation technology society with individual membership. Such societies already exist in North America - RESNA [7] - and Japan - RESJA - and have been very successful. Europe certainly has a sufficient population base. The society should be open to all actors in the field.

Such an initiative should as much as possible take advantage of and be based on existing movements and forces. At present there are two important forces of such nature: the ECART Foundation and conference and the TIDE Programme within the Commission of the European Community.

**References**

[1]     Rehabilitation Engineering Technology: Demand, Priorities and Future Directions. Proceedings of REHAB-1. United Nations Economic and Social Council, Economic Commission for Europe. Geneva, Switzerland, 1991.

[2]     TIDE, Technology Initiative for Disabled and Elderly People. 2nd Phase Workplan. Commission of the European Communities, Directorate-General XIII. Brussels, February 1992.

[3]     CORE Consortium, Actor Issues and Requirements That Have an Impact on the Rehabilitation Technology Market. Deliverable #1. Hoensbroek, The Netherlands, 1992.

[4]     G. Fagerberg, International Cooperation in Rehabilitation Engineering. In: J. Persson (Ed.) Innovation Assessment in Rehabilitation. Proceedings from a workshop at the VIIth Nordic Meeting on Medical and Biological Engineering. ISSN 0283-1228. CMT Report 1988:1. Center for Medical Technology Assessment, Linköping, Sweden.

[5]     European Conference on the Advancement of Rehabilitation Technology. Proceedings. ECART, Hoensbroek, The Netherlands, 1990.

[6]     TIDE News. No 1, December 1992. The Swedish Handicap Institute, Vällingby, Sweden.

[7]     RESNA Directory 1991-92. RESNA National Office, Washington, D.C., U.S.A.

# Evaluation Methodologies for Rehabilitation Technology

Ian Craig, Paul Nisbet, Phil Odor, Marion Watson

*Call Centre, University of Edinburgh, 4 Buccleuch Place, Edinburgh, Scotland*

**Abstract.** We consider what sorts of evaluation are appropriate when the rehabilitative technology under development interacts in complex ways with the society it serves. Issues are related to an outline of a project on the design and use of Smart Wheelchairs. The case is made for a multiple measures, systems approach to evaluation, based on formative techniques. Those employed in this particular case include both subjective and objective measures of process and product. The paper describes how such data-gathering is integrated into the development cycle itself.

## 1. Introduction : Evaluation and the Smart Wheelchair project

Independence is a powerful motivator. Without independent mobility, for instance, children have reduced opportunity for exploration and general learning, less social contact, and poorer chances of developing those broader aspects of independent living, like communication and assertiveness which lead to a full democratic role in society, and possibly a vocation. For people who cannot even operate conventional powered wheelchairs the resulting cycle of deprivation is at its worst. Such a person is denied both the chance to practice exactly those skills which are needed to improve mobility, and the motivation to do so.

Our project aims to break this destructive cycle, by providing a range of augmentative extensions to a basic electric wheelchair chassis which should ensure that it can be safely used by even the most disabled newcomer, and can be adapted to reflect and capitalise on their emerging skills as they learn and grow. It is a fundamental part of the project to provide not just the hardware and software, but to design individualised programmes of training which bring out positive aspects of independent mobility in a motivating way. Here is a pen portrait of one of the children in the project.

"Steven is a 16 year old spastic quadriplegic youth whose voluntary physical control is limited to some gross movement in his left hand, and in particular flexion and tension over his left index finger. Little was know about his functional vision, hearing or cognitive skills. Concepts of cause and effect had previously been introduced via a range of different switch-controlled learning aids, but all had proved unreliable in use: his experience of such technologies only extends over the last three years of his life. His concentration span in these tasks was around 20 minutes. Steven is difficult to seat because of his postural deformities. His communication was constrained to (unreliable) eye pointing, crying, smiling or laughing.

Preparation for the Smart wheelchair involved: building a custom seating system for him; devising a reliable input device (a specially-designed 'hall effect' finger switch mounted on a glove); devising an introductory programme; and training staff and parents.

The initial results were dramatic. A gentle introductory phase designed to go at the child's own pace and envisaged to take several weeks progressed so rapidly, that Steven was independently operating his Smart Wheelchair within one week. He quickly demonstrated previously unknown levels of assertiveness and exploratory behaviour, and rapidly took over functionality from the chair, until the limits of his single switch control made it imperative to move to a scanning or coding system to provide richer independent control options. Such systems were also available on his previous learning technologies, but never taken up by him.

The Smart Wheelchair is designed to develop physical, cognitive, social and communicative skills and encourage their transfer to other areas of the school curriculum, for example communication therapy. Steven had no previous experience of using augmentative communication aids. As part of the control choice extensions, communication functions are now being integrated into his Smart wheelchair design. Since his vision and perception were difficult to assess, as were his ability to track, a two-choice scanner with digitised visual and audible cues was built using HyperCard on an Apple Macintosh PowerBook laptop computer. Again, he quickly demonstrated that he could select either chair movement or sound as appropriate and the system was extended to give six options: forward, left or right movements, and three communicative messages. At the time of writing this system is about to be delivered to the school."

In situations like this (and they are increasing with the range of augmentative systems of all kinds, from interpersonal communication to vocational aids), it is not sufficient either to develop or to evaluate the hardware and software in isolation from the broader systems of use. Many potentially useful tools never make it into general use because their inventors either did not recognise the variety and complexity of the environment in which their devices had to work, nor the forms of service and support infrastructure needed to make them effective. In this paper, we will describe the dual nature of our evaluation of the Smart wheelchair, monitoring its effectiveness in bringing about beneficial changes in individuals, and the effect on the professional and personal practices of those who initiate, plan and support those personal developments.

## 2. Evaluation Issues

### 2.1 Why evaluate?

Given the evidence from other studies and from our own pilot projects [1, 2, 3, 4], we believe in the effectiveness of the Smart Wheelchair in encouraging forms of personal development which go well beyond mobility per se. Of course, our belief is not sufficient (and not very informative to newcomers), and the first and most obvious reason for spending scarce resources on evaluation is to test out the system in real settings, and document the results for others to use. Because we are an engineering team, we take a rather practical view of such a process, and expect not only to find flaws in our thinking and design, but to act on them immediately.

Many evaluative designs seek to test and inform about products or techniques in this way. Nevertheless many demonstrably effective techniques and systems fail to come into general use. Difficulties often arise not from technical design flaws, but because the development and evaluation projects failed to also set up and test those social conditions which support effective use of the new technologies. Aspects include product manufacture and marketing, training and service support and (in our case) tailoring and continuing refinement of the Smart Wheelchair to meet continued personal development. The project recognises that a complex collection of social and professional factors determines individual success or failure, and that to deliver effective support for users of the Smart Wheelchair, we need to take a broad systems view of both person and environment.

Our evaluation therefore also aims to judge the Smart wheelchair product and its associated services against the special needs of both disabled individuals, and the organisations which serve them. Evaluation includes testing correctness of design (including safety aspects), measuring effectiveness in use, reporting on effectiveness of training and support services, and estimating costs.

### 2.2 What is to be evaluated?

As the case study shows, there are many issues involved. Some are clearly technical, being either individualisation or engineering issues. It is an evaluation design aim that such technical problems should be identified and distinguished from each other in time for action to be taken well within the project timeframe. Other aspects which need to be understood centre around how best to encourage development of a variety of skills in particular children, and (closely related) how to generalise and disseminate these findings, and to whom they should be disseminated. Distinct from staff training needs are the day - to - day management problems of staff and carers as they try to exploit new technologies. It is thus an evaluative goal to understand these needs and to translate them into costed plans for new training and support services.

Each of these issues involves many inter-related variables. It is not a trivial task to choose evaluative techniques which will capture the broad range of information we need, within a modest budget.

*2.3. How do we evaluate?*

Despite the richness of modern evaluation methods, one technique - exemplified by clinical trials - shapes the dominant popular stereotype of how scientific judgments are formed. Such an approach suits the large-scale testing of mainly single - function products or technologies. However, to achieve our multiple goals, we have had to distance ourselves from that restrictive approach. Although clinical trials are appropriate in many situations, they are not meaningful where the trial population exhibits wide variations (of, in our case, cognitive, communication, sensory and perceptual skills, and physical abilities), and where the target population of potential users will be even more varied. Yet this is the situation for our users, and why Special Education is so named - it deals with individuals *each* with special needs. Nor are mass trials possible where part of the project is aimed at encouraging environment-specific developments around each user: controls, in these situations, become unwieldy and unconvincing, and detract from larger issues. There are both ethical and practical problems of design. Finally, there are issues of cost. Project design, for most evaluators, hinges on getting the most, and the most usable information, for a fixed cost. Even had we chosen to deal with the kind of very restricted group of children and environments which might have achieved some form of homogeneity (at the expense of breadth of usefulness of the results), the price of accurate measurement along some restricted dimension would have been too high in comparison with what could have been learned, and would have prejudiced observation of too many other important dimensions of development.

Our project takes the form of a *Formative Evaluation*, in which one of us (MW) acts as a team member in both school and engineering project teams. The case study above shows that she has responsibilities for traditional evaluative observation, and for formative aspects such as training of staff and parents, contributing to the design of individualised programmes, and fault and progress chasing.

Several things contribute to the success of a formative evaluation. Firstly, being an active participant in the school teams helps the evaluator to encourage openness in the team community, and keeps her in touch with practical issues which would escape other evaluative designs. Secondly, at least part of her effectiveness comes from her prior experience in schools (in her case, as a therapist). The evaluator must be trusted. We feel that, whatever their personal skills, employing one of our engineers as evaluator would have been much less productive. Lastly, the project has to have a payoff for the schools and individuals. Any project like this is intrusive, and promises of great public good in the future are not so persuasive to busy staff as demonstrations of effective interventions now. This in turn means an evaluation must be responsive to suggestions, and must react quickly when problems occur. No formative evaluator in this kind of project can work without the resources of the engineering group always on hand.

Abandoning clinical trial models in favour of a formative evaluation does not imply either accepting less rigour in our design, nor abandoning objective in favour of subjective data. What is important is that the data which *is* collected, matches the intermediate and long-term aims of the project community as a whole. To this end, it is important to distinguish between those situations where immediate feedback is needed (implying rapid collection of information and continuous public scrutiny of the results by the project community), from those where issues will only emerge over time (and where, therefore, more traditional data collection methods can be incorporated into longer formative cycles of development). We'll consider three time-frames: technical system design and refinement, assessment of individual performance, and the development of a support infrastructure. The distinctions are convenient, but artificial, since each element activity both informs and depends on the others. Let us take the broadest view first.

### 2.3.1. Service Development

The longest timescales in our study emerge from our attempts to determine how the Smart wheelchair can make the transition from research project to service. To provide practical experience on which to base future plans and proposals, the project was set up as a small - scale simulation of one possible service model: a 'mini-service'. This had several elements :
- a multi-disciplinary assessment service for children,
- design services for both specialised components (especially controls), and for appropriate intervention plans for the child
- small-scale manufacturing of common hardware subassemblies (around a commercial chassis)
- adaptation to meet the individual designs above, including seating, switching, and software
- initial and continuing training of staff and carers
- support for child and carers during subsequent cycles of intervention and assessment

This simulation was set up between the project partners: the CALL Centre at Edinburgh University, the Bioengineering Unit at Princess Margaret Rose Hospital, and the three schools - Graysmill, Westerlea, and Oaklands. We chose children and situations which would stretch the capabilities of the service. For the children, this meant ensuring a wide spread of age; ability and disability; and developmental goals. In the schools, we looked for representative styles of provision and management.

Generating the evaluative outcomes we need involves all team members in a continual review of those school and home management and environments which services will need to support; the level and form of training needed; and the costs of each element. To help focus discussions about these issues, we have outlined a tentative service model [5] and are currently relating cost measures and management issues to it. This process moves slowly throughout the project from informal data gathering and localised changes to the simulated service system's practices (decided by reviews of day to day discussions about specific problems), through more specific interviews with staff (now underway) to more formal proposals about workable solutions (which we are now embarking on).

Of course, any technical research group has to support its subjects. What made a difference to our ability to judge the long-term service needs was the explicit prior decision to observe, cost, and develop our support system as an object in its own right, rather than treating support issues as a side effect of the 'main' R & D effort.

## *2.3.2. Effectiveness of the Smart Wheelchair*

Although we have described the service evaluation first, the most important aspect of the evaluation is nonetheless to test the effectiveness of the wheelchair in use. However, it should now be clear that there are tensions between the demands of evaluating possible service structures (requiring breadth of potential application and environment) and those of evaluating individual performance (where similarity between subjects would have been most helpful. There are also specific problems in capturing children's developmental processes, which in one child might be a slow progressive skill - learning measured over months, and in another might be an insightful experience happening in seconds. Our compromise solution was to design each child's case observations individually (matching the evaluation regime to the individualised intervention design), but also to collect common data where possible, so as to maximise the possibility of cross comparisons.

One of our claims is that skills learned through mobility transfer to other areas - communication, social assertiveness, and education. This brings into sharp focus the difficulties which surround single case study designs such as matched internal-reference (in which there are assumed to be related developmental variables not affected by the intervention which can act as benchmarks for the supposedly isolated controlled variable). Our approach here is to ensure that the data collected on each child is sufficient for us to make comparisons between the period of intervention, and that immediately before.

In conjunction with the school teams, we designed single case studies so as to collect both long-term and short term information. Each study had two components -

*product measures* - These are generated by comparison between pre- & post- study profiles of a broad range of abilities, chosen to include features directly associated with mobility, and those which would indicate successful transfer of skills. Written profiles were negotiated with the schools, and a common format agreed across each of them. Pre - intervention video records in home and school were taken and coded (see below). Each child's initial profile was then related to their individualised intervention plan, and the project team agreed when to target particular observation effort during the child's planned staged developments. We tried to ensure that our assessment exercises complemented those normally undertaken by the school.

*process measures* - a major part of the process measures have are derived from video sequences (of both structured and unstructured tasks). These are used in two ways. In their raw state, they help the project teams re-examine and interpret behaviours. Coded into computer - readable form, they allow objective measurement and comparisons of important behavioural sequences.

The profiles, assessments, and video records above contain a rich mixture of subjective and objective measures, designed to be accessible to the whole project community. They were supplemented by diary observations kept by staff and carers, and a macro-level overview of major events maintained by the evaluators. This latter document (also a process measure) shows time on task, illness and absence, major achievements and goals attained, system unreliability, and the like. By opening up observations to public scrutiny as far as possible without overstepping the bounds of acceptable personal privacy (different in different cases), we ensured that we had good opportunities for triangulation of reports from teachers, therapists, parents and ourselves, and that our own evaluative role was seen to be at the same 'level' as other aspects of the project, and just as open to criticism and comment.

## *2.3.3. Evaluation of Smart Wheelchair system design*

Once the data-gathering systems were in place for the service simulation and the observations of childrens use of the wheelchair, progress-chasing for design refinement was almost automatic. Because the evaluator worked as part of the school teams, immediate feedback of technical problems was possible, with the evaluator acting as first-line technician and fault analyst. The video record also served in fault monitoring and system refinement.

In some ways, the problems have been to deal effectively with the volume of information and the pace of demands from an increasingly sophisticated project community. The engineering team have tried to exercise control where possible by the staged introduction of new features, (although this is difficult when a child makes unexpectedly rapid progress, outpacing what sometimes emerge as conservative intervention plans).

## 3. Conclusions

Since this paper focuses on the effectiveness of systems - based evaluative methodologies, rather than the effectiveness of the Smart Wheelchair or its service delivery, we will resist reporting the outcomes beyond saying that the children's use of the wheelchair greatly encourages us; that the main problems are human and economic (such as ensuring continuity of trained key staff); and that we now have the makings of a plan for introducing the chair into broader service which is much different from what we would have proposed at the project outset. As to the evaluation itself, we believe that:

- it is vital to provide developers of new technologies with resources for appropriately staffed, systems-based, open evaluation as an integral part of the design process.
- such evaluations should encompass the broad social settings into which the product will migrate, and should test the support services which will be needed
- where the combination of environmental variety, breadth of client need, and technological complexity is great, and where safety is not compromised, developers should not be afraid of adopting mixed - measures approaches such as the one we have outlined here.
- financial constraints are not the only reason to abandon clinical trials with restricted dimensions: you may, as we do, believe that the community of users has much to teach you about your own design, and you need to find ways to encourage their inventiveness.

Our grateful thanks are due to Nuffield Foundation for their generous support during this project. We should also like to thank our colleagues in the three schools for their enthusiasm and patience, and to the Scottish Home and Health Department and the Scottish Office Education Department for their joint support for the development project itself.

## 4. References

[1] RESNA- Association for the Advancement of Rehabilitation Technology , *Selected Readinsg on Powered Mobility for Children and Adults with Severe Physical Disabilities* (1986), eds. Trefler E., Kozole, K., Snell E., pub. RESNA, Suite 700, 1101 Connecticut Avenue NW, Washington, DC 20036.

[2] RESNA- Association for the Advancement of Rehabilitation Technology, *Childhood Powered Mobility: Developmental, Technical and Clinical Perspectives.* (1988), pub. RESNA, Suite 700, 1101 Connecticut Avenue NW, Washington, DC 20036.

[3] Nisbet P.D., Odor J.P., Loudon I.R., *The CALL Centre Smart Wheelchair.* Proc. 1st International Workshop on Robotic Applications to Medical and Health Care, Ottawa. 9.1-9.10.

[4] Rosie, R. *Jeff and the Smart Wheelchair*, ISAAC UK Newsletter, No. 12, Winter 1990, 1990.

[5] CALL Centre *Interim Formative Evaluation Summary Report*, CALL Centre Advisory Paper SW5.3, 1992.

# User Requirements Capture for Adaptable Smarter Home Technologies

Simon J Richardson, David F Poulson, C Nicolle
HUSAT Research Institute
Loughborough University of Technology
The Elms  Elms Grove Loughborough
Leicestershire LE11 1RG United Kingdom

**Abstract.** The ASHoRED (TIDE 101) project has developed methodologies for the specification, development and assessment of adaptable smarter home technology with an emphasis on the needs of the visually impaired and the elderly. The approach has been user driven, supplemented by expert opinion, direct observation and prototyping. The approach has facilitated the development of innovative technologies and in particular the design of three different smart home demonstrators based in three different member states of the EEC. This paper describes the approach used within ASHoRED to develop the user requirements from 'wish lists' into low level product definition and actual requirements. It concludes that in the design of such technology user centred design involving domain experts and other stakeholders are necessary but not sufficient pre-requisites for success. Hands on experience using prototyping and systematic assessment techniques are also invaluable.

## 1  Introduction

Opportunities to support people who are physically and/or psychologically disadvantaged in some way are increasing with the increased functionality and flexibility of new technology.  This increased potential offers the possibility of independent living and can providedthe basis for an increased quality of life.  In addition to individual benefits new technology shows great promise in tackling the widespread care crisis, reducing the financial burden on central and regional government and other hard pressed care providers [1].

These potential benefits have long been recognised.  Many developments throughout the world have sought to exploit the full potential of integrating functions and devices within the home and to providing new forms of communication within and outside the home environment.  Typically these initiatives seek to achieve some degree of 'intelligent' or 'smart' home.  In the past this intelligence has been applied to energy conservation and security, more recently applications have been expanded to include other areas of home activity.

Initiatives have been taken in Japan and the USA and within Europe [2].  A major problem in the take up of these technologies stems from the fact that, for a number of reasons, they are technology led.  This approach carries with it a high risk of poor acceptability and low or inappropriate usage.  Such risks undermine the advantages to be gained and significantly affect the possibility of commercially exploitable adaptable smarter home systems and devices.

The ASHoRED project (Adaptable Smarter Homes for Residents who are Elderly or Disabled People) is a systems integration project within TIDE involving three adaptable smarter home demonstrators located in Germany, Spain and Finland.  The demonstrators extend previous research in this area and seek to show the benefits of adaptable smarter homes by combining support services and devices adapted for use with telecommunications and internal buses to control the appliances and the environment. An essential characteristic of the project is that it is, within certain constraints, user led.

For adaptable smarter homes to be successful they need to match the needs of the users.  To achieve this, particular emphasis must be given to the formulation of requirements and to the specification and design of the interfaces between the user and the technology as well as to the functionality of the technology itself. These requirements are particularly important for the heterogeneous and diverse characteristics of the disabled, the visually impaired and the elderly.

This paper reports the approach used within the ASHoRED pilot project to capture user requirements and the translation of these into practical products to support the independent living of the elderly and visually impaired.

## 2  Problems with User Requirement Capture

The process of innovation can be described in an number of ways and one useful distinction is between processes which are technology led and those which are user/customer led. Technology led innovation is characterised by systems which are created on the basis of technical feasibility, with little attention to incorporating the needs of users into the design cycle. User/customer led processes however begin from user requirement analysis and continue into prototyping before design solutions are generated. The former is a high risk strategy in the sense that a if a product fails to meet user needs it stands a higher risk of inappropriate use or rejection and can generate undesirable acceptability problems. Thus much reported research underlines the need to adopt user/customer led strategies for design and innovation.

The capture of user requirements remains however a problem area within systems analysis and design, and it is acknowledged that few systems are created which adequately match the needs of their users [3]. There are a number of well documented reasons for this:

- problems with identifying a valid and representative sample, especially for the large and heterogeneous consumer market for domestic appliances.
- a lack of knowledge on the part of developers of how to capture and integrate user needs into design.
- an erroneous assumption that designers can identify needs for other users based on their own expert knowledge and experience.
- lack of user knowledge about new products and options and difficulty in conceptualising the potential value of innovative products that might assist them with their daily lives.

In addition it was observed during the ASHoRED project that:

- elderly users had problems articulating their requirements for future products, partly through a lack of familiarity with the potential that technology might have for solving their problems, and also in some cases through lack of capability. Thus an elderly person beginning to suffer from mild dementia may not be able to say what they need from technology, and may not even be fully aware of the problems they face in everyday living.
- the elderly may also underestimate their difficulties, and may not be able to clearly identify what their real problems are despite the fact that the home environment is no longer appropriate to their reduced capabilities. In some circumstances they are not able to anticipate the benefits of changing their home environment even at the simplest level.
- in some situations a fear of stigmatisation rather than a lack of ability impeded conventional forms of requirements capture. Some physically disabled people, for example, were concerned not to reveal their dependency on others, and therefore under-reported their problems. This was particularly apparent in the young visually impaired who did not wish to appear as different in any way from the normally sighted population.

There are therefore limits to the extent to which user requirements capture for future products can be determined by simply asking the users to report the problems they experience at home in an attempt to identify what their true needs and requirements are. These have to be supplemented with other methods including observation, the involvement of other people, domain experts and in particular prototypes that can be demonstrated to users or enable them to have hands on experience.

## 3   *The ASHoRED approach*

In seeking to identify the requirements of the elderly and the visually impaired, the ASHoRED project adopted an innovative approach involving several levels of analysis with an opportunity at each level to reformulate/modify/fine tune these requirements. This approach followed as far as possible an iterative, user centred design process. An important and valid constraint on the process (in the context of designing demonstrators) was that there were limitations on the devices that could be used and on the extent to which these could be modified.

In general terms the approach used was to formulate the perceived, baseline requirements, from interview and group discussion techniques with key stakeholders and users without any 'hands on' experience of the technology itself. Subsequent stages of the development of the demonstrators, including a detailed assessment at the end of the project, would result in the refinement, and in some cases the re-definition of these baseline requirements such that they represented more precise 'actual' requirements. Three methodologies were created to achieve these goals. The first concerned requirements capture, the second the development of usage scenarios and the third an assessment strategy for the demonstrators.

The requirements capture process used here can be loosely likened to some of the principles of the 'cascade model' of organisational information flow where information is relayed from one point to another in increasingly lower levels of detail. At each point the information is reviewed, validated and extended before being passed forward. For ASHoRED the model provided a means for moving from high level, perceived requirements to low level, actual requirements and specifications. This approach has subsequently been developed and used elsewhere [4].

### *Intelligence*

Within the ASHoRED project the initial definition of requirements took place by interviewing end users. In the absence of a suitable methodology one was developed specifically for the ASHoRED project. A limited sample of elderly and visually impaired users were interviewed in the UK and in Norway, with a view to identifying the problems they faced in their current household tasks.

Panels of experts were also consulted. Panel participants included care providers and social services personnel as well as a small number of users themselves. In open discussion these groups identified the scale and nature of everyday problems experienced in the home and through this defined high level requirements that any form of new technology should possess. The result of these activities was the production of a 'wish list' of the functional areas needing support in the home. This 'wish list' represented the perceived, base line, requirements.

For example two of the functional areas identified included 'access to the home', and 'receiving visitors'. The elderly and visually impaired had major concerns about home security and would therefore welcome products which assisted in this area. Products would be needed which assisted the user in gaining entry to the home, and once in the home to be able to identify and give access to visitors. Other particular problems areas included food preparation, the washing and care of clothes, medical care and taking of medicines, home administration, personal hygiene and use of the bathroom, and the operation of electrical fittings and controls.

### *Definition*

The next phase of the development cycle was to identify the areas of convergence between the needs for products identified, and what would be feasible to produce. This was an iterative process where the basic products that would be demonstrated in the three demonstrator sites were first identified and then the details of their functionality assessed against the base line requirements. Some of this functionality had been defined in the original ASHoRED specification eg. a totally automated washing machine, whilst other features of the functionality arose directly from the user requirements eg. the use of a door camera to assist in the identification of visitors.

The integration process between requirements capture on the one hand and the technological possibilities on the other took place by a process of consultation involving human factors specialists and designers within the consortium. This was facilitated by the production of descriptions of the tasks that it was anticipated the users would be able to perform with the equipment produced at each of the three sites.

For example, it was feasible to include technology to assist in identifying and admitting a visitor in one of the demonstrator sites. In consequence, a door opening device along with an intercom and door camera for identifying visitors in this demonstrator was included in the specification. To meet the previously defined requirements it was necessary that this technology should be operable through a number of control units in the home, specifically designed for use by the elderly and visually impaired.

The agreed functionality of each of the demonstrators was then translated into usage scenarios which were based partly on a modified version of the scenario building methods defined in the RACE [5] programme where the implications of the market, service, activity and user characteristics are explored . These scenarios described the everyday tasks that it was anticipated users would be able to perform with the available equipment subject to any technical modifications previously or subsequently defined.

A methodology for compiling the scenarios was designed to document not only the usage but also the assumptions which were behind the various factors involved. The methodology enabled the analysis to move from the high to the low level by first documenting the objectives, user groups and constraints of each of the sites, progressively moving to lower levels of task detail. This generated detailed matrices which related task activities to devices, controls and displays as well as defining priorities for development and assessment. Over 120 scenarios were finally formulated spread across each of the three sites.

The objective of these scenarios were to define what could be demonstrated at each of the three sites, what functionality the smarter homes should possess, what devices and control systems would be used and to contribute to the further definition of user requirements. These scenarios also acted to fix the specification of the demonstrator products (including interface and display specifications), and provide part of the framework for subsequent assessment of the products with the users.

*Assessment*

Following the formulation of the perceived requirements, the development of usage scenarios and the specification and engineering of the demonstrators, an assessment strategy was developed to evaluate the results of the demonstrators against project objectives and usability and acceptability criteria. The methodology involved the participation of human factors specialists, experts from relevant domains and users and was divided into four phases. The assessment followed 'constructive' as distinct from 'traditional' forms of technology assessment [6].

In the first phase, and prior to the installation of the configured technology an expert usability panel assessment was undertaken to examine the separate devices, components, control systems and the interactions between them. The second part of the assessment involved, amongst other things, the development of tools to assess user characteristics and care needs and the extent to which the demonstrators could be used to meet the usage scenarios previously defined. During this phase certain laboratory studies were carried out. Systematic and detailed field trials were also conducted. In the third phase, user panels were convened (where appropriate) to examine the value of the demonstrators and in the final phase 'expert' panels were again convened to examine the wider implications and acceptability issues arising from experiences with the three demonstrator sites [7].

Assessment of the demonstrator products then took place by a combination of end user trials and expert assessment. These approaches served to provide information about the validity of the user requirements previously identified, they helped to identify other products needed to support users in their everyday living, and provided essential data on the improvements that needed to be made to the configured demonstrators. The importance of this approach cannot be under estimated. It is only through having tangible prototypes and products that users and other experts can assess the full implications of the technology and articulate their 'actual' long term requirements.


## 4   Conclusions

The ASHoRED project has focused its attention on the development of adaptable smarter home technologies to assist and support the elderly and visually impaired within their home. The initial difficulty was to find appropriate ways of determining 'actual' requirements for future innovative products and services and translating these into usable specifications.

The use of the cascade principle and the development of three specific methodologies has been of great importance to achieving these goals. It is clear that in a technology application area which is highly innovative, there is a need to involve users and other stakeholders in the initial description of requirements. The initial description of requirements however can only be a base line from which to begin development. Further development will also need to include 'hands on' experience and user participation in an iterative, evolutionary design process.

It is anticipated that the procedures and methods developed within this project can be applied to a much wider range of design projects and problems.


## 5   Acknowledgements

The authors are grateful to the CEC for the funding received within the TIDE programme and acknowledge the contributions of other members of the ASHoRED Consortium for their inputs into this development process and enthusiasm in testing out the techniques developed.


## 6   References

[1]   Eason, K.D. (1988) Information Technology and Organisational Change. Taylor and Francis. London.
[2]   Haddon, L. (1990) International Round-up. *The Intelligent Home* 1, No. 2.
[3]   Poulson, D.F, Richardson, S.J. (1993) Issues in the Uptake of Adaptable Smarter Home Technology. European Conference on the Advancement of Rehabilitation Technology. ECART 2. Stockholm, May 26-28, 1993.
[4]   Nicolle, C., Ross, T., Richardson, S.J. (1993) Identification and Grouping of Requirements for Drivers with Special Needs. European Conference on the Advancement of Rehabilitation Technology. ECART 2. Stockholm, May 26-28, 1993.
[5]   URM Consortium (1991) Usage Reference Model: URM Conceptual Framework. RACE Project R1077: Usage Reference Model for IBC.
[6]   Cronberg, T., Dueland, P., Jensen, O.M., Qvortrup, L. (eds.) (1991) Danish Experiments - Social Constructions of Technology. New Social Science Monographs - Copenhagen.
[7]   Richardson, S J,. Poulson, D., Nicolle, C., (1993) Supporting Independent Living through Adaptable Smart Home (ASH) Technologies. HUSITA 3. Information Technology and the Quality of Life and Services. Maastricht, 15-18 June 1993.

# An Integrated Research Strategy for Improving Communication Systems for Severely Physically Impaired Non-speaking People

Norman ALM, Alan F. NEWELL, John L ARNOTT
*MicroCentre, Department of Mathematics and Computer Science*
*University of Dundee*
*Dundee, Scotland, U.K.*

**Abstract.** Efforts to provide technical assistance to enable severely physically impaired non-speaking people to be able to communicate as effectively as unimpaired speakers have thus far been limited in their results. This is because human communication is a complex and rapid process, the physical mechanisms of which are not controlled consciously. Also the rules of human interaction through language are only imperfectly understood. There are a number of implications from this position for research to improve the situation. Such research must be multidisciplinary, it must involve potential users as consultants and evaluators at all stages of the process, and it must take into account the whole range of social and personal functions which a communication system should assist with. This paper describes a research strategy which takes these points into account.

## 1. Introduction

Despite several years of technical development and significant increases in portable and reasonably-priced computing power, the goal of creating a communication system for severely physically impaired non-speaking people which allows them to communicate with an effectiveness approaching that of unimpaired people is still far from being reached. The usual communication rate achievable with an augmentative or alternative communication system (AAC) can be as low as one or two words per minute, or even less. Rates of 2-10 words per minute have been cited as representative [1]. By comparison unimpaired speech proceeds at 120-200 words per minute [2]. Speaking partners of AAC users tend to control the conversation, and ask a large number of yes/no questions. Non-speakers initiate less frequently, and tend to use restricted language forms, such as one-word responses. They typically spend more time interacting with people where there is an unequal relationship, such as parents, therapists, and teachers, and less time interacting with peers [3,4]. True, a number of exceptional non-speaking people have managed to break out of this pattern to varying degrees. However, from their own reports, non-speakers say they often feel marginalised, considered unintelligent, or just invisible [5,6].

## 2. Redefining the Goals

It may be that achieving complete parity between AAC users and natural speakers will always be impossible, given the low input rate which is achievable with the general degree of impairment which most non-speakers have. Research effort should thus be directed at identifying those communicational situations in which significant improvements in performance can be made. The goals could thus be redefined. Instead of trying to help a severely physically impaired non-speaker to produce speech in the same way us an unimpaired person, we should concentrate efforts on the impact and effectiveness of their communication, however it is produced [1,7]. Taking this approach may be lead to entirely new ideas for communication methods. It has been pointed out that 'It was only after we stopped trying to copy nature's design criteria for birds that we began to fly -- perhaps the same may be true of AAC devices.' [7]

It should be noted that, as well as technical innovation, non-technical improvements would also make a considerable difference to non-vocal people, and research in this direction would also be valuable. For instance, teaching listeners better strategies for speaking with aided communicators, or training frequent contacts to understand the speaker's dysarthric speech. However, it would be naive to assume that such social changes can be made easily, or on a very wide scale. This leaves the non-speaker still needing technical help to communicate outside their immediate circle of family and close friends. This wider social world includes commercial and work-related contacts which are vital in ensuring that non-speakers play a full part as citizens.

## 3. Requirements for Successful Research

The difficulties which have been encountered in improving augmentative and alternative communication systems demonstrate that the research effort must incorporate non-technical as well as technical expertise. The research must be truly multidisciplinary and should be aimed at achieving the social and interactional goals of potential users -- not merely solving technical problems. Relevant technical skills for this research are computer science, software engineering, human factors engineering, and electronics. In addition to these disciplines, this research should call on expertise and knowledge from psychology, sociology, linguistics, teaching, social work, philosophy, and the arts (particularly graphic design and drama). Effective human communication research is required to be multidisciplinary by its very generality and complexity. Also, it frequently happens that the answers to a difficult research problem in one field are available and general knowledge in another field. Thus innovation can often be achieved by moving knowledge across the boundaries of disciplines.

Research into improving communication systems for non-vocal people should involve potential users as consultants and research helpers at all stages of the research. In the past, simpler systems could be developed, and when completed, tested with potential users. As systems become more complex, they should be evaluated in functional situations, as the behaviour of complex systems and their human users cannot be completely predicted until they are in use. A more subtle but no less important result of frequent contact with potential users by researchers is that the intuitive skills of the researcher may be improved. It is recognised that research proceeds by making hypotheses and then testing them. The empirical results are the test of the ideas, but it is equally important that the hypotheses be good ones. The process is not one of random searching. This, of course is difficult to plan for, but it seems reasonable that frequent exposure to the successful and unsuccessful strategies employed by non-vocal people will be an aid to the imaginations of researchers.

## 4. A Coordinated, Multidisciplinary Research Strategy

In the research being done in the MicroCentre at Dundee University, we have followed the guidelines given above, and have also devised a coordinating strategy which we would recommend for consideration by other AAC researchers. At the MicroCentre we have a team of seventeen researchers and four Ph.D. students working on a number of individual research projects concerned with improving augmentative and alternative communication. Each project is investigating a particular aspect of the problem. The disciplines represented in this group include computer science, software engineering, electronic engineering, human factors engineering, psychology, linguistics, special and general education, social work, and philosophy. A number of members of the team combine two or more of these disciplines in their background, which makes the multidisciplinary approach quite a natural one. Also a number of physically impaired non-speaking people have helped us in the development of research ideas and test new prototypes. One AAC user has been a member of our research group on a weekly basis for the past three years.

The primary goal of our current research is to make three areas of communication possible and more efficient for severely physically impaired non-speakers. These areas are social conversation, writing, and performing at work. Each research area has a number of projects working on different aspects of the problem, and all of the projects are contributing towards the construction of a multi-purpose communication system. Examples of this research work are given below :

### 4.1 Facilitating social conversation by non-vocal people

A number of research projects have explored the possibility of facilitating social conversation by non-vocal people by means of modelling conversation patterns and providing predictions for the user as to what they might want to say next. These projects have all involved developing software to be run on commercially available portable computers with synthetic speech output. The fields of discourse analysis and computational linguistics provided useful insights in the development of a number of these systems. Opening and closing phases of a conversation and providing feedback to another speaker were facilitated in the CHAT prototype [8]. The TOPIC prototype was based on a commercially available text-database which was used to store and retrieve conversational material for speaking through a speech synthesiser [9]. The TalksBack prototype included techniques derived from artificial intelligence to provide sentence prediction through modelling the semantics of the discussion, and also the user's and conversation partner's social situation [10]. The PROSE system used similar computational techniques to assisted the user to tell stories, and to predict when a stored text might be relevant in the conversation [11]. To experiment with the interface for a text-retrieval system, the FloorGrabber system was developed and tested with a non-vocal research helper, using a hypertext storage method and a graphical interface [12].

What all these projects share is an approach to helping non-vocal people communicate which takes fully into account the social dimension of human communication. Advanced computational techniques are used in order to model the user's social purposes and thus simulate what a natural speaker is doing at a non-conscious level.

### 4.2 Assisting motor-disabled and language-disabled people with writing

Software which provides word prediction to assist motor and language disabled children and adults is under development at the MicroCentre. The PAL (Predictive Adaptive Lexicon) system was developed originally to help children and adults with motor dysfunction to create written text more easily. PAL works by exploiting the redundancy in natural language to reduce the number of keystrokes necessary to produce a piece of text. The user is continuously given a short menu of word predictions which may be selected with a single key press. The predictions are produces from a dictionary of words containing statistical information relating to frequency and recency of use. PAL is now a commercial product, and can offer severely physically impaired people between 30% and 60% savings in keystrokes needed to create text. Trials of PAL showed that it significantly reduced the effort necessary in writing, and so increased the amount of writing which physically impaired people were able to do [13]

Current research on the PAL system is investigating its effectiveness in helping children and adults with language dysfunctions and spelling problems. It is known that a large number of physically impaired non-speakers also have language dysfunctions, so the PAL system would be useful for them as part of an overall AAC provision, because of its assistance in overcoming their motoric problems, and also their language difficulties.

### 4.3 A Multi-modal Workstation in a Work Environment for a Severely Physically Impaired Person

A multi-modal input system is being developed at the MicroCentre in the ECHO (Extra-Ordinary Computer Human Operation) project. [14] This project is exploring ways in which a multi-modal system might enable a severely physically disabled person to use an office workstation in a work environment. The intention is to widen the band-width of control between the user and the computer. In addition to control with a keyboard and mouse, and specialised switch inputs, the ECHO system includes control of the computer with eye-gaze, speech recognition, and gesture. Output from the computer can be through text, in a standard windows-based interface, or through a speech synthesiser. The system is being evaluated with a small set of physically impaired users, who will be performing simulated office tasks using multiple input modes to control a number of applications. In the first instance, the efficiency of multi-modal input is being compared with the single mode input. Further evaluations and extensions of the system are being planned.

## 5. Conclusion

Although the projects described above are all independent pieces of research, they are all related by being possible contributors to a proposed multiple function communication system. This system would be internally complex, and able to operate on multiple levels, but to the user, would be an easy system to use, because much of the cognitive effort in using it would be taken over by the system itself. As the research programme proceeds, some projects will produce potential components for such a system and others will produce negative findings. As each project makes its contribution, the realisable characteristics of an ideal communication system become clearer. In the meantime, each project provides useful individual outcomes, both theoretical and technical insights, and also commercial products. The results of this coordinated research strategy have been useful theoretical and practical insights, which have been reported to the wider research community. In addition two commercial products have resulted from this work, and a further product is under discussion with a manufacturer.

The improvement of communication systems for severely motor and speech impaired people will require multidisciplinary research. This research can be coordinated by assuming that each prototype system could form, part of a multi-level communication system which would provide a user with help, in some cases, approaching that of a human assistant. Important issues for this research will be facilitating the users' social purposes, and developing simple and easy to sue interfaces for complex and powerful systems.

## References

[1] Kraat, A. (1985) *Communication Interaction Between Aided and Natural Speakers: A State of the Art Report*. Toronto: Canadian Rehabilitation Council for the Disabled.

[2] Foulds, R. (1980) Communication rates for non-speech expression as a function of manual tasks and linguistic constraints. In *Proceedings of the International Conference on Rehabilitation Engineering* (Toronto, Canada, 16-20 June), Toronto : Rehabilitation Engineers Society of North America, pp83-87.

[3] Light, J. (1988) Interaction involving individuals using augmentative and alternative communication systems: state of the art and future directions. *Augmentative and Alternative Communication*, Vol 4 No 2, pp66-82.

[4] Blackstone, S. (1991) Intervention with the partners of AAC consumers: Part I - Interaction. *Augmentative Communication News,* Vol 4 No 2, pp 1-3.

[5] Eulenberg, J. (ed.) (1984) *Conversations with Non-speaking People*. Toronto: Canadian Rehabilitation Council for the Disabled.

[6] Sienkiewicz-Mercer, R, Kaplan, S. (1989) *I Raise My Eyes to Say Yes*. Boston : Houghton-Mifflin.

[7] Newell A.F. (1992) Today's dream - tomorrow's reality (Phonic Ear *AAC* Distinguished Lecture). *Augmentative and Alternative Communication*, Vol 8 No 2, pp81-88.

[8] Alm, N., Arnott, J.L., Newell, A.F. (1992a) Prediction and conversational momentum in an augmentative communication system.

[9] Arnott, J.L., Alm, N,. Newell, A.F. (1988) A text database as a communication prosthesis. *Proceedings of the International Association for the Advancement of Rehabilitation Technology*. Montreal: Association for the Advancement of Rehabilitation Technology, pp 76-77.

[10] Broumley, L., Arnott, J.L., Cairns, A.Y., Newell, A.F. (1990) TalksBack: An application of artificial intelligence techniques to a communication prosthesis for non-speaking people. *Proceedings of the European Conference on Artificial Intelligence*. Stockholm, 6-10 August 1990, pp117-119

[11] Waller, A. (1992) Providing narratives in an augmentative communication system. Ph.D. Thesis, University of Dundee, Dundee, Scotland, UK.

[12] Alm, N., Arnott, J.L., Newell, A.F. (1992) Evaluation of a text-based communication system for increasing conversational participation and control. *Proceedings of the 15th Rehabilitation Engineers Society of North America International Conference*. Washington, D.C. The RESNA Press. pp 366-368.

[13] Newell, A.F., Arnott, J.L., Booth, L., Beattie, W. Brophy, B., Ricketts, I. (1992) The use of the PAL word prediction system on the quality and quantity of text generation. *Augmentative and Alternative Communication*. Vol 8 No 4, pp 304-311.

[14] Cairns, A.,Y., Peddie, H., Filz, G., Arnott, J.L., Newell, A.F. (1990) ECHO : a multimodal workstation for ordinary and extra-ordinary human computer interaction. *Proceedings of the IEE Colloquium on Multi-Media: The Future of User Interfaces*. London, 26 November 1990

# Evaluation of Products which are Intended to Ease the Lives of Elderly People: The Hi-Riser Chair

Bernard Isaacs, Tamara Barnea, Netta Bentur, Ilana Mizrahi, Ariel Simkin.
JDC-Brookdale Institute of Gerontology and Human Development,
POB 13087, Jerusalem, Israel

**Abstract**. The evaluation of a prototype of a new chair, the Hi-Riser chair, equipped with an innovative mechanism for assisting the user to rise and sit, has proved beneficial to the manufacturer, and raised critical issues that relate to applied industrial research. In this paper we use data from the research to illustrate key examples of these issues. Special emphasis is given to the involvement of the potential consumer in the evaluation process.

## 1. Introduction

Rising and sitting are basic activities for independent functioning. About 8% of elderly people who live within their own community in the United States report difficulty in getting up from a chair or a bed[1].

This paper is based on the experience of the Technology and Aging Research Team at the JDC-Brookdale Institute, whose work is in collaboration with ESHEL, the Association for Planning and Development of Services for the Aged in Israel, Tzora Furniture and the Kossel Center for Physical Education. The focus of this paper is the methodology of the research and not the function of the experimental chair itself.

## 2. Research Objectives

The aims of the research were to assist the manufacturer in developing an assistive chair for people who experience difficulty in rising from and sitting down on an ordinary chair and to deepen the understanding of the physical and cognitive processes used by elderly people in the course of learning to rise from and sit down in an assistive chair.

These aims might also be expressed as determining the suitability of the chair for elderly people, and the suitability of elderly people to the chair.

## 3. Research Design

### 3.1. Research Chair:

The chair incorporates a piston mechanism which raises the seat upward and forward during rising, and which retards descent during sitting. The mechanism locks automatically when the user sits down, and is released before rising by pressing a button, located under the seat at the front and side. The strength of the piston can be adjusted by moving a lever under the seat, to one of eight applied force positions. The experimental chairs were of two piston strengths, one of 1,000N and the other of 1,400N. They were suitable for subjects weighing 50 - 100 kg. The angle of rise of the seat can be adjusted between 0° and 45°. In the experimental chair the angle was fixed at 30°. The chairs were of two heights (44 cm, 49 cm). As a control chair in the research we used the experimental chair with its mechanism locked.

### 3.2. Research Population:

The research was conducted with the participation of 33 elderly subjects, who had different degrees of difficulty in rising and sitting. Seven had no difficulty, 10 had moderate difficulty, and 16 had severe difficulty. Twelve were residents of a sheltered housing project for elderly people and 21 were regular visitors at a day center for the disabled elderly. Most of them were females. The age range was 60 - 97, and the median was 76. None of them needed human assistance in mobility, but twenty-eight subjects used mobility assistive devices - mainly walkers (15) and tripods (7). In their activities of daily living (ADL) - eating, dressing, bathing, and using the toilet - 10 of them were independent and 23 were limited in 1-3 activities.

Subjects' difficulties in using an ordinary chair were characterized by the following medical problems: musculoskeletal (14 subjects), neuromuscular (10), cardiorespiratory (2), overweight (2), weakness, other symptoms (5). All, but one participant were able to communicate with the researchers. All agreed voluntarily to participate in the research.

### 3.3. Evaluation Process:

The process started with preliminary screening of potential subjects suitable for the research. Prior to the experiment the new chair was presented to the staff of the facilities from which the research population was drawn. They were approached for consultation and consent to conduct the research. After subjects were selected and gave their consent, background data was collected. This included: sociodemographic data, usual use of chair, anthropometric and performance measures, and functional data.

The research was conducted in three stages:

Stage 1: Trial of 22 subjects; performance on experimental chair compared with performance on control chair.

Stage 2: Trial of seven subjects who experienced difficulty in stage 1; modification of procedure; modification of chair.

Stage 3: Trial of modified version of the chair, with 11 new subjects.

*3.4. Research Protocol:*

The research was carried out according to the following protocol:
Trial of control chair, filmed performance on control chair, interview,
explanation and demonstration of experimental chair, trial of experimental
chair, adaptation of piston applied force if required, second interview, filmed
performance on experimental chair. The interdisciplinary research staff was
composed of a geriatrician, bio-mechanics engineer and researchers in the
fields of gerontology, rehabilitation and elderly consumers, assisted by a
technician from the manufacturing team.

*3.5. Research Instruments:*

The qualitative and quantitative research instruments included:
1) Questionnaires with closed and open questions about subject performance
with the chairs and their attitude toward them: ease, comfort, aesthetics,
appropriateness, willingness to use the chair.
2) Closed and open questions for analysis of subject performance with the
chairs by observers. The videotapes were observed simultaneously by the five
researchers, who judged performance after reaching consensus. Based on the
literature[2][3] and the research team's clinical experience, units of analysis
were: ease of rising and sitting, smoothness of movement, completeness of
movement, safety, learning to operate the chair, fitness of chair to the person,
fitness of person to the chair.
3) Case study analysis played an important role in understanding the
interaction between subject and chair.
4) Bio-mechanical analysis was made of the movements of markers which
were fitted on prominent body points of the subjects. This data was collected
for validation of the subjective data, and to identify the contribution of bio-
mechanics to the evaluation process.


## 4. Findings

The findings presented here are partial and serve only as examples.

*4.1. Preliminary Screening of Research Population:*

Since we did not know before undertaking the experiment what were the
potential benefits and disadvantages of the chair, we decided to test it on subjects
who presented a wide range of difficulty in using an ordinary chair.
However, problems still remained in determining how to screen people
according to this characteristic as there is no value for "normal" rising and sitting
in old age and no established measurement or measure of difficulty.
In this research we used three information sources - the care staff, self-
assessment by the subject, and assessment by the researchers while observing the
subject rising and sitting on the control chair. "Difficulty" was established by the
independent identification of problems in rising and sitting by at least two sources.

The compatibility between the three sources is low. The highest compatibility is between the observation by the researchers and reporting by the care staff. It relates to 14 subjects out of 33. The lowest compatibility is between subject reporting and staff reporting, 6 subjects out of 33. The results related to the other 27 subjects were split as follows: subjects reported more difficulty than staff in 12 cases, and staff reported more difficulty in 15 cases. A similar level of compatibility existed also between subjects and researchers. It relates to 25 subjects, but the results show a different trend than the above: subjects assessed 18 persons as having more difficulty while the researchers assessed 7 persons as having more difficulty. In general, subjects assessed more persons as having difficulty than other data sources.

Based on our experience it is advisable to use the care staff assessment for preliminary screening, but to use the elderly's self-assessment and the researcher's observation for the grading of difficulties of the potential participants in the research.

*4.2. Contribution of the New Device to Subjects:*

Performance of the subjects on rising from and sitting down on the experimental chair was assessed by the researchers and by the subjects who graded their own performance on a four-point scale: no difficulty, slight difficulty, moderate difficulty, severe difficulty. Based on the subject reporting we learned that those who benefit most from the Hi-Riser chair were those who had moderate and severe difficulties in rising (11 out of 13) and sitting (4 out of 8) on the control chair. The chair assisted more of them in rising than in sitting. It created difficulties in sitting for one subject (see Table 1).

Table 1: Effect of the Hi-Riser Chair on Performance of Subjects with Moderate and Severe Difficulty in Rising and Sitting on Control Chair (Subject's Self-Report)

| Degree of Difficulty in Rising & Sitting on Control Chair | Performance with the Hi-Riser Chair | | | |
| --- | --- | --- | --- | --- |
| | Improved | No Change | Deteriorated | Total |
| Rising: Total | 11 | 2 | 0 | 13 |
| Moderate | 7 | 1 | 0 | 8 |
| Severe | 4 | 1 | 0 | 5 |
| Sitting: Total | 4 | 3 | 1 | 8 |
| Moderate | 2 | 3 | 1 | 6 |
| Severe | 2 | 0 | 0 | 2 |

*4.3. Contribution of Applied Research to the Manufacturer:*

The research contribution to the manufacturer involved: improved design of the chair and its assistive mechanism, improved adaptation process of chair to the user and user to the chair, definition of instructions for use by sales people or caregivers, improved definition of the target population and the appropriate marketing strategy.

To illustrate these types of benefits we present two examples.

Piston strength: While originally the manufacturer planned to produce two types of chair with different piston strengths (1,000N and 1,400N), the research taught us that there is no need for more than one strength of piston (1,000N) with 8 degrees of applied force to adapt to the weight of the user (between 50-100 kg). We were able to provide the manufacturer with a new scale of piston strength, which is appropriate for elderly people with difficulty in rising and sitting. The video analysis showed that it is preferable to fix the degree of the piston strength in order to achieve successful sitting rather than successful rising, since in most cases sitting required a lower piston strength than rising.

Favorable and unfavorable effects: At the developmental stages, several unfavorable effects were identified. Most of these effects were resolved later, but in presenting this study, and with the permission of the manufacturer, we would like to point them out. Our analysis is based on about 280 observations on individual subjects' 5 - 10 trials of sitting on and rising from the Hi-Riser chair.

*Unfavorable effects.* In Rising: Excessive upward force, instability, "fragmented" movement, incomplete rise, slipping of the feet, movement of chair. In Sitting: Difficulty in activating mechanism to lower the seat, tendency to slip off the opened seat, failure to lock the mechanism on completion of sitting, slipping of the feet, falling into the seat. In the Locking Mechanism: Forgetting to activate the release button, difficulty in locating the release button, inefficient use of the release button.

*Favorable effects.* In Rising: Reduction of effort, relief of pain, improvement of stability. In Sitting: Reduction of effort, reduction of tendency to fall into chair, prevention of movement of the chair, prevention of need for assistance.

## 5. Summary

This research has demonstrated the need to explore further a number of methodological issues in the scientific evaluation of an innovative commercial product. These include: identification of target population; evaluation of performance; validation of qualitative measurements; the balance between advantages and disadvantages; the involvement of the potential consumer in the research; and the interaction between commercial and scientific imperatives.

### References
[1] National Center of Health Statistics. *Vital and Health Statistics*, USA, 1991.

[2] M. Schenkman, R. Berger, P. O'Rilley, R. W. Mann, and W. A. Hodge, Whole-body Movements During Rising to Standing from Sitting, *Physical Therapy* 70 (10): 51 - 61, 1990.

[3] A. Karalj, R.J. Jaeger, and M. Munich, Analysis of Standing Up and Sitting Down in Humans: Definitions and Normative Data Presentation, *Journal of Biomechanics* 23 (11): 1123-1138, 1990.

# Index of Authors